Adverse Drug Effects

A Nursing Concern

Adverse Drug Effects

A Nursing Concern

JENNIFER KELLY

BA (Hons), MSc, RGN, Dip N, Dip Ed
Senior Lecturer Practitioner Wound Care
at
Addenbrooke's Hospital and Homerton College, Cambridge

W
WHURR PUBLISHERS
LONDON AND PHILADELPHIA

First published 2000 by
Whurr Publishers Ltd
19b Compton Terrace, London N1 2UN, England and
325 Chestnut Street, Philadelphia PA 19106, USA

Reprinted 2001

British Library Cataloguing in Publication Data
A catalogue record for this book is available from the British Library.

ISBN: 1 86156 191 1

Printed and bound in the UK by Athenaeum Press Ltd,
Gateshead, Tyne & Wear

Contents

PART 3 THE PRACTICE — 12 CASE STUDIES

Preface

Nurses have always had to have knowledge of drugs as they have been involved with their administration both in the hospital and the community setting, and they have also been involved in the education of patients in regard to drug therapy. However, with the advent of nurse prescribing, albeit from a limited list of drugs, and the increasing use of drug protocols, the need for nurses to have a good understanding of drug therapy, rather than just a basic knowledge, has become vital. This book has been written to achieve this aim.

Unlike most books on the subject of pharmacology, this book looks at drug therapy from the angle of adverse effects. The reason for this is that adverse reactions are the main concern from the patient's perspective of drug usage, and one of the main reasons why they frequently choose not to take the medications that they are prescribed. Due to the close relationship which nurses have with their patients, they are well placed to detect adverse drug effects early and take action to deal with them before harm comes to the patient. Furthermore, if nurses are aware of the broad spectrum of adverse reactions that drugs can produce, they can help to monitor them and report back to the Committee on Safety of Medicines, so that unsafe drugs can be withdrawn from usage earlier rather than later.

The book is written chiefly for qualified nurses working in all specialities, and nursing students coming to the end of their training. However, it will also be of interest to others who have an inquisitive mind and want to know why drugs have the adverse effects they do.

Please note Directive 92/27/EEC requires use of the Recommended International Non-proprietary Name (rINN) for medicinal substances. In the majority of cases, the British Approved Name

(BAN) and rINN are identical, but in some cases the BAN and rINN are totally different. This book has anticipated the directive being put into force in the near future, and so where drug names do differ this book gives the name of the rINN with the old BAN in brackets. The reader is advised to consult the British National Formulary (BNF), which is published six monthly by the British Medical Association in conjunction with the Royal Pharmaceutical Society of Great Britain, for up-to-date information about this issue and any other concerns regarding the use of medicines.

Acknowledgement

I would like to thank Debrae Ward-Walsh, Senior Lecturer at Homerton College, and a practising Aromatherapist and Remedial Masseur for her contributions to the book, Chapter 18 and a case study in Chapter 19.

Jennifer Kelly
May 2000

Introduction

This book is not intended to be a comprehensive overview of individual drugs and their adverse effects as this is already available in the admirable form of the British National Formulary (BNF), and other pharmacopoeia. Instead this book attempts to explain the how and why of adverse drug reactions, so that the reader has a working understanding of the principles behind adverse reactions. The advantage of comprehending what is happening when you give a patient a drug, is that when you meet a new drug, if you know what type of drug it is, then you can deduce its actions and adverse effects. This saves you having to learn individual drugs by rote, or, alternatively, having to carry the BNF around all the time. However, the understanding which you will gain from reading this book will not mean that you will not have to check the details of your knowledge in the BNF or an alternative pharmacopoeia occasionally, especially as our knowledge of adverse drug reactions is forever increasing.

This book is divided into three parts. The first two parts echo nursing in that they look at the art and science of pharmacology. At a time when nursing is moving into academia, and proudly declaring that it is research based and hence a scientific discipline, it is sobering to remember that nursing is also an art. Knowledge is not enough; there must also be creativity, intuition and skill. Thus the first part of this book looks at the pharmacology of drugs, i.e. what the body does to drugs (pharmacokinetics), what the drug does to the body (pharmacodynamics), and how adverse reactions can arise from these two processes. Less predictable, idiosyncratic effects are examined next, before looking at the three client groups - the child, the pregnant women and her foetus, and the elderly - where due to their different physiology adverse effects are particularly prevalent and problematic. Part 1 finishes with a systems approach to looking at adverse effects, which is the converse to most pharmacology texts that map the drugs to their adverse effects. In line with the approach of this book which examines principles rather than specifics, this review of adverse effects is not all encompassing, but instead it aims to demonstrate the scope of the problem.

Part two looks at the art of putting the scientific knowledge into action, through its examination of nurse administration and prescribing, drug development and the involvement of the nurse, and the thorny issue of patient compliance and empowerment. The final chapter in part two looks at complementary and alternative therapies. This is in recognition that nurses are becoming increasingly involved in complementary therapies. Furthermore, it is a response to the popularly held belief that 'natural' remedies are 'safe' and free of adverse effects, when compared with drugs produced by pharmaceutical companies. This is not necessarily the case, as the chapter reveals.

Part three consists of 12 case studies grouped together into four chapters. These present scenarios based on real cases, in which drugs have led to adverse effects, and examines prescribed drugs as well as over-the-counter medications, and complementary therapy. At the end of each case study the reader is given a series of questions in order to test his or her knowledge and understanding of the events before the text explains what has actually happened. The case studies allow the theory to be embedded in practice.

The book has been laid out with lots of headings and tables enclosing essential points so that the reader can dip in as necessary to find answers to a particular problem. Throughout the book, concepts have been explained utilizing examples, so that you the reader can relate the theoretical concepts to the drugs that you are familiar with. As the book is concerned with general principles of adverse drug reactions, generic names of drugs are used throughout. The book ends with a glossary, as although all the pharmacological terms are explained in the text, readers who dip into sections of the book, might not be familiar with terms that have been defined elsewhere.

Part 1
The Science of Adverse Drug Effects

Chapter 1 Pharmacokinetic effects – absorption and distribution

Introduction

A drug is a chemical substance used in the prevention or treatment of a disease in order to improve a patient's condition. Drugs range from vitamins through to narcotics, and include complementary medicines such as herbal remedies and aromatherapy. Unfortunately, it is a truism to say that any drug that can do you good also has the potential to do you harm. Thus when drugs are used the aim is to maximize their therapeutic effects while minimizing their harmful effects. This involves a cost-benefit analysis which should be carried out by the patient and prescriber in partnership, as only the patient knows what risks they are prepared to tolerate in return for which benefits. Thus for example where there are minor therapeutic gains; e.g. reducing the discomfort of hayfever, then minor adverse effects may be tolerated in the form of slight drowsiness. However, if the adverse effect is severe drowsiness and the patient is a machine operator the risks of harm are likely to outweigh the benefits. In contrast, if the therapeutic benefits of the drug are very significant, as in the treatment of a malignancy such as leukaemia, then the patient may accept much more extensive and severe adverse effects.

In 1977, Rawlins and Thompson devised a convenient method of classifying adverse drug reactions into two principal kinds, namely type A and type B effects (Table 1.1). Type A reactions account for at least 80% of adverse drug effects, are dose related and usually result from the pharmacology of the drug (deShazo and Kemp, 1997). They are frequently referred to as side-effects in recognition of the fact that drugs do not simply interact with their site of intended action, but indiscriminately affect all the receptors or binding sites with which they are compatible. Thus, for example atropine may be used as a premedication to dry up secretions before surgery. However, atropine does not just bind to the acetylcholine receptors of the mouth, it also antagonizes those of the eye leading to pupil dilation and blurred vision, which is consequently a side-effect. Conversely, the atropine may be given to dilate the pupil in order to visualize the retina. Then the pupil dilation becomes the therapeutic effect and the dry mouth the side-effect.

Side-effects can be reduced in a number of ways (Table 1.2). Reduction of drug dosage is one method. The smallest effective dose should always be given, and then if need be the dose gradually increased to maximize the therapeutic effect. The oral contraceptive

Table 1.1 Type A and B reactions

Type A reactions	
Side-effects	The unwanted effects that occur as a result of the pharmacology of the drug
Secondary effects	The indirect consequences of a primary drug action, e.g. opportunistic infections that may develop after antibiotic treatment
Overdose or toxicity effects	Exaggerated but characteristic pharmacological effects produced by administering supratherapeutic doses of a drug
Teratogens	Drugs capable of producing developmental defects in the foetus
Drug interactions	Unwanted effects that occur due to the simultaneous pharmacological activity of two or more drugs
Type B reactions	
Intolerance	Undesirable pharmacological effect that occurs at subtherapeutic drug dosages
Idiosyncrasy	A qualitative abnormal reaction to a drug, usually due to a genetic abnormality
Allergic or hypersensitivity reaction	Any immunological response to a drug or its metabolites that results in adverse effects

Table 1.2 Methods of reducing side-effects

- Reducing drug dosage
- Restricting drug access
- Drug targeting

pill illustrates the positive benefits of reducing the dosage of a drug. Here a reduction in drug dosage has minimized the risk of deep vein thrombosis while maintaining protection against conception.

A second possibility for reducing side-effects is to restrict the access of the drug, so that it is only administered to the site of required action. In the case of the atropine example above, administration of the drug as eye drops would allow pupil dilation but would limit significantly the drug's systemic effects. Similarly in the treatment of asthma, the administration of steroids as aerosols rather than as an oral medication has led to a considerable reduction in side-effects. However, there are exceptions to the rule; topical therapy is not generally recommended in the case of antibiotics as this is likely to increase the risk of bacterial resistance developing (Cooper and Lawrence, 1996; Cullum and Roe, 1995).

A third possibility for limiting side-effects is the use of drug targeting, i.e. the use of drugs that are specific in their effect rather than broad spectrum. Thus in the case of treating a bacterial infection, it is better to identify the causative organism and then choose an appropriate and specific drug, rather than simply opt for broad-spectrum antibiotics. Another example is the use of salbutamol to treat asthma in preference to isoprenaline. Both drugs have the required effect on bronchial smooth muscle, i.e. relaxation, but isoprenaline is not as selective as salbutamol (it is an agonist at both β_1 and β_2 adrenoceptors, while salbutamol is active mainly at β_2 adrenoceptors – see Chapter 3), and so produces side-effects in the form of tachycardia.

Drug interactions are an important form of Type A reaction. They occur whenever the effect of one drug is modified by the prior of concurrent administration of another pharmacologically active substance (Finley, 1992). Such interactions may result in an antagonist, synergistic or unexpected response. They can be beneficial or harmful. Examples of beneficial interactions include the concurrent use of an opioid and a non-steroidal anti-inflammatory drug in the treatment of pain in order to gain maximum analgesia with minimal adverse effects, or the combination of a diuretic and a β-blocker to treat hypertension. Most clinically significant adverse drug interactions result in either a decreased therapeutic response to one or both drugs or enhanced toxicity, and the interaction can be severe enough for the drug to be withdrawn from use, e.g. Roche voluntarily withdrew mibefradil (Adams, 1998). As is to be expected adverse drug interactions become more common the more drugs a person takes.

Type B reactions only occur in some people. They are generally unpredictable and not related to drug dosage, and consequently they are difficult to prevent. However, if a person or their family has a history of a particular reaction to a drug, every effort must be made to ensure that they are not put in contact with the drug a second time. Type B reactions include unwanted effects due to inherited abnormalities, i.e. idiosyncratic reactions, and immunological processes, i.e. drug allergy (see Chapter 5).

As well as the two main classifications of unwanted drug reactions there are also three subordinate groupings recognized (Table 1.3). Type C reactions are the result of chronic or long-term drug usage.

Table 1.3 Classification of adverse effects (Page et al., 1997)

Type of effect	*Explanation*	*Examples*
Augmented effects	Unwanted effects that occur as a result of the pharmacology of the drug. Also termed side-effects. Relatively common and usually minor	Hypotension due to anti-hypertensives. Haemorrhage due to anticoagulants
Bizarre effects	Unpredictable unwanted effects that are not dose-related. Relatively uncommon, but they have a high rate of morbidity and mortality.	Anaphylaxis due to penicillin. Hyperpyrexia due to halothane
Chronic effects	Unwanted effects that occur after prolonged treatment.	Parkinsonism with phenoth-iazines. Colonic dysfunction with laxatives
Delayed effects	Unwanted effects that do not occur for years after treatment or that affect the next generation.	Secondary cancers after treatment with cytotoxics. Carcinoma of the vagina in daughters of women who took diethylstilbestrol during pregnancy
End-of-use effects	Unwanted effects that occur when the drug is stopped suddenly, i.e. withdrawal effects	Adrenocortical insufficiency after stoppage of glucocorticoids. Delirium tremens after ceasing heroin intake

Type D reactions occur some years after treatment has finished and may in fact occur in the offspring of the person given the therapy. Finally, type E effects occur where discontinuation of therapy is too abrupt. More recently Wills and Brown (1999) have proposed a very different means of classifying medicines in which B reactions are classified into seven categories and there is also the addition of an unclassified group (Table 1.4).

Table 1.4 A new classification for adverse drug effects (Wills and Brown, 1999)

Type of effect	*Explanation*	*Examples*
Augmented	Pharmacologically predictable. Dose related. Improves if medicine withdrawn. Common.	Bradycardia due to digoxin. Respiratory depression due to diamorphine.
Bugs	Pharmacologically predictable. Involves interaction with microbes. Improves if medicine withdrawn.	Dental caries due to sugar-containing medicines. Bacterial resistance due to antibiotic use.
Chemical	An irritant reaction related to drug concentration.	Extravasation reactions due to irritant action of medicine. Gastrointestinal damage due to local irritant reaction of aspirin.
Delivery	Caused by method of administration or nature of formulation. Improves if medicine is withdrawn or delivery method changed.	Inflammation and fibrosis around drug implants. Fat hypertrophy around insulin injection site.
Exit	Pharmacologically predictable. Begins only when medicine is stopped or dose reduced. Improves if medicine re-introduced.	Delirium tremens with withdrawal of opioids. Benzodiazepines, tricyclic antidepressants, ß-blockers, clonidine.
Familial	Only occurs in those genetically predisposed. Improves if medicine is withdrawn.	Haemolysis with quinine in those suffering with glucose-6-phosphate dehydrogenase deficiency.
Genetotoxicity	Causes irreversible genetic damage.	Mutation and tumour formation.
Hypersensitivity	Requires activation of the immune system. Improves if medicine is withdrawn.	Anaphylaxis, allergic skin rashes, Stevens-Johnson syndrome.
Unclassified	Mechanism not understood.	Drug-induced taste disturbances. Nausea and vomiting after a general anaesthetic.

Adverse drug reactions are defined by the World Health Organisation (1966) as any noxious, unintended and undesired effect of a drug which occurs at doses used in humans for prophylaxis, diagnosis or therapy. A meta-analysis of 39 prospective studies carried out in the United States over a period of 32 years identified the overall incidence of adverse reactions as 6.7% and of fatal adverse reactions as 0.3% of hospitalized patients (Lazarou et al., 1998). The authors estimated that in 1994, 2 216 000 hospitalised patients had serious adverse drug reactions and 106 000 had fatal adverse drug effects, making these reactions between the fourth and fifth leading cause of death. However, a recent study by Jha et al. (1998) suggests that the incidence of adverse drug events may be higher than previously reported, and that the method used to collect the data affects the number and type of adverse reactions identified.

When adverse effects occur Smith (1984) suggests that there 'is either something wrong with the drug, something wrong with the patient or something wrong with the doctor or prescriber. Thus, these three factors should always be analysed when dealing with adverse effects (Table 1.5). The drug classes most frequently implicated in adverse reactions are shown in Table 1.6. As far as patient variables are concerned, extremes of age (see Chapter 6), gender, genetic polymorphism (Chapter 2) and race (Chapter 5), and intercurrent disease (Chapter 2) can all predispose to adverse reactions. As far as gender is concerned in general, women appear to be at greater risk of adverse drug reactions than men are, and increased drug exposure does not account completely for the difference (Lee and Beard, 1997). For example, women are reputed to be more susceptible to blood dyscrasias, with phenylbutazone and chloramphenicol, to histaminoid reactions to neuromuscular blocking drugs, and to reactions involving the gastrointestinal tract.

Pharmokinetics

Pharmokinetics is the study of what the body does to a drug over time. It explores the processes of absorption, distribution, metabolism and excretion (Table 1.7). Each of these processes will occur at a specific rate characteristic for that drug, and the overall action of the drug - be it therapeutic or toxic - will be dependent on these processes. This chapter and the next will examine each of the four processes in turn.

Table 1.5 Causes of adverse effects

Cause	*Possible reasons*
The drug	Narrow therapeutic window, components of the formulation have a tendency to cause allergy.
The patient	Age, genetic constitution, disease, personality, lifestyle.
The prescriber	Drug given for inappropriately long time, withdrawn too rapidly, or given with other drugs leading to interactions.

Table 1.6 Drug classes most frequently implicated in adverse effects (Bates et al., 1995)

• Analgesics	• Cardiovascular drugs
• Antibiotics	• Cytotoxics
• Anticoagulants	• Electrolytes
• Anti-diabetic drugs	• Sedatives

Table 1.7 The processes of pharmacokinetics

Absorption	The passage of a drug from its site of administration into the blood or plasma.
Distribution	The movement of the drug from the blood to its site of action.
Metabolism	The chemical transformation of a drug.
Elimination	The removal of a drug or its metabolite from the body.

Absorption

Absorption can be defined as the passage of a drug from the site of its administration into the blood or plasma. As most drugs are taken orally they must pass through the gut wall to enter the blood. Drugs can cross cellular membranes by simple diffusion, facilitated diffusion, filtration, active transport and endocytosis, although diffusion is the most important method. The cell membrane being a lipid bilayer can act as a barrier to some drugs. The effectiveness of a drug will depend upon its rate of absorption, as this will determine its peak effect. Thus a drug that is absorbed very slowly may be metabolized and excreted as fast as it is absorbed, and thus it may fail to reach therapeutic concentrations. Conversely the drug may be absorbed very rapidly and reach toxic levels which can result in adverse effects.

As well as considering the rate of absorption, drugs vary in the extent of their absorption or bioavailability. Bioavailability refers to the amount of drug that reaches the systemic circulation, such that a drug that is poorly absorbed from the gut will have a low bioavailability, while a drug administered intravenously will have a 100% bioavailability. Drugs with a low bioavailability can be problematic, as large amounts of drug may have to be given before a therapeutic effect is achieved. However, low bioavailability can also be put to good use. For example, the antibiotic neomycin is poorly absorbed from the gut, and so it can be used to cleanse the gut of bacteria before gastro-intestinal surgery. As it is not absorbed, systemic adverse effects are minimal.

The chemical properties of the drug itself together with physiological variables will affect drug absorption (Table 1.8).

Table 1.8 Chemical and physiological variables affecting drug absorption

Chemical variables	• Molecular weight • Partition coefficient • Formulation of drug • Drug chemistry
Physiological variables	• pH at the site of absorption • Enzymatic activity • Gut motility • Presence or absence of food • Presence of other drugs • Blood flow

Molecule size and lipid solubility

The chemical nature of the drug itself will affect absorption (Table 1.9). Since the diffusion coefficient of a drug is inversely related to the square root of the molecular weight, small molecules will diffuse more easily across a membrane than larger molecules. Lipid solubility, which is often indicated by a ratio termed the 'partition coefficient', can play a major role in drug absorption. It reflects the solubility of a drug molecule in a lipid relative to its solubility in water. The higher the partition coefficient the more rapidly the drug can diffuse across the lipid membrane. Drugs that are lipid soluble tend to be uncharged molecules, in other words they do not ionize easily and so do not carry an electric charge or act as electrolytes. Furthermore, the molecules are non-polar. This means that they do not have a positive charge at one end of the molecule and a negative charge at the other end, as water does.

Table 1.9 Characteristics of drug molecules that will promote movement across membranes

- Low molecular weight
- Uncharged
- Non-polar
- High lipid solubility

Formulation

The formulation of a drug refers to the components that make up a medicine. These include the active drug as well as bulking agents, binders and coaters, disintegrants, colours and flavourings. The formulation can affect the rate of absorption, as illustrated by liquid formulations which generally afford a faster onset of action because the drug is either in solution and therefore available for absorption, or in a suspension of fine particles (Taylor and Helliwell, 1992). More sophisticated methods of altering absorption rates are through the application of an enteric coating that prevents the drug from dissolving until it is in a suitable alkaline environment, or the use of a modified release preparation which releases the drug slowly and continuously. Modified release preparations have the benefit that they can prolong the action of a drug whose effect would otherwise be rapidly lost. They also minimize fluctuations in the amount of drug in the body, and this can help to reduce adverse effects. Thus, the patient who gets a headache with a standard formulation of nifedipine may not get it with a modified release preparation. When prescribing modified release formulations it is best to use the brand name, since different brands of modified release formulations do not necessarily have the same absorption characteristics (Aronson, 1993).

The particle size of the formulation can also make a difference and unintentionally affect the rate of absorption. This was clearly demonstrated in a study in which a group of normal volunteers were given standard oral digoxin tablets from different manufacturers. The volunteers were found to have grossly different plasma concentrations of the drug, with one product's peak serum level being seven times that obtained with another, even though the digoxin content of the tablets were identical (Lindenbaum et al., 1971). Furthermore, significant variations were found between different batches of digoxin tablets prepared by a single manufacturer. Discrepancies in the bioavailability and the therapeutic effect of other drugs have also been observed, for example chloramphenicol (Glazko et al., 1968), oxytetracycline (Blair et al., 1971), phenylbutazone (Searl and Pernarowski, 1967), prednisone (Campagna et al., 1963), and tolbutamide (Varley, 1968). This has implications for changing the brand of drug that a patient is taking, especially in the case of drugs with a narrow therapeutic index; i.e. where the difference between the therapeutic and toxic dose is small. For this reason, some states and health insurers in the United States want to make it harder to substitute generic drugs for about 25 drugs that will only work properly in precise doses (Anon, 1998).

The formulation of a medicine is designed by the manufacturer for a purpose, and nurses must consider this seriously before grinding tablets up to enable their administration through nasogastric tubes or to ease their administration to elderly patients. Grinding up tablets can have serious adverse effects. This is illustrated by the peripheral vasodilator naftidrofuryl (Praxilene). These tablets have local anaesthetic properties, and so there is the danger that if they are administered in a ground up form and then not swallowed properly, the patient may loose their gag reflex and aspirate when given a drink. Enteric-coated, sublingual chewable, modified-release (including sustained release, long-acting and retard) preparations should not be crushed, and caution should be exercised and advice sought before crushing cytotoxics, hormone preparations, antibiotics and prostaglandin analogues (Naysmith and Nicholson, 1998).

Gut pH and enzymes

Most drugs are taken orally and they have to contend with the adverse conditions of the gut, which can have major effects on their absorption. Many drugs that are protein in nature, for example insulin, cannot be taken orally because the gut enzymes digest them and hence they are absorbed as amino acids rather than as active drug. Similarly, the strong acidity of the stomach inactivates some drugs, for example the antibiotic benzylpenicillin, and hence alternative routes of administration have to be used.

Most drugs are small molecules with a molecular weight of less than a 1000 and are absorbed via simple diffusion. Molecules cross the lipid bilayer that makes up the cell membrane in a non-ionized form. As most drugs are either weak acids, bases or amphoteric, the pH of the environment where the drug formulation disintegrates and dissolves will determine the fraction of drug in solution that is in the non-ionized form, and hence the amount of drug that can diffuse across the cell membranes. The general rule is that drugs will exist in the non-ionized form when exposed to a pH-same chemical environment. Thus aspirin, and other weakly acidic drugs, are best absorbed from the stomach, while alkaline drugs, such as morphine, are best absorbed from the small intestine.

Concurrent use of medications that affect gut pH can alter drug absorption. For example, the antifungal drug ketoconazole requires an acidic environment for adequate dissolution, and commonly used acid suppressors such as H_2-receptor antagonists, e.g. cimetidine, and proton pump inhibitors, e.g. omeprazole, can dramatically reduce ketoconazole absorption (Hansten, 1998). Fortunately, alteration in gastrointestinal pH is not a common cause of clinically important drug interactions, because the absorption of most drugs is not markedly affected by pH changes in the gut.

Gut contents and motility

The presence of food in the gut may alter absorption responses in 72–93% of drugs (Murray and Healey, 1991), usually with total drug absorption being significantly reduced (Table 1.10). Drugs and nutrients can interact directly in what is termed a chelation or complexing reaction to produce an inactive complex that is poorly absorbed. An example of a chelation reaction is the combination of tetracycline with divalent cations such as calcium in dairy products or antacids, leading to decreased absorption of both. Complexing reactions can occur when iron binds with fluoroquinolone antibiotics such as ciprofloxacin, and this has been shown to reduce bioavailability by 52% (Polk et al., 1989). A second type of interaction between a drug and food occurs when the food acts as a mechanical barrier that prevents drug access to the mucosal surfaces. This is illustrated by the antibiotic azithromycin, which if taken with food results in a 52% reduction in the maximum plasma concentration and a 43% reduction in bioavailability (Kirk, 1995). Spacing food and drug intake about two hours apart will usually minimize drug food interactions.

Table 1.10 Examples of drug-nutrient interactions

Drug	*Nutrient type*	*Effect of interaction*
ACE inhibitors, e.g. captopril	Food generally. Potassium salt substitutes	Delay in blood pressure lowering. Hyperkalaemia
Antibiotic		
• Erythromycin, penicillins	Acidic fruit juices and beverages, citrus fruits	Inactivation by increased gut acidity
• Ciprofloxacin, ofloxacin	Iron	Decreased absorption
• Azithromycin	Food generally	Decreased absorption
• Tetracyclines	Calcium-containing foods, e.g. cheese, ice cream, milk, yoghurt	Decreased absorption
Antivirals		
• Zidovudine	High fat meals	Decreased bioavailability
Anticoagulants, e.g. heparin, warfarin	Vitamin K containing foods, e.g. beef liver, green leafy vegetables	Decreased anticoagulation if intake increased. Bleeding if intake decreased
Antifungals		
• Griseofulvin	High fat meal	Increased absorption
Antihypertensives		
• Felodipine, nifedipine	Citrus juices	Decreased diastolic blood pressure
Immunosuppressants		
• Cyclosporin	Milk and food generally	Increased bioavailability
Iron	Ascorbic acid. Phosphates, phytates, tannates	Increased absorption Decreased absorption
Levodopa	Amino acids	Decreased absorption
Monoamine oxidase inhibitors, e.g. isocarboxazid, phenelzine, tranylcypromine	Foods with high tyramine content, particularly those that have undergone ageing and or fermenting, pickling, smoking or bacterial contamination; e.g. aged meat, beer, sherry, red wine, anchovies, avocados, bananas, chicken liver, chocolate, meat tenderizers, pickled herring, raisins, sausage, sour cream, soy sauce, yeast extract, yoghurt	Hypertensive crisis
Non-steroid anti-inflammatory drugs, e.g. indometacin (indomethacin)	Food or milk	Decreased gastro-intestinal irritation

A third type of interaction is illustrated by levodopa, which is commonly used to treat Parkinson's disease. The drug utilizes an active transport mechanism in the gut that is normally used for the absorption of amino acids, so concurrent administration of protein and levodopa will result in competition for the carrier. Consequently, if protein intake is reduced, drug absorption will be increased, and the action of the drug enhanced.

Drug absorption can in some cases be increased by the presence of nutrients in the gut. This is illustrated by the interaction between iron and vitamin C. Ascorbic acid stimulates iron absorption partly by forming soluble iron-ascorbate chelates and partly by reducing ferric iron to the more soluble ferrous form. Another example is the antifungal griseofulvin, the absorption of which is promoted if administered with a high fat meal.

The presence of other drugs can also affect drug absorption. This is illustrated by the antiemetic metoclopramide, which speeds up gastric emptying and hence can promote absorption of drugs like paracetamol. This is particularly useful in the management of migraine, where gut motility is slowed. Conversely, drugs with anticholinergic effects, such as atropine, decrease drug absorption. Drug interactions do not only affect drug absorption when medications are administered orally. The combination of adrenaline (epinephrine) with lidocaine (lignocaine) is very useful when suturing small wounds, as the adrenaline (epinephrine) causes peripheral constriction and slows the removal of the lidocaine (lignocaine) from its site of action, hence prolonging its anaesthetic effects. A further bonus is that bleeding at the wound site is minimal, making visualization easier. The effect of the adrenaline (epinephrine) is so powerful that it must not be injected into fingers and toes, otherwise gangrene may occur.

The motility of the gut will also affect absorption. Slowed gastric emptying can be a significant determinant of drug response affecting the ability to achieve therapeutic levels and reducing the effectiveness of the drug. Alternatively, increased gut motility may cause the drug to pass through the gut too rapidly to be effectively absorbed. For this reason women taking the oral contraceptive pill are advised to take extra precautions if they have a bout of diarrhoea.

Blood flow

The blood flow to the site of administration will affect absorption as the process depends on the presence of a concentration gradient between the site of administration and the blood. If blood flow to the administration site is poor a concentration gradient is not maintained by the continual removal of the drug by the flowing blood, and so absorption will be poor. This explains why the administration of an intramuscular injection of analgesics to a patient in pain and in a state of shock is ineffective. In shock the blood is retained in the vital centres. The periphery, including the muscle of the buttocks, receives little blood, so the concentration gradient between the muscle and blood is small, and consequently drug absorption is poor.

Distribution

Once a drug has been absorbed into the blood it is distributed throughout the body by the blood. Drug distribution can be defined as the movement of the drug from the blood to the site of action. The rate at which a drug reaches the different areas of the body depends upon the ability of the drug to cross the capillary walls. Drugs, which are lipid-soluble readily cross capillary walls, whereas lipid-insoluble drugs take longer to arrive at their site of action. However blood flow, and hence cardiac function, also affects the rate and extent of drug distribution. Thus organs that normally have a good blood supply, for example the liver and lungs, will receive the drug first, followed by those tissues that have a poor blood supply, for example bone, muscle and fat. Poor distribution of drugs to tissues means that getting a sufficiently high concentration of drug to the site of action can be problematic, and hence treating diseases like osteomyelitis can be difficult. The problem can be increased in heart disease, e.g. congestive cardiac failure.

The body tissues can act as reservoirs and allow a drug to accumulate through binding to specific tissues in the body. This prolongs the pharmacological effect of the drug. The body's reservoirs result from plasma protein binding and tissue binding.

Plasma protein binding

Some drugs are distributed simply dissolved in plasma water, while many others are transported with some proportion of their molecules bound to plasma proteins. The main carrier protein is albumin which has a strong affinity, but low capacity, for carrying acidic drugs. Other carriers include lipoprotein and α_1-acid glycoprotein which both carry basic drugs such as chlorpromazine, imipramine and quinidine. The proportion of a drug that is dissolved in the plasma is termed free drug and the proportion attached to plasma proteins is termed 'bound' drug. The extent of this binding varies considerably, with some drugs like warfarin being 99% bound. Other highly bound drugs include diazoxide, etacrynic acid (ethacrynic acid), methotrexate, nalidixic acid, phenylbutazone and the sulphonamides (Stockley, 1996).

The binding of a drug to a plasma protein is reversible, with a dynamic equilibrium being established between those molecules that are bound and those that are free. Thus at any moment in time a molecule of drug can be bound, and the next moment it can be free; its movement on and off the carrier being random. The unbound molecules are free to interact with the tissues, and thus they are pharmacologically active. In contrast the bound drug acts as a circulating reservoir, but is pharmacologically inactive. It is also protected from metabolism and excretion by its attachment to the plasma protein. The free drug is not so protected, and hence is metabolized. As this happens the equilibrium between bound and unbound drug is upset, and to correct it more bound drug becomes free and active, and is subsequently metabolized in turn.

As plasma proteins are important for transferring drugs, a fall in the level of plasma proteins, i.e. hypoalbuminaemia, can lead to adverse drug effects. This can occur as a result of poor nutrition or as a result of disease. Diseases of the liver can result in decreased protein synthesis as well as an increase in endogenous substances like bilirubin that compete for the binding sites on the plasma protein. Some kidney diseases can result in excessive loss of plasma proteins into the urine, while drainage of fistulas and ascites can significantly decrease plasma protein levels. Table 1.11 gives some examples of the changes in bound drug levels that can occur as the result of liver and renal disease. It is therefore important that the response to protein bound drugs is monitored carefully in patients who have liver and kidney disease, and that drug dosage is adjusted accordingly.

Table 1.11 Examples of drugs that are plasma protein bound, indicating how disease can alter the degree of binding (Laurence et al., 1997)

Drug	*Percentage of bound drug - in health*	*Percentage of bound drug - in disease*
Diazepam	98%	94% in liver disease
Furosemide (frusemide)	98%	94% in nephrotic syndrome
Clofibrate	96%	89% in nephrotic syndrome
Phenytoin	91%	81% in renal disease
Triamterene	89%	60% in renal disease
Theophylline	65%	29% in liver disease
Digoxin	25%	18% in renal disease

Depending on their concentrations and their relative affinities for binding sites, one drug may compete with another drug and displace it from its binding site. The displaced, active free drug enters the plasma where its concentration can rise to produce adverse effects. However, the displacement is only likely to increase the number of free active molecules significantly if the majority of the drug is within the plasma rather than the tissues, i.e. drugs with an apparent low volume of distribution. Some examples are shown in Table 1.12.

The adverse effects caused by drug displacement from plasma proteins is often overstated, and is usually short lived. The reason for this is that as the drug becomes displaced, it becomes available for metabolism and excretion, and so the amount of total drug present in the plasma rapidly falls, reducing the risk of toxicity.

Tissue binding

Some drugs have a special affinity for some tissues. Lipid-soluble drugs, particularly general anaesthetics and the benzodiazepines, have a high affinity for adipose tissue, which is where these drugs are

Table 1.12 Examples of drugs likely to be displaced from plasma proteins and to cause adverse effects (Stockley, 1996)

Drug	*Percentage bound*	*Volume of distribution*
Anticoagulants, e.g. warfarin	99%	9 litres
Phenytoin	90%	35 litres
Sulphonylureas, e.g. tolbutamide	96%	10 litres

sequestered. Due to the relatively low blood flow through fatty tissue, it becomes a stable reservoir for the drug.

Body fat is not the only tissue in which drugs can accumulate. As a result of specialized transport mechanisms iodine is concentrated in the thyroid gland. The affinity of iodine for thyroid tissue is so strong that radioactive iodine can be given orally, and it will concentrate to such an extent in the thyroid that it can be utilized to destroy a malignancy of the gland without causing significant radiation damage elsewhere in the body. Other examples of tissue binding include the phenothiazines and chloroquine that bind to melanin-containing tissues, including the retina, which may explain their ability to cause retinopathy, and the tetracyclines which bind to growing bones and teeth resulting in mottling of the teeth and increased bone fragility in children.

Carrier-mediated transport

Cell membranes frequently contain carrier molecules, i.e. trans-membrane proteins, which bind to a specific particle and move it to the other side of the membrane. These transporters can act passively and move particles along their concentration gradient, in a process termed facilitated diffusion. Alternatively the carrier may be coupled to an energy source and so can move the particle across the membrane against its concentration gradient. Drugs can utilize these carriers for distribution purposes and important sites for this process are the gastrointestinal tract, the biliary tract, the renal tubule and the blood-brain barrier. For example, in the gut, levodopa, which is used to treat Parkinson's disease, is taken up by a carrier that normally transports phenylalanine, while the cytotoxic drug fluorouracil is transported by the system that carries the natural pyrimidines, i.e. thymine and uracil (Rang et al., 1995).

Barriers to drug distribution

Some of the membranes in the body can act as barriers to drug distribution. Two examples of this are the blood-brain barrier and the placental barrier (see p 67 for the latter).

Blood-borne substances within the capillaries of the brain are separated from the interstitial space and nerve cells by a continuous layer of endothelial cells. These cells are joined by tight junctions, are supported by a relatively thick basement membrane, and form the blood-brain barrier. Only lipid soluble drugs such as ethanol, barbiturates, general anaesthetics, and nicotine can pass easily through this anatomical structure. This can make treatment of diseases of the brain, e.g. malignancy, difficult, as the drugs cannot reach their target in sufficiently high concentrations to be effective. Consequently, the drug may need to be given directly into the cerebrospinal fluid, i.e. intrathecally. However, inflammation in the form of meningitis can disrupt the integrity of the blood-brain barrier allowing normally impermeable substances like penicillin to be given systemically to treat bacterial meningitis. Some parts of the central nervous system are functionally outside the blood-brain barrier and so are easily accessible to drugs, e.g. the chemoreceptor trigger zone which is involved in the vomiting reflex.

Volume of distribution

Once in the blood a drug disperses throughout the body compartments (Table 1.13) until equilibrium is achieved. The pattern of drug distribution is characteristic for each drug, and varies between drugs. Precise information on how a drug distributes requires biopsy samples and these are generally unacceptable for drug monitoring in patients. However, blood samples can be easily obtained and the concentration of the drug in the plasma measured. Knowing this and the dose of drug given it is possible to calculate the apparent volume of distribution. This is a theoretical volume and is defined as the volume in which the drug appears to distribute (or which it would require) if the concentration throughout the body were equal to that in the plasma (Laurence et al., 1997). If a drug remains mainly in the plasma its volume of distribution will be small, while if it is dispersed throughout the tissues its apparent volume of distribution will be large (Table 1.14). The value of this knowledge is that in the case of poisoning for example, haemodialysis will be useful in removing drugs like aspirin which have a small volume of distribution and hence remain in the plasma, but of less use for drugs like digoxin that distribute into the tissues.

A few drugs such as heparin are confined to the plasma, as the molecules are too large to traverse the capillary wall. However, drugs

Table 1.13 The main body fluid compartments of a 70 kg person.
Total body water ~ 40 litres or 50–70% of body weight, being less in women than men

Fluid compartment	*Components of fluid compartment*	*Percentage of body weight*
Intracellular fluid (~28 litres)		35–40%
Extracellullar fluid (~12 litres)	Blood plasma (~2.5 litres)	~4.5%
	Interstitial fluid (~6.5 litres)	~16%
	Lymph (~1.2 litre)	~1.2%
Transcellular fluid (~1.8 litres)	Cerebrospinal, digestive, foetus, intraocular, peritoneal, pleural, synovial (~1.8 litres)	~2.5%
Fat		~20%

Table 1.14 Apparent volume of distribution of some drugs (Laurence et al., 1997)

Drug	*Apparent volume of distribution (litres)*
Heparin	5
Aspirin	11
Gentamicin	18
Furosemide (frusemide)	21
Amoxicillin (amoxycillin)	28
Atenolol	77
Diazepam	140
Pethidine	280
Digoxin	420
Nortriptyline	1 000
Chloroquine	13 000

are more often kept in the blood because they are strongly bound to plasma proteins, as in the case of warfarin. Polar drugs such as tubocurarine, gentamicin and carbenicillin have an apparent volume of distribution similar to that of the extracellular space. This is because polar molecules are not very lipid soluble and so they are unable to enter the cells, nor can they cross the blood-brain barrier or the placental barrier. Distribution values more than the theoretical value, i.e. 0.2 L/kg result either from a limited degree of penetration into cells or from binding of the drug in the extravascular compartment. Lipid-soluble drugs such as phenytoin, ethanol and diazepam are able to enter cells and so their apparent volume of distribution relates to total body water. Binding of the drug anywhere outside the plasma compartment as well as partitioning in fat can increase the apparent volume of distribution beyond the value of total body water, e.g. morphine, tricyclic antidepressants and haloperidol.

References and further reading

Adams P (1998) Drug interactions that matter (1) Mechanisms and management. The Pharmaceutical Journal 261: 618-21

Anon (1998) Take that. New Scientist 157: 19

Aronson J (1993) Drug absorption: achieving optimal clinical response. Prescriber 4: 77-80

Bates DW, Cullen, DJ, Laird N, Petersen LA, Small SD, Servi D, Laffel G, Sweitzer BJ, Shea BF, Hallisey R, Vliet MV, Nemeskal R, Leape L (1995) Incidence of adverse drug events and potential adverse drug events. Implications for prevention. Journal of the American Medical Association 274: 29-34

Blair DC, Barnes RW, Wildner EL, Murray WJ (1971) Biological availability of oxytetracycline HCl capsules. Journal of the American Medical Association 215: 251-4

Campagna FA, Cureton G, Mirigian RA, Nelson (1963) Inactive prednisone tablets. Journal of Pharmaceutical Sciences 52: 605-6

Cooper R, Lawrence J (1996) The role of antimicrobial agents in wound care. Journal of Wound Care 5: 374-80

Cullum N, Roe B (1995) Leg Ulcers. Nursing Management: a Research-Based Guide. London: Scutari Press

deShazo RD, Kemp SF (1997) Allergic reactions to drugs and biologic agents. Journal of the American Medical Association. 278: 189-906

Finley RS (1992) Drug interactions in the oncology patient. Seminars in Oncology Nursing 8: 95-101

Glazko AJ, Kinkel AW, Alegnani WC, Holmes EL (1968) An evaluation of the absorption characteristics of different chloramphenicol preparations in normal human subjects. Clinical Pharmacology and Therapeutics 9: 472-83

Hansten PD (1998) Understanding drug-drug interactions. Science and Medicine 5: 16-25

Jha AK, Kuperman GJ, Teich JM, Leape L, Shea B, Rittenberg E, Burdick E, Seger DL, Vander Vleit M, Bates DW (1998) Identifying adverse drug events: development of a computer-based monitor and comparison with chart review and stimulated voluntary report. Journal of the American Medical Informatics Association 5: 305-14

Kirk JK (1995) Significant drug-nutrient interactions. American Family Physician 51: 1175-82

Laurence DR, Bennett PN, Brown MJ (1997) Clinical Pharmacology. 8th edn. Edinburgh: Churchill Livingstone

Lazarou J, Pomeranz BH, Corey PN (1998) Incidence of adverse drug reactions in hospitalised patients. Journal of the American Medical Association 279: 1200-5

Lee A, Beard K (1997) Adverse drug reactions. (1) Pharmacovigilance and the pharmacist. The Pharmaceutical Journal 258: 592-5

Lindenbaum J, Mellow MH, Blackstone MO, Butler VP (1971) Variation in biologic availability of digoxin from four preparations. New England Journal of Medicine 285(24): 1344-7

Murray JJ, Healy MD (1991) Drug-mineral interactions: a new responsibility for the hospital dietician. Journal of the American Dietetic Association 91: 66-70

Naysmith MR, Nicholson J (1998) Nasogastric drug administration. Professional Nurse 13: 424-7

Page CP, Curtis MJ, Sutter MC, Walker MJA, Hoffman BB (1997) Integrated Pharmacology. London: Mosby

Polk RE, Healy DP, Sahai J, Drwal L, Racht E (1989) Effect of ferrous sulfate and multivitamins with zinc on absorption of ciprofloxacin in normal volunteers. Antimicrobial Agents and Chemotherapy 33: 1841-4

Rang HP, Dale MM, Ritter JM (1995) Pharmacology. 3rd edn. Edinburgh: Churchill Livingstone

Rawlins MD, Thompson JW (1977) Pathogenesis of adverse drug reactions. In: Davies DM (ed). Textbook of adverse drug reactions. Oxford: Oxford University Press.

Searl RO, Pernarowski M (1967) The biopharmaceutical properties of solid dosage forms: I. an evaluation of 23 brands of phenylbutazone tablets. Canadian Medical Association Journal 96: 1513-20

Smith S (1984) How drugs act. 3. Side-effects. Nursing Times 80: 46-7

Stockley IH (1996) Drug Interactions. 4th edn. London: The Pharmaceutical Press

Taylor D, Helliwell M (1992) Liquid preparations for oral administration. Professional Nurse 8: 163-6

Varley AB (1968) The generic inequivalence of drugs. Journal of the American Medical Association 206: 1745-8

Wills S, Brown D (1999) A proposed new means of classifying adverse reactions to medicines. The Pharamaceutical Journal 262: 163-5

World Health Organisation (1966) International Drug Monitoring: The Role of the Hospital. Geneva: WHO. Technical Report Series No 425

Chapter 2 Pharmacokinetic effects – metabolism and excretion

Metabolism

Metabolism describes the chemical transformations that a drug undergoes, and occurs mainly in the liver. However, some metabolism occurs in a number of other tissues, for example suxamethonium in the plasma, insulin and vitamin D in the kidneys, tyramine and salbutamol in the walls of the intestine. Metabolism changes drugs in two principal ways. Firstly, many lipid-soluble, weak organic acids and bases are not readily eliminated from the body. They must therefore be metabolized to compounds that are polar, and hence more water soluble, in order that they can be excreted in the urine. Metabolism also alters the biological behaviour of drugs in one of three ways. In the case of most drugs, metabolism converts a pharmacologically active substance into an inactive substance. Alternatively, metabolism can convert a pharmacologically active substance into another active substance. For example the painkiller codeine is metabolized to morphine which is itself a powerful painkiller. Thirdly a pharmacologically inactive drug, or pro-drug as it is termed, can be converted to an active substance. For example benorilate (benorylate), which is found in many cough remedies is converted to salicylic acid (a relative of aspirin) and paracetamol.

Phase I reactions

The biochemical reactions involved in drug metabolism occur in two phases. Phase I reactions include oxidation, reduction and hydrolysis, and the products are often more reactive and sometimes more toxic than the parent drug.

Drug oxidation is the most common metabolic reaction and involves the addition of oxygen to, or the removal of hydrogen from, a drug. The smooth endoplasmic reticulum in many organs, especially the liver, contains membrane-associated enzymes, the primary components of which are the mixed function oxidases, or cytochrome P450 isoenzymes. Because it is not possible for organisms to anticipate every chemical and drug that they will encounter in their lifetime, they have had to develop systems to detoxify chemicals that they have never seen before, and this is the role of this enzyme group. The substrate specificity of this enzyme complex is very low, i.e. the enzymes are not very finicky, and so it is responsible for the oxidation of a wide variety of drugs, as well as for the oxidation of fatty acids and endogenous steroids. Because fewer than 10 cytochrome P450 isoenzymes are involved in the biotransformation of most drugs used clinically, it is not surprising that bottlenecks occasionally occur, and drugs interfere with each other's metabolism. This is one of the most common ways in which clinically important drug interactions occur.

Not all drug oxidation reactions involve the mixed function oxidase system. Some involve soluble enzymes that are found in the cytosol and mitochondria of a variety of cells and are responsible for the non-microsomal oxidation of a few drugs. For example, ethanol is metabolized by a soluble cytoplasmic enzyme, alcohol dehydrogenase, while the mitochondrial enzyme monoamine oxidase is involved in the metabolism of catecholamines and serotonin.

Reduction reactions occur in both the microsomal and non-microsomal metabolizing systems, and involve the addition of hydrogen or the removal of oxygen from the drug. Reduction reactions are much less common than oxidative ones, but are important for the metabolism of drugs such as warfarin and cortisone.

Hydrolysis is the process in which water is used to split a drug into smaller components. These reactions do not involve hepatic microsomal enzymes, but occur instead in the plasma and many body tissues.

Phase II reactions

In Phase II reactions, drugs or Phase I metabolites that are not sufficiently polar to be excreted in the urine are made more hydrophilic by conjugation. For this to occur, a drug requires a large functional polar group – usually added or unmasked during Phase I – suitable for conjugation with an endogenous substrate and the presence of transfer enzymes. Phase II reactions can involve glucuronidation, acetylation, ethylation, sulphation and conjugation with amino acids such as glycine (Finlayson, 1994). The conjugate, which is usually pharmacologically inactive and less lipid soluble than its parent molecule, is excreted in the urine or the bile.

Route of administration

Metabolism is affected by a number of factors (Table 2.1), including the route of drug administration. Any drug that is swallowed is absorbed from the gut and taken via the portal vein directly to the liver. Here the hepatic enzymes may inactivate the drug, or part of it, before it reaches its site of action. This is called first pass or presystemic metabolism. A good example of this process involves the vasodilator glyceryl trinitrate. If this is taken orally rather than sublingually, the drug is completely inactivated by the liver and no active drug reaches the systemic circulation, i.e. its oral bioavailability is zero. However, when the drug is taken sublingually the glyceryl trinitrate is absorbed through the oral mucosa directly into the systemic circulation and so it is able to have an effect on the heart before it reaches, and is broken down by, the liver. Other drugs undergoing substantial first pass metabolism are shown in Table 2.2.

Table 2.1 Factors affecting drug metabolism

Factor	*Comment*
Administration route	See text
Age	The liver cannot detoxify drugs such as chloramphenicol as well in neonates as it can in adults
Chemical properties of the drug	See text
Circadian rhythm	In rats and mice, the rate of hepatic metabolism of some drugs follows a diurnal rhythm. This may be true in humans as well (Jacob, 1992)
Diet	Starvation can deplete glycine stores and so alter glycine conjugation
Disease	See text
Gender	Young males are more prone to sedation from barbiturates than females
Genetics	See text

Table 2.2 Drugs undergoing substantial presystemic metabolism (Rang et al., 1995)

• Aspirin	• Morphine
• Clomethiazole	• Nortriptyline
• Chlorpromazine	• Pethidine
• Glyceryl trinitrate	• Propranolol
• Imipramine	• Salbutamol
• Levodopa	• Verapamil

A number of drugs form conjugates with glucuronic acid during Phase II metabolism and are excreted in the bile. The conjugates are too polar to be reabsorbed and so they remain in the gut. Here they are hydrolysed by enzymes and bacteria to release the parent drug, which is then reabsorbed into the portal circulation and reconjugated in the liver. This enterohepatic recycling is important in maintaining the effect of the NSAID sulindac, and ethinylestradiol (ethinyloestradiol), which is found in many contraceptives (Laurence et al., 1997). The recycling of drugs by the enterohepatic circulation can be adversely affected by the use of antibiotics, which may kill the bacteria in the gut so that the parent drug is not regenerated and is not available for recycling (Adams, 1998). Certainly unwanted pregnancies have been documented in patients who combined the oral contraceptive and penicillin antibiotics (Stockley, 1996).

Chemical properties of the drug

The ability of the body to metabolize drugs can be altered by the drugs themselves. In the process of enzyme induction there is an increase in the quantity of microsomal oxidase and conjugating systems following chronic exposure to chemicals such as tobacco smoke, ethanol, barbecued meats, insecticides, industrial pollutants and some drugs (Table 2.3). Some inducing agents such as phenobarbital (phenobarbitone) cause a non-selective increase in many of the metabolic enzymes, whereas drugs like ethanol produce effects that are more selective. The importance of induction arises because it can lead to clinically important drug interactions. For example, the antituberculous drug rifampicin has a relatively selective effect on the activity of steroid metabolizing enzymes, which can reduce the effectiveness of the oral contraceptive pill. The low-dose oestrogen pill relies on a minimum concentration of oestrogen to maintain

Table 2.3 Induction and inhibition of cytochrome P450 isoenzymes (Hansten, 1998)

Isoenzyme	*Examples of substrates*	*Examples of inhibitors*	*Examples of inducers*
CYP1A2	Clozapine Theophylline Tacrine	Ciprofloxacin Fluvoxamine Mexiletine	Barbiturates Carbamazepine Smoking
CYP2C9	Phenytoin Tolbutamide Warfarin	Amiodarone Cimetidine Fluconazole	Barbiturates Carbamazepine Rifampicin
CYP2C19	Diazepam Lansoprazole Omeprazole	Fluoxetine Fluvoxamine Omeprazole	Barbiturates Rifampicin
CYP2D6	Codeine Dextromethorphan Metoprolol	Cimetidine Paroxetine Quinidine	Not very susceptible to induction
CYP2E1	Alcohol Isoniazid Paracetamol	Alcohol intoxication Disulfiram Isoniazid**	Alcohol abuse (person sober)* Isoniazid**
CYP3A4***	Cisapride Cyclosporin Vinca alkaloids	Erythromycin Grapefruit Verapamil	Griseofulvin Phenytoin Primidone

* Acute alcohol intoxication tends to inhibit CYP2E1, while chronic alcohol abuse leads to enzyme induction when the individual is sober.
** Isoniazid tends to inhibit CYP2E1 while it is in the body, but induces it several hours later.
*** Highly susceptible to induction.

adequate contraception, and enzyme induction substantially increases the risk of pregnancy (Waller, 1993).

Enzyme induction may also partially explain drug tolerance. Tolerance is defined as a decreased physiological response to a drug due to prior exposure. Thus, the patient needs more drug in order to get the same effect. It can occur when repeated administration of a drug reduces its concentration at its receptor sites by increasing the drug's rate of metabolism (metabolic tolerance). In the case of barbiturates, for example, enzyme induction results in increased metabolism so that a given dose of barbiturate produces a reduced effect. Alternatively, tolerance can occur where repeated drug administration brings about adaptive changes at the receptor or closely related systems (cellular or pharmacodynamic tolerance). Tolerance to the sedative effects of benzodiazepines is an example of pharmacodynamic tolerance and results from changes in the responsiveness of the central nervous system (Edwards, 1997).

Enzyme inhibition is the opposite of enzyme induction. It occurs when one drug inhibits the metabolism of a second drug. Inhibition of enzyme-catalysed reactions occurs more rapidly than induction, and can occur even after a single dose. Widely used enzyme inhibitors include allopurinol, dextropropoxyphene (a constituent of coproxamol), quinidine and cimetidine. Enzyme inhibition can cause toxicity effects. For example, if a patient is prescribed both the NSAID azapropazone and the anti-diabetic drug tolbutamide, the azapropazone may inhibit the metabolism of the tolbutamide so that the tolbutamide is not broken down, continues being active, and possibly precipitates a hypoglycaemic coma. Andreasen et al. (1981) found that azapropazone increases the serum half-life of tolbutamide threefold.

Enzyme induction does not just lead to drug interactions, it can also lead to interactions with dietary nutrients. For example, anti-epilepsy drugs increase the breakdown of dietary and endogenously formed vitamin D, producing an inactive metabolite. This can be severe enough to lead to osteomalacia. The accompanying hypocalcaemia can increase the tendency to fits and a convulsion may lead to fractures of the demineralized bones.

The effect of inducers and inhibitors on drug metabolism can be quite complex, as can be illustrated by alcohol. The effects of ethanol on drug metabolism vary depending on the amount, duration and timing of alcohol ingestion relative to the drug. Acute alcohol intoxication tends to inhibit drug metabolism, thus increasing the serum concentration and pharmacodynamic effects of concurrently administered drugs. This is why it is dangerous to ingest alcohol together with other central nervous system depressants such as the benzodiazepines. The alcohol adds to the depressant effects of the benzodiazepine, whilst at the same time inhibiting the ability of the body to metabolize and inactivate the drug. Conversely, chronic alcohol abuse tends to result in enzyme induction. However, this alcohol-induced increase in drug metabolism is only observed when the individual is not intoxicated, i.e. when the enzymes are not being utilized to metabolize alcohol. Thus, in a chronic alcohol abuser the metabolism of drugs can be slower than normal when he is intoxicated or faster than normal when he is sober. Furthermore, long-term alcohol abuse can lead to liver damage, which impairs drug metabolism and further complicates the picture.

Genetics

Genetic differences and abnormalities can affect metabolism. There are two distinct types of the enzyme cholinesterase, namely acetylcholinesterase or true cholinesterase, and butyrylcholinesterase or pseudocholinesterase. The former is membrane-bound and is found in the synaptic cleft of cholinergic synapses where it breaks down the released neurotransmitter. Pseudocholinesterase in contrast is found in a variety of tissues as well as in the plasma. It has broader substrate specificity than true cholinesterase, and is responsible for metabolizing drugs such as procaine and suxamethonium. About 1 in 3000 people have a deficiency of pseudocholinesterase, as a result of having two copies of the recessive gene responsible for the deficiency. Consequently, they have difficulty metabolizing suxamethonium. This widely used short acting neuromuscular blocking agent is normally inactivated within a few minutes by plasma cholinesterase. In people with cholinesterase deficiency, the neuromuscular block lasts for several hours, and the patient requires ventilating until it has worn off. Relatives of an affected individual should be sought out, checked to assess their own risk, and told of the result.

Disease

The liver is the major site of drug metabolism, and so it is to be expected that diseases affecting the liver are likely to affect drug metabolism. Diseases that have been shown to affect metabolism include alcoholic liver disease, cirrhosis, hepatoma, porphyria (see Chapter 12), and viral hepatitis. With the notable exception of chronic ethanol exposure, diseases of the liver decrease its ability to metabolize drugs. Possible reasons for this decreased capacity are decreased liver enzyme activity, altered hepatic blood flow and hypoalbuminaemia. The picture however is complex as the metabolism of some drugs is affected, whilst those of others is not, as shown in Table 2.4.

Other non-hepatic diseases can also affect metabolism. These particularly include the hormonal diseases such as hyperthyroidism, pituitary insufficiency (dwarfism), adrenal insufficiency, pituitary, thyroid or adrenal tumours, diabetes and the genetic abnormalities

Table 2.4 The effect of liver cirrhosis on drug metabolism (Gibson and Skett, 1986)

Drugs affected	*Drugs not affected*
• Barbiturates	• Lorazepam
• Chlordiazepoxide	• Morphine
• Diazepam	• Oxazepam
• Methadone	• Paracetamol
• Salicylates	

of sexual development (Gibson and Skett, 1986). The importance of hormonal control is well established in rats and mice but has been little regarded in clinical practice, perhaps due to lack of research in this field in humans.

Drug elimination

Drug elimination is the process by which a drug or its metabolite is excreted from the body, and is considered to have occurred when 95% of the drug is excreted. Elimination generally takes five plasma half-lives (Lovejoy and Matteis, 1996). The drug can be excreted via any body fluid, including urine, bile, sweat, saliva, faeces, breast milk and across the placenta. Some drugs such as anaesthetic gases are eliminated in expired air; this route is also utilized for medico-legal purposes in the breathalyser test to identify the alcohol concentration in the expired air of vehicle drivers. However, the kidneys together with the gall bladder are the most important organs for drug excretion. Depending on metabolism the excreted drug may be active or inactive. If the drug is still active then elimination is important in getting rid of the drug and preventing it from building up in the blood and becoming toxic. If the drug is in an inactive non-harmful state then the process of elimination is not quite so crucial. However, whether excreted in an active or inactive state concern is being expressed because the excreted drugs are 'turning up in tap water at concentrations to rival those of pesticides' (Pearce, 1999).

Glomerular filtration

The term clearance is used to express removal of a drug from the blood, and is usually associated with the kidney. Renal clearance is dependent upon three processes, the first being glomerular filtration, in which small molecules (those with a molecular weight less than 10000) are forced from the blood in the glomerular tuft into the Bowman's capsule of the nephron. Water soluble and polar compounds, once they are in the kidney tubule, are unable to diffuse back into the circulation and so are excreted unless there is a specific transport mechanism for their reabsorption.

The process of filtration decreases with renal disease and decreases quite considerably with age. Thus, the elderly have a reduced ability to clear drugs from their body, which partly explains why this age group is particularly prone to developing side-effects from drugs. The problem in the elderly is complicated by the fact that many of the drugs that they take have a narrow therapeutic window. This means that the difference between the dose that causes a therapeutic effect and that which causes a toxic effect is small. Thus, a small decrease in excretion can result in the rapid development of side-effects.

Renal tubular reabsorption

The glomerular filtrate contains the same concentration of drug as is found free (unbound) in the plasma. As the filtrate passes along the nephron, the filtrate is progressively concentrated so that the concentration of drug in the filtrate becomes higher than that in the blood. If the kidney tubule is freely permeable to the drug then about 99% of the filtered drug will return to the blood, which means that clearing a drug from the body would take a long time. Whether a drug diffuses down its concentration gradient and returns to the blood depends upon how lipid soluble it is, and, as already indicated, metabolism transforms drugs so that they are not lipid soluble, and so they remain in the filtrate.

Drugs are lipid soluble when they are non-ionized; whether they are ionized or not depends to some degree on the relative acidity or alkalinity of the filtrate in the nephron. Thus, as the filtrate becomes more alkaline, any acidic drug present will become more ionized and so less lipid soluble, and so its reabsorption into the blood will decrease. Similarly, a basic drug will become more ionized in an acidic environment. This knowledge can be utilized to speed up the process of drug elimination in the case of drug overdose. The administration of sodium bicarbonate will make the urine more alkaline and this will hold acidic drugs, such as aspirin and barbiturates, in the kidney tubule and prevent them being reabsorbed. Similarly, acidification of the urine will speed up the excretion of alkaline drugs like amphetamines. This process is called forced diuresis.

Renal tubular secretion

Mechanisms for active tubular secretion exist in the proximal tubule. The cells lining the kidney tubule perform this energy requiring process, which allows the body to excrete normal waste products like creatinine and uric acid against their concentration gradients. Although there are no active transport mechanisms designed by the body to get rid of specific drugs, the proteins that carry out the shunting process can be utilized by some drugs. Two transport mechanisms move chemicals from the blood into the tubular filtrate. Firstly the hippurate system, which transports organic acids and is used by drugs such as penicillins and probenecid, and, secondly, a carrier system for organic bases which is utilized by drugs such as quinidine and amiloride (Table 2.5).

Tubular secretion is potentially the most effective mechanism for drug elimination by the kidney, especially as unlike glomerular filtration, carrier mediated transport can achieve maximal drug clearance even when most of the drug is bound to plasma proteins. This is because the carrier transports drug molecules unaccompanied by water, unlike filtration that involves isosmotic movement of water and solutes. Thus as drug molecule is removed from the plasma by

Table 2.5 Examples of drugs that are actively secreted into the proximal kidney tubule (Rang et al., 1995)

Acids	*Bases*
• Cephalosporins	• Amiloride
• Furosemide (frusemide)	• Amfetamine (amphetamine)
• Indometacin (indomethacin)	• Dopamine
• Methotrexate	• Morphine
• Penicillins	• Pethidine
• Phenobarbital (phenobarbitone)	• Quinine
• Probenecid	• Triamterene

the carrier, the concentration of free drug falls. This causes a net dissociation of bound drug from its plasma protein, making it available to the carrier for transport into the kidney tubule. Thus, all of the drug, both bound and unbound is effectively available to the carrier.

Knowledge of the active transport process can be utilized to alter drug excretion. Thus, when penicillin was first discovered in 1928 it was not possible to manufacture it in sufficient quantities to meet demand, although the urine of patients treated with the drug was collected and the drug extracted for reuse. One solution to this problem was to give the penicillin in conjunction with the drug probenecid, which is used to treat gout. This drug uses the same transport molecule as penicillin, and so the probenecid molecules and penicillin compete for sites on the transport molecule, with the result that less penicillin is excreted in the urine. Thus, smaller doses of penicillin are required to achieve the same therapeutic effect. However, competition between drugs can also result in adverse effects. It is suggested that the amantadine toxicity observed when it is administered with triamterene or trimethoprim is the result of competition for the basic drug transport system (Hansten, 1998).

Biliary excretion

The liver, like the kidneys, has two active transport systems, one for acids and one for bases. In addition, a carrier system transports non-ionized molecules like digoxin into the bile. Small molecules tend to be reabsorbed by the bile canaliculi and generally only compounds that have a molecular weight greater than 300 are excreted in bile.

Half-life

The four components of pharmokinetics do not work alone, but in concert. Firstly, metabolism and excretion work together to affect a drug's half-life. This is the time taken for the concentration of a drug in the blood to fall by half, and can range from minutes to days (Table 2.6). The relevance of half-life is that drugs with long half-lives have the potential to accumulate and reach toxic levels. This is of concern with drugs like digoxin, which already have a narrow therapeutic window. Any increase in length of half-life can quickly turn a therapeutic dose of drug into a toxic one.

Table 2.6 Half-lives of a selection of drugs (Mucklow, 1993)

Drug	*Half-life (t1/2)*
Isoprenaline	3 minutes
Naloxone	1–1.5 hours
Gentamicin	2–4 hours
Morphine	2.5 hours
Atenolol	5–9 hours
Imipramine	8–20 hours
Digoxin	20–50 hours
Phenobarbital (phenobarbitone)	17–120 hours
Thyroxine	6–7 days
Mefloquine	21 days
Amiodarone	50 days

Steady state

The level of a drug in the bloodstream and in the body as a whole depends on the relative rates of absorption of the drug and its elimination. If drug is administered faster than it is eliminated, it will accumulate as time goes by. The concentration increases until a steady state is attained. The concentration does not carry on rising indefinitely because the body responds to the increasing blood levels and increases metabolism and excretion. Steady state may take several weeks in the case of drugs such as the anti-epileptic drug phenytoin. This means that there is no point in frequently changing drug doses if they do not have an effect immediately. Furthermore, patients need to be made aware of this if they are not going to discontinue the medication because they falsely believe that the drug is not effective.

The idea of steady state underpins good pain control. After major surgery patients tend to have considerable pain for which they are given strong analgesia. If this is given every four to six hours by intramuscular injection, the client has to wait for the drug to be absorbed before he experiences any benefit. Thus, the client experiences peaks and troughs in his pain control. If the client is given the same drug by intravenous infusion then the drug does not have to be absorbed; it is already in the blood. Furthermore, if a very small dose of the painkiller is infused continuously, drug levels remain at a steady state and the client's pain is effectively controlled with minimal side-effects.

References and further reading

Adams P (1998) Drug interactions that matter (3) Antibiotics. The Pharmaceutical Journal 261: 779-83

Andreasen PB, Simonsen K, Brocks K, Dimo B, Bouchelouche P (1981) Hypoglycaemia induced by azapropazone-tolbutamide interaction. British Journal of Clinical Pharmacology 12: 581-3

Edwards J (1997) Guarding against adverse drug events. American Journal of Nursing 97: 26-30

Finlayson NDC (1994) Drugs and the liver. Medicine International 22: 455-9

Gibson GG, Skett P (1986) Introduction to Drug Metabolism. London: Chapman and Hall

Hansten PD (1998) Understanding drug-drug interactions. Science and Medicine 5: 16-25

Jacob LS (1992) Pharmacology. 3rd edn. Pennsylvania: Harwal Publishing Company

Laurence DR, Bennett PN, Brown MJ (1997) Clinical Pharmacology. 8th edn. Edinburgh: Churchill Livingstone

Lovejoy NC, Matteis M (1996) Pharmacokinetics and pharmacodynamics of mood-altering drugs in patients with cancer. Cancer Nursing 19: 407-18

Mucklow J (1993) What effect does half-life have on drug response? Prescriber 4: 58-61

Pearce F (1999) Something in the water. New Scientist 161: 18-19

Rang HP, Dale MM, Ritter JM (1995) Pharmacology. 3rd edn. Edinburgh: Churchill Livingstone

Stockley IH (1996) Drug Interactions. 4th edn. London: The Pharmaceutical Press

Waller D (1993) How relevant is drug metabolism to prescribing? Prescriber 4: 53-7

Chapter 3 Pharmacodynamics and receptors

Pharmacodynamics is the study of how drugs exert their effects on the body, be the effects therapeutic or toxic. An understanding of how drugs produce their effects is important as it enables those dealing with drugs to predict adverse effects, it reminds them when not to combine drugs with the same mode of action, and it allows them to anticipate some types of drug interactions. It also allows them to understand the likely time course of response and, in some cases, it may help them to identify how to treat drug toxicity (Aronson, 1993). Most drugs exert their effects by interacting with the macromolecules of a cell or organism to initiate biochemical and physiological changes that lead to the drug's observed effect. The main macromolecules targeted by drugs are receptors, ion channels, enzymes, and carriers. These will be looked at in this and the following chapter. However, a few drugs owe their activity to purely mechanical or chemical effects, and it is worth briefly looking at a couple of examples of this first.

Mechanical and chemical agents

Drugs that work simply because of their chemistry or mechanical properties make up some of the most commonly used drugs. For example, antacids are all alkalis or bases that reduce gastric acidity by chemically neutralizing hydrochloric acid in the stomach. By raising the pH they also inactivate the proteolytic enzyme pepsin, which only functions at a pH of less than 5.The alkali most commonly used is a hydroxide, but also carbonates, bicarbonates, and trisilicates are utilized. The therapeutic and adverse effects of an antacid depend upon the metal ion with which the alkali is combined, and this is usually aluminium, magnesium or sodium. The advantage of aluminium and magnesium is that they themselves inactivate pepsin. However, magnesium salts act as purgatives, while aluminium salts tend to cause constipation. Aluminium salts may also cause encephalopathy in patients with chronic renal failure, and by binding phosphates so that they are not absorbed from the gut, they may cause hypophosphataemia.

The laxatives consist of four groups of drugs that all act purely mechanically. The bulk laxatives such as methylcellulose and ispaghula work by increasing the volume of faecal material in the large intestine, and in so doing they stimulate the stretch detectors in the bowel promoting peristalsis in the large intestine. The osmotic laxatives, which include magnesium salts and lactulose, exert an osmotic pressure that serves to retain fluid within the bowel. This fluid keeps the stool soft, and the increased bulk stimulates peristalsis. The third group is the faecal softeners such as docusate sodium that lower the surface tension of fluids in the bowel and so allow more water to remain in the faeces. Finally, the stimulant laxatives such as dantron (danthron) and senna increase gut motility.

Receptors

Receptors are proteins found mainly in the phospholipid bilayer that makes up cell membranes. As the receptors are on the cell surface the chemicals with which they interact do not need to be lipid soluble, as they do not have to enter the cell in order to initiate a response. Some receptors are found within the cytoplasm and these are utilized by lipid soluble chemicals such as steroids (Kelly, 1995).

Receptors are the targets for the body's own chemical messengers, namely hormones and neurotransmitters. When an endogenous chemical interacts with a receptor, it does so through a lock and key mechanism. The binding of the small molecule, or ligand, with the receptor results in a conformational change in the receptor, which is in turn coupled to a cascade of events within the cell that eventually lead to a response. Only cells with the appropriate receptor can respond to a particular ligand, and the response triggered is dependent upon the cell itself. Thus, for example the response to noradrenaline (norepinephrine) of the non-sphincter smooth muscle of the gastro-intestinal tract is to relax, while the sphincter smooth muscle cells of the gut respond by contracting. Drugs interact with receptors in one of three main ways, by acting as agonists, antagonists or partial agonists.

Agonists

Agonists are molecules that bind to a receptor, activate it, and produce a biological response. They do so because they resemble the endogenous chemical. The response produced is the same as that which the endogenous chemical would produce, or at least reproduces some of the effects of the endogenous compound. This means that all the hormones and neurotransmitters produced by the body can be classified as agonists. For example, adrenaline (epinephrine) is an agonist at adrenoceptors (adrenaline receptors) whether it is produced as a consequence of watching a horror movie or as a result of an injection of the chemical as a drug, and its effect will be the same regardless of the source.

It might be thought that all agonists are simply the endogenous chemicals of the body given as drugs, but this is not entirely true. Morphine is an example of an agonist that has been used to relieve pain for thousands of years. However, until recently it was not known how morphine worked. Receptors have now been found in the brain and spinal cord to which morphine binds, and in 1975 the endogenous chemicals that normally bind to these receptors were also found. They are called endogenous opioid peptides and consist of three groups, i.e. endorphins, enkephalins and dynorphins. Both morphine and the opioid peptides work in the same way, i.e. they bind to receptors in the brainstem and spinal cord and reduce the activity of the dorsal horn relay neurones. As a result, they produce analgesia. Morphine is an agonist despite the fact that its effect is to reduce or inhibit neurotransmission, because it is having the same effect as the endogenous chemical when it acts at the same site.

Receptor subtypes

Researchers have found that all the receptors for a particular hormone or neurotransmitter are not identical, and that there are receptor subtypes. This can be illustrated with the neurotransmitter and localized hormone, histamine. When histamine receptors were examined by molecular biologists, they were found to differ slightly from each other, and they were classified accordingly - H_1, H_2 and H_3. Histamine binds to all these receptor subtypes and brings about its appropriate biological response. However, as the receptors are slightly different, drugs can be produced which fit one receptor subtype but not another. The benefit of this is that the desired effect can be obtained with minimal unwanted effects. Thus, for example, if one wanted for some reason to cause the stomach to produce more acid you could give an H_2-agonist that will bind to H_2-receptors, leading to acid production, but not to H_1-receptors. Thus, you would get the effect you wanted - production of stomach acid, without the side-effects, i.e. an allergic response. As more receptor subtypes are identified, drug companies can produce drugs that are more specific. This will help to minimize adverse drug effects, although, it must be noted that selectivity is not usually 100%.

Drug specificity

For a drug to be therapeutically useful it must act selectively on particular cells and tissues, i.e. it must show a high degree of binding site specificity. Similarly, receptors that act as drug targets generally show a high degree of ligand specificity, i.e. they recognize only ligands of a certain type and ignore closely related molecules. However, it must be emphasized that no drug acts with complete specificity. Thus, antihistamines that can be shown to have a greater affinity for H_1-receptors than for other sites, produce many effects such as sedation and suppression of vomiting, which do not appear to depend on histamine antagonism. In general the lower the potency of the drug and the higher the dose needed to bring about an effect, the more likely it is that sites of action other than the primary one will assume significance. In clinical terms, this is often associated with the appearance of unwanted side-effects. For example, the β_2-agonist salbutamol, which is used to promote bronchial dilation, may activate β_1-adrenoceptors in the heart causing tachycardia and palpitations.

Antagonists

Antagonists are drugs that prevent an agonist from binding to a receptor. Antagonists do not themselves have any pharmacological actions mediated by the receptors. Antagonists exert their effect by preventing the endogenous chemical from interacting with the receptor and bringing about a response. For example, if a patient was suffering from excess stomach acidity, an alternative to using an antacid to neutralize the acid would be to utilize a drug that was an antagonist at histamine H_2-receptors. This type of drug exists in the form of cimetidine and ranitidine, and they block or antagonize the histamine receptors on the stomach involved with gastric acid secretion, but have a minimal effect on the other receptor subtypes.

Another example of an antagonist is propranolol, which is an antagonist at adrenoceptors. If a person is suffering from the symptoms of stress before taking an examination, they may be prescribed propranolol. This will bind to the adrenoceptors and stop the adrenaline (epinephrine) from having its effect; i.e. it will stop the person having palpitations and feeling stressed. However, if a person was not stressed by examinations, they would not release any endogenous adrenaline (epinephrine) or noradrenaline (norepinephrine) and so the propranolol would not have any effect, as there would be no endogenous chemical to antagonize, or block from reaching the receptor. This is an important property of antagonists; they will only have an effect if there is endogenous chemical present available to bind to receptors.

A third example of an antagonist is the drug tamoxifen. This is used to treat breast cancer. It binds to receptors in the cytoplasm of breast cells. Not all receptors are in the cell membrane, some are in the cytoplasm itself, and so the drug molecules have to pass through the cell membrane to reach their target. In order to do this they must be lipid soluble, like the steroidal hormones, of which oestrogen is an example. Tamoxifen binds to receptors in breast tissue and blocks the oestrogen that normally binds to the receptor. As the oestrogen is important in stimulating the breast cell to grow and multiply, the blockage of the receptor slows the growth of the cancer. Table 3.1 gives some further examples of agonists and antagonists.

Partial agonists

It would appear from the discussion so far that a drug either activates a receptor, i.e. it acts as an agonist, or it causes no activation, i.e. it acts as an antagonist. In reality however, the ability of a drug to activate a receptor is graded, rather than an all-or-nothing property. Some drugs bind to a receptor and produce a maximal response, i.e.

Table 3.1 Examples of agonists and antagonists working at different receptor subtypes

Receptor subtype	*Agonist*	*Antagonist*
Acetylcholine–muscarinic	Acetylcholine	Atropine
Acetylcholine–nicotinic	Nicotine	Tubocurarine
Adrenoceptor–α_1	Phenylephrine	Prazosin
Adrenoceptor–α_2	Clonidine	–
Adrenoceptor–β_1	Dobutamine	Atenolol
Adrenoceptor–β_2	Salbutamol	–
Dopamine–D_2	Bromocriptine	Chlorpromazine
$GABA_A$	Diazepam	Flumazenil
$GABA_B$	Baclofen	–
Histamine–H_1	Histamine	Terfenadine
Histamine–H_2	Histamine	Cimetidine
Serotonin–$5HT_{1D}$	Sumatriptan	Ergotamine
Serotonin–$5HT_3$	Serotonin	Ondansetron

the largest response that the tissue is able to give. These are known as full agonists. Other drugs, known as partial agonists, produce a response that falls short of the full response. However, while these partial agonists are bound to the receptor they are blocking the access of the endogenous chemical to the receptor. As the endogenous molecule will normally produce a greater degree of receptor activation than the partial agonist, these drugs have both agonistic and antagonistic actions. Oxprenolol and pindolol are partial agonists at ß-adrenoceptors.

An agonist's strength of action depends on two parameters. Firstly, its affinity, i.e. its tendency to bind to receptors, and, secondly, its pharmacological efficacy, i.e. its ability once bound to initiate changes which lead to effects. However, of greater concern to clinicians is the therapeutic efficacy or effectiveness of a drug. Thus if one drug can produce a therapeutic effect that cannot be obtained with another drug, no matter how much of that drug is given, then the first drug has a greater therapeutic efficacy. Laurence et al. (1997) illustrate this concept with three diuretics. Amiloride has a low therapeutic efficacy as it can cause no more than 5% of filtered sodium to be excreted in the urine. Bendroflumethiazide (bendrofluazide) is of moderate efficacy because the maximum sodium it can cause to be excreted is 10%, no matter how much drug is administered, while furosemide (frusemide) has high efficacy as it can cause 25% or more of filtered sodium to be excreted.

Receptor regulation

Chronic exposure to drugs can lead to an alteration in receptor response. Some receptors, when exposed to an agonist repeatedly, can become desensitized. For example, bronchodilators that act on ß-adrenergic receptors and are used to treat asthma can become less effective when repeatedly administered at the same concentration. An explanation for this change in response could be that the signal generated by the stimulated receptor has become depressed, or that the receptor itself has been altered. Radioligand binding studies demonstrate that receptor numbers do not remain constant over time, but that they can change according to circumstances. Chronic exposure to an agonist can result in a decrease in the number of receptors in the cell membrane, or down-regulation, as it is termed. The superfluous receptors are taken into the cytoplasm of the cell.

Supersensitivity of receptors to agonists can occur with chronic administration of an antagonist. For example, abrupt discontinuation of propranolol in a patient who has been taking it chronically can precipitate dysrhythmias. Supersensitivity may result from the synthesis of additional receptors (up-regulation).

References and further reading

Aronson J (1993) How drugs produce their pharmacological effects. Prescriber 4: 21-5

Kelly J (1995) Pharmacodynamics and drug therapy. Professional Nurse 10: 792-6

Laurence DR, Bennett PN, Brown MJ (1997) Clinical Pharmacology. 8th ed. Edinburgh: Churchill Livingston.

Chapter 4 Pharmacodynamics, enzymes, ion channels and carriers

Ion channels

Ion channels are proteins found in cell membranes that act as pores and allow the movement of ions, or small charged particles, down their electrochemical gradient. The opening of an ion channel is controlled either by the membrane electrical potential (voltage-gated) or by the binding of a molecule to a binding site on the ion channel (ligand-gated). Some ion channels, like the calcium-channels in the heart, are both voltage and ligand sensitive. There is a variety of ion channels (Table 4.1); drugs interact with them either as blockers or modulators.

Table 4.1 Examples of drugs that act as blockers and modulators at different ion channels (Rang et al., 1995)

Ion channels	*Blockers*	*Modulators*
Voltage-gated Ca^{2+}-channels	–	Dihdropyridines, e.g. nifedipine
GABA-gated Cl^--channels	–	Benzodiazepines, e.g. diazepam
Glutamate-gated Cl^--channels	Ketamine	–
Voltage-gated Na^+-channels	Local anaesthetics, e.g. lidocaine (lignocaine)	–
Renal tubule Na^+-channels	Amiloride	Aldosterone
ATP-sensitive K^+-channels	–	Sulphonylureas, e.g. tolbutamide
Voltage-gated K^+-channels	4-aminopyridine (not used clinically)	–

Blockers

The simplest form of interaction between a drug and an ion channel involves a physical blocking of the mouth of the channel by a drug molecule so that ions cannot move through. Examples of this blocking action are the local anaesthetics, such as lidocaine (lignocaine), on the voltage-gated sodium channel, or the blocking of sodium entry into renal tubular cells by the diuretic amiloride.

Modulators

The second way in which drugs can interact with ion channels is as modulators. This means that the drug either increases or decreases the ease with which ion channels open. This effect can be illustrated with the example of diazepam. This well-known drug is a tranquillizer that interacts with a neurotransmitter called GABA (gamma-amino butyric acid). GABA is an example of an inhibitory neurotransmitter, which means that when GABA is released at a synaptic junction it will diffuse across the synaptic cleft and affect the post-synaptic nerve so that it becomes hyperpolarized and is unable to conduct a nervous impulse. When GABA is released from a nerve terminal it diffuses across the synaptic gap and binds to a binding site on the ion channels on the post-synaptic membrane. This causes the ion channels to open and chloride ions to enter. If a patient has taken some diazepam, this binds to another binding site on the ion channel. In so doing the diazepam makes it easier for the GABA to bind to its binding site, and therefore more likely for chloride ions to enter the nerve. If more chloride ions move into the post-synaptic nerve, it becomes inhibited. It is this general inhibition of the nervous system that brings about the tranquillizing effects of the benzodiazepines.

Enzymes

Enzymes are highly specialized proteins that are found embedded in plasma membranes, inside cells, and in tissue fluids. They act as biological catalysts, which means that they speed up the rate of chemical reactions without themselves being changed. Enzymes convert one molecule, termed the substrate, to another molecule, termed the product, in either anabolic or catabolic reactions. The substrate, which is considerably smaller than the enzyme, reacts with a particular area on the enzyme called the active site. Most enzymes appear to function according to an induced-fit principle whereby the binding of the substrate to the enzyme causes a change of shape in the latter so that the substrate can fit exactly into the active site. Enzymes are very efficient, with some enzymes metabolizing substrate at the rate of 1012 molecules per second (Martin, 1983), and as such, they make a valuable target for drug therapy.

Inhibitors

One way that drugs can interact with enzymes is as inhibitors. The drug binds either reversibly or irreversibly to the active site of the enzyme and so prevents the substrate from binding. A good example of an enzyme inhibitor is the drug aspirin.

When tissue is damaged, the phospholipids of the cell membrane are converted to arachidonic acid by the enzyme phospholipase A_2. The arachidonic acid is in turn converted to a common prostaglandin precursor, PGH_2, by the enzyme cyclooxygenase, and this in turn is finally converted to various types of prostaglandins by cell-specific synthases.

Prostaglandins are a complex group of chemicals that have a variety of effects. One of their functions is to cause the symptoms of inflammation, i.e. redness, swelling, pain and fever. A drug that can inhibit the enzyme cyclooxygenase can prevent prostaglandins being formed, and thus reduce the symptoms that they evoke. This is in fact what aspirin and related drugs such as paracetamol and ibuprofen do – they attach to the active site of the enzyme, prevent the formation of prostaglandins, and so reduce the symptoms of inflammation. However, as prostaglandins have so many different roles (Table 4.2) inhibition of prostaglandin synthesis can result in many side-effects. In the 1980s, it was found that there are two cyclooxygenase enzymes, COX-1 and COX-2. COX-1 is continuously expressed in almost all tissues; it is required to convert arachidonic acid to prostaglandins for homeostatic functions. COX-2, however, appears to be produced only during the inflammatory response when it regulates the synthesis of prostaglandins involved in this process. Thus, compounds that inhibit COX-2 but not COX-1 would be expected to be effective anti-inflammatory drugs whilst producing minimal side-effects; selective COX-2 inhibitors are at present being developed.

Table 4.2 Physiological functions of prostaglandins (Needleman and Isakson, 1998)

- Protect the stomach mucosa from acid
- Promote platelet aggregation
- Increase renal blood flow
- Regulate salt and water balance
- Relax bronchial smooth muscle
- Contract uterine smooth muscle
- ? Participate in memory and other cognitive functions in the central nervous system

Activators

As well as inhibiting enzymes drugs can also activate them, or are themselves enzymes (Aronson, 1993). For example, the proteins involved in the clotting cascade and the fibrinolytic pathway are enzymes, and some drugs that act on clotting and fibrinolysis do so by increasing the activity of these enzymes. Thus, heparin acts as an anticoagulant by activating the enzyme prothrombin III, whilst the drugs streptokinase, alteplase, and anistreplase are activators of plasminogen, converting it to the enzyme plasmin, which digests clots. Clotting factor deficiencies can be treated by replacing deficient enzymes, as in the case of factor VIII, which is given to haemophiliacs. Similarly, children with cystic fibrosis who do not secrete pancreatic digestive enzymes into their gut can be given replacements in tablet form.

False substrates

A drug is described as a false substrate when it interacts with an enzyme and undergoes chemical transformation to form an abnormal product that subverts the normal metabolic pathway. An example of a drug that acts in this way is the antihypertensive methyldopa. Chemically this drug is very similar to dopa, which is converted to noradrenaline (norepinephrine) in adrenergic neurones. Due to its similar chemical structure the methyldopa is able to fit into the active site of the enzymes that act on dopa, but instead of being converted to noradrenaline (norepinephrine), methyldopa is converted to α-methylnoradrenaline. The false transmitter tends to collect in the neurone, as it is not broken down in the same way as noradrenaline (norepinephrine) is. Thus when the neurone is stimulated to release neurotransmitter, α-methylnoradrenaline is released instead of noradrenaline (norepinephrine). Because α-methylnoradrenaline is less active at adrenergic receptors than noradrenaline (norepinephrine) it causes less vasoconstriction and consequently reduces peripheral resistance and so helps to lower blood pressure. Furthermore, α-methylnoradrenaline is more effective than noradrenaline (norepinephrine) at stimulating the inhibitory feedback mechanism that controls the amount of transmitter released by the neurone. Thus, the amount of transmitter released is less than normal, which further adds to methyldopa's antihypertensive effects.

Pro-drugs

Pro-drugs are inactive drugs, which rely on enzymes in the body to activate them. It might appear more logical to give the active drug in the first place, but some drugs are unpalatable, irritable to the stomach or poorly absorbed from the gut, and these problems can be reduced by utilization of a pro-drug. The active drug is linked to another chemical group in order to render it more palatable, less irritant, or better absorbed. The drug is then converted to its active derivative either on its first pass through the liver or by other tissue enzymes. For example, the antibiotic ampicillin has a variable and low bioavailability. Consequently, large doses of the drug are required to achieve adequate tissue concentrations, with the result that considerable amounts of ampicillin reach the colon unabsorbed, leading to disturbances of bowel flora and a high incidence of diarrhoea (Waller, 1993). Pro-drug derivatives of ampicillin, such as pivampicillin, are more completely absorbed, therefore they are effective at lower oral doses, and so there is reduced risk of bowel upset.

Another example of the use of pro-drugs is in the treatment of Parkinson's disease. In this disease there is a lack of dopamine in a part of the brain called the basal ganglia, which controls movement, resulting in a person with Parkinson's disease suffering with tremor, muscular rigidity, difficulty in initiating motor activity, and loss of postural reflexes. The obvious way to treat Parkinson's disease would be to give dopamine. This does not work however, because the dopamine is unable to pass from the circulatory system into the brain due to the blood-brain barrier. The blood-brain barrier is a boundary consisting of specialized capillaries that have tight junctions between the cells, and astrocytes that prevent the passage of materials from the blood to the cerebrospinal fluid and the brain. As dopamine cannot cross this barrier, the pro-drug levodopa is given which can. The levodopa enters the brain, where the enzyme dopa decarboxylase converts it into dopamine. This would appear to solve the problem of Parkinson's disease. There is now dopamine in the brain so the symptoms of the disease are ameliorated. Unfortunately, dopa decarboxylase is also found in the rest of the body and so levodopa is converted to dopamine in the peripheral nervous system. There is now an excess of dopamine in the peripheral tissues, and this results in unpleasant side-effects, including nausea, postural hypotension, dizziness, tachycardia, arrhythmias, and involuntary choreiform movements. Giving a decarboxylase inhibitor that is unable to cross the blood-brain barrier, e.g. carbidopa, can prevent this. Thus by giving a mixture of levodopa to replace the missing dopamine in the brain, and carbidopa to prevent the formation of dopamine in the peripheral nerves, the symptoms of Parkinson's disease can be reduced and the side-effects minimized (Kelly, 1995). Sinemet is an example of this drug combination.

Carriers

Carriers, or transporters, are proteins in the cell membrane that move specific substances, for example amino acids, across the membrane by changing shape. Carriers can move molecules with their concentration gradient in a process termed facilitated diffusion, or against their concentration gradient by utilizing adenosine triphosphate (ATP) as their energy source in a process called active transport. In the latter case, the carrier protein is often referred to as a pump. Carriers form an important target for drug therapy with the drugs acting either as inhibitors or as false substrates.

Inhibitors

An inhibitor, as its name suggests, prevents a carrier from doing its job. A good example of a drug that is an inhibitor is omeprazole, which is used to reduce stomach acidity. Secretion of acid into the gastric lumen results from the activity of the proton pump located in the parietal cells of the fundus of the stomach. This pump, also called the hydrogen-potassium adenosine triphosphate enzyme system (H^+/K^+ATPase), moves hydrogen ions into the gastric lumen where they combine with chloride ions to form hydrochloric acid. Omeprazole binds irreversibly to the proton pump and incapacitates it permanently. Acid production only resumes after the synthesis of new H^+/K^+ATPase by the parietal cells.

Omeprazole is of particular interest because it was thought to be a 'magic bullet', i.e. a drug that deals with the root cause of the problem rather than the effects of the problem. Until recently, the belief was that peptic ulceration was the result of excess acid and pepsin production. Initially treatment was with antacids that simply neutralized the acid. Then it was identified that acid production by the parietal cells is stimulated by the parasympathetic nervous system and by histamine acting through H_2-receptors. Thus, treatment consisted of either antagonizing the parasympathetic nervous system with drugs like pirenzepine, or antagonizing histamine H_2-receptors with drugs like cimetidine. These drugs have side-effects, and they were not tackling the perceived root of the problem. Hence, the development of omeprazole, which does go to the heart of the problem, and because of doing so should have minimal side-effects. Ironically at the time that omeprazole was being developed research revealed that in reality the root cause of most peptic ulcers is infection with the bacterium *Helicobacter pylori*, which can easily be treated with antibiotics.

False substrates

Drugs can interfere with carriers as false substrates. This means that they mimic the normal chemical that the carrier transports and so 'fool' the carrier into moving it across the membrane. This is how amphetamines function.

After a neurotransmitter has been released into the synaptic cleft, it is inactivated, either by being broken down by enzymes in the synaptic gap or by being taken up by carriers on the synaptic membrane. In the case of neurones using the neurotransmitter noradrenaline (norepinephrine), carriers are used to take up the chemical into the presynaptic neurone. Here it is stored in vesicles until the nerve is next stimulated and needs to release the transmitter. Amfetamine (amphetamine) deceives the carrier into taking it into the nerve terminal. In the presynaptic neurone, the amfetamine (amphetamine) displaces noradrenaline (norepinephrine) from its storage vesicle, causing it to be released into the synaptic cleft where it diffuses across and binds to the postsynaptic receptors. The stimulant effects of amphetamines thus result from excess release of noradrenaline (norepinephrine) in the central nervous system.

References and further reading

Aronson J (1993) Drug action via enzymes and transport systems. Prescriber 4: 64-8

Kelly J (1995) Pharmacodynamics and drug therapy. Professional Nurse 10: 792-6

Martin EA (ed) (1983) Macmillan Dictionary of Life Sciences 2nd edn. London: Macmillan Press

Needleman P, Isakson PC (1998) Selective inhibition of cyclooxygenase 2. Science and Medicine 5: 26-35

Waller D (1993) How relevant is drug metabolism to prescribing? Prescriber 4: 53-7

Chapter 5
Idiosyncratic effects and drug allergy

Introduction

Drug allergies or hypersensitivity reactions are adverse reactions resulting from immunological responses to drugs, their metabolites, or a non-drug element in the formulation. The risk of an allergic reaction is between 1% and 3% for most drugs, with reactions ranging from mild to life threatening and accounting for between 6% and 10% of observed adverse drug reactions (deShazo and Kemp, 1997). Patients with allergic diseases such as asthma and eczema are more likely to develop drug allergies. Allergic reactions share the five characteristics shown in Table 5.1.

Antigens trigger hypersensitivity reactions, and high molecular-weight drugs, for example insulin and antisera, are complete antigens and thus are more likely to produce allergic reactions. Low molecular-weight drugs and their metabolites are unable to trigger an immune response on their own, and are termed haptens. However, if haptens combine with body proteins, they can then induce an immune response. This response may be harmful, i.e.

Table 5.1 Characteristics of allergic or hypersensitivity reactions

1. They occur in only small numbers of patients using the drug
2. There is no linear relation between the drug dose and the reaction, so very small doses may trigger severe effects
3. They require previous exposure to the same or a chemically related drug
4. They develop rapidly after re-exposure
5. They produce clinical syndromes that are commonly associated with immunological reactions, e.g. rashes, angio-oedema, serum sickness syndrome, anaphylaxis

allergy, or harmless. Many patients produce antibodies to drugs such as penicillin, but comparatively few react clinically to re-exposure. Those that do react clinically to one member of a group of drugs are likely to react to other members of the group, which is termed cross-allergy. Thus if allergy is established to a particular drug other drugs in the group should be avoided. Drugs commonly causing allergic reactions are shown in Table 5.2.

Table 5.2 Drugs commonly implicated in allergic reactions (deShazo and Kemp, 1997)

- Allopurinol
- Anaesthetics, e.g. halothane
- Antiepileptics, e.g. carbamazepine, phenytoin
- Antimalarial drugs, e.g. chloroquine, mefloquine
- Antisera and vaccines
- Antithyroid drugs, e.g. carbimazole
- Antituberculous drugs, e.g. isoniazid, rifampicin
- Aspirin and other non steroidal anti-inflammatory drugs
- ß-lactam antibiotics, e.g. penicillin
- Enzyme preparations, e.g. streptokinase
- Gold
- Griseofulvin
- Hydralazine
- Methyldopa
- Neuroleptics, e.g. chlorpromazine, clozapine
- Nitrofurantoin
- Penicillamine
- Procainamide
- Quinidine
- Sulphonamides
- Sulphonylureas, e.g. chlorpropamide, glibenclamide

Hypersensitivity reactions

Drug allergies can be classified to some extent according to the Coombes and Gell classification of hypersensitivity reactions. The first three types are antibody-mediated, while T cells and macrophages primarily mediate the fourth type.

Type I

In type I reactions the drug or its metabolite acts as an antigen and stimulates the production of corresponding antibodies of the IgE class by B-lymphocytes. These bind to receptors on mast cells and basophils. When the patient encounters the drug at a later date, the drug or its metabolite, forms cross bridges between the bound IgE antibodies. The cross-linking triggers the release of chemical mediators, including histamine, serotonin, and kinins, from the mast cells and basophils. The chemical mediators produce vasodilatation, increase vascular permeability, stimulate smooth muscle contraction, and promote glandular hypersecretion. This physiological response manifests itself classically as urticaria, rhinitis, bronchial asthma, angio-oedema and anaphylactic shock. As histamine causes contraction of gut and pelvic smooth muscle, it can also cause abdominal pain, nausea, diarrhoea, pelvic pain and abortion (Khrais and Ouellette, 1995). Type I reactions are also known as immediate hypersensitivity reactions as the allergy develops within minutes of second exposure, and lasts one to two hours. Drugs likely to trigger this response include penicillins, streptomycin, vaccines, local anaesthetics, and radio-opaque iodine contrast media.

Type II

In type II reactions, also called cytotoxic reactions, haptens become bound to cell membrane proteins so that the body no longer recognizes the proteins as 'self'. The apparent foreign protein acts as an antigen and stimulates the production of antibodies of the IgG, IgM or IgA class. On re-exposure, the antibodies bind to the antigen to form a drug-protein-antibody complex, which activates the complement system. The activation of this group of serum proteins results in cell lysis, particularly of blood cells, and tissue damage because of cytotoxic chemicals released by phagocytes and natural killer cells. Penicillins, methyldopa, rifampicin, quinine and quinidine can induce lysis of red blood cells and so cause haemolytic anaemia. Lysis of white cells and agranulocytosis can occur with phenylbutazone, carbimazole, tolbutamide, antiepileptics, chlorpropamide and metronidazole, whilst quinidine, digoxin, and rifampicin can induce platelet damage and thrombocytopenia.

Type III

In type III, or immune complex-mediated hypersensitivity, first exposure to the drug or its metabolite results in sensitization and formation of IgG antibodies. On re-exposure, either soluble or insoluble antigen-antibody complexes are formed. If circulating antibody swamps the antigen, then insoluble complexes form and precipitate where the antigen first encounters the antibody – the so called

Arthus reaction. Alternatively, if there is an excess of antigen in relation to antibody, the complexes formed remain soluble, giving rise to serum sickness, so called because it used to occur as a reaction to the injection of foreign serum, e.g. anti-tetanus serum. Both types of complex can activate macrophages, aggregate platelets, initiate the complement cascade, and so cause tissue damage. Circulating immune complexes can lodge in the blood vessels of many organs to give a vasculitis, principally affecting the skin and joints. Clinical symptoms include fever, arthritis, enlarged lymph nodes, urticaria, and maculopapular rashes. Penicillins, streptomycin, sulphonamides and antithyroid drugs are common causes of this type of reaction. Another example of type III reaction is acute glomerulonephritis, which may be triggered by penicillins and some NSAIDs.

Type IV

Unlike the other forms of hypersensitivity, which involve antibody, type IV, or cell-mediated, reactions require T lymphocytes. These are initially sensitized by a drug-protein antigenic complex. When the lymphocytes encounter the antigen on re-exposure, an inflammatory response ensues. When the responsible antigen enters via the skin, as in contact sensitivity, an eczematous rash with oedema develops at the site. Type IV reactions are exemplified by contact dermatitis triggered by local anaesthetic creams, antihistamine creams and topical antimicrobial drugs. Type IV reactions are also called delayed-type hypersensitivity reactions because they take 24–72 hours to develop.

The Mantoux test, which is used to confirm immunity against tuberculosis, relies on the type IV hypersensitivity reaction. When tuberculin protein is injected into the skin of a sensitized person, it induces a response, which leads to the accumulation of macrophages and inflammatory exudate at the site. Depending on the degree of hypersensitivity response, which may range from little tissue damage through to massive necrosis and ulceration of the skin, the person's immunity to tuberculosis can be gauged.

Pseudo-allergic reactions

Pseudo-allergic effects mimicking type I reactions are called anaphylactoid and occur with aspirin and other NSAIDs, morphine, tubocurarine, dextran, and iodine contrast media. As the name suggests, these reactions resemble hypersensitivity reactions but no immunological basis can be found, and they are largely genetically determined. They are due to the release of chemical mediators, which are triggered either directly or indirectly by the drug. For example, in the case of aspirin sensitivity it is believed that because aspirin inhibits the enzyme cyclooxygenase, arachidonic acid is preferentially converted to leukotrienes. Leukotrienes are slow-reacting substances of anaphylaxis and induce vasoconstriction, bronchoconstriction and increased vascular permeability, accounting for some of the symptoms of aspirin sensitivity (Small and Allen, 1995). Unlike true allergic responses, pseudo-allergic reactions are dose dependent, so a larger dose of drug causes a more severe reaction. Furthermore, the reaction can occur on first exposure to the drug (Campbell, 1997).

Type II reactions are mimicked by the haemolysis induced by drugs such as antimalarials, sulphonamides, and foods such as broad beans in subjects with inherited abnormalities of erythrocyte enzymes or haemoglobin, while type III reactions are mimicked by nitrofurantoin (pneumonitis) and penicillamine (nephropathy). Lupus erythematosus due to drugs such as procainamide, isoniazid and phenytoin may be pseudo-allergic.

In reality, it is not always possible to fit drug reactions into Coombe and Gel's classification system because they present as clinical syndromes. It is therefore useful to examine drug allergies from a clinical perspective.

Anaphylactic and anaphylactoid reactions

Although these two reactions differ in their underlying pathophysiology, the clinical manifestations and treatment are the same in both cases. The onset of the reaction can be within minutes of exposure to the triggering substance, or delayed for up to half an hour. The severity of the reaction can vary from skin irritation and a feeling of unease right through to collapse. The manifestations depend not only on the amount and type of mediator released, but also on the relative sensitivity of the target organs, such as the airway and heart. The sensitivity of these organs may be determined by underlying diseases, e.g. asthma, and concomitant medications such as ß-blockers. Classical symptoms include diffuse erythema, pruritus, urticaria, angio-oedema, bronchospasm, laryngeal oedema, vomiting, hypotension, and cardiac arrhythmias. The management of anaphylactic and anaphylactoid reactions must be prompt, and is outlined in Table 5.3.

Table 5.3 Management of anaphylactic and anaphylactoid reactions

- Identify and discontinue the causative agent
- Lay the patient down with legs raised on a pillow to promote venous return
- Insert an airway if the patient loses consciousness and give 100% oxygen via a mask
- Administer appropriate drugs, e.g. adrenaline (epinephrine), chlorphenamine (chlorpheniramine), hydrocortisone, salbutamol
- Resuscitate if there is no cardiac output

The key to successful treatment of anaphylactic and anaphylactoid reaction is adrenaline (epinephrine). Early administration of adrenaline (epinephrine) by deep intramuscular injection, repeated every 10 minutes up to a maximum of three doses, not only reverses the bronchoconstriction and peripheral vasodilatation that may be life threatening but has the extra benefit of inhibiting further release of mast cell derived mediators. As adrenaline (epinephrine) can irritate the myocardium the lowest therapeutic dose possible should be administered (Table 5.4) and cardiac rhythm should be monitored.

Once the patient has recovered from the acute attack, advice on how best to avoid the precipitating factor is needed. Skin-prick tests may be helpful in confirming sensitivity, but they are generally more useful in the case of food allergy and insect bites than drug-induced allergy (Youlten, 1996). Patients' notes should be indelibly marked to

Table 5.4 Guidelines on dosages of adrenaline (epinephrine) by deep intramuscular injection for different age groups (DoH, 1996)

Age	*Dose 1:1000 (1 mg per mL)*
Less than one year	0.05 mL
One year	0.1 mL
Two years	0.2 mL
Three–four years	0.3 mL
Five years	0.4 mL
Six–ten years	0.5 mL
Adults	0.5–1 mL

indicate drug allergies, and nursing assessments should always inquire into the possibility of allergy. In addition, where drugs or vaccines are suspected of having caused the allergy the reaction should be reported to the Committee on the Safety of Medicines.

It is possible to desensitize a patient by a course of injections of a weak solution of the offending allergen. However, this approach is not without its risks and should only be carried out where there are facilities for full cardio-respiratory resuscitation as anaphylaxis may result from injection of the allergen. One group of patients which may particularly benefit from desensitization are patients with HIV who are 100 times more likely to suffer from hypersensitivity than immunocompetent or HIV-negative immunodeficient patients (Carr, 1997). The drug class most commonly observed to cause hypersensitivity in these patients is the sulphonamides, in particular co-trimoxazole, sulfadiazine (sulphadiazine), and dapsone, drugs commonly used in the treatment or prophylaxis of *Pneumocystis carinii* pneumonia and toxoplasmic encephalitis. Desensitization may be appropriate if there is persistent hypersensitivity and no suitable alternative therapy, especially if rechallenge is unsuccessful.

Drug fever

Fever may be the sole or most prominent feature of an adverse drug reaction. Drug fever can be defined as a fever that coincides with the administration of a drug, for which no other cause for the fever can be ascertained after careful physical examination and appropriate laboratory study, and which disappears after discontinuation of that drug (Mackowiak and LeMaistre, 1987). It has been suggested that any drug has the capacity to induce fever, but some drugs are more likely than others (Table 5.5).

Drug-induced fevers can range from 38–43°C and may be accompanied by rigors. The patients generally have few signs or symptoms of serious systemic toxicity. The mechanism of drug fever is unknown, but it may be associated with eosinophilia, leucocytosis, elevated erythrocyte sedimentation rate (ESR), myalgia, and possibly a rash. Withdrawal of the responsible drug results in resolution of symptoms within 48–72 hours. In the case of penicillins, it can sometimes be difficult to distinguish drug fever from a fever that persists because of resistant infection.

Table 5.5 Examples of drugs commonly responsible for causing drug fever (Mackowiak and LeMaistre, 1987)

• Amphotericin	• Methicillin
• Ampicillin	• Methyldopa
• Bleomycin	• Nitrofurantoin
• Cloxacillin	• Penicillin G
• Iodine	• Procainamide
• Isoniazid	• Quinidine
• Lysergic acid (LSD)–overdose	• Tetracycline

Erythema multiforme and Stevens-Johnson syndrome

Erythema multiforme is a red polymorphic skin eruption that is caused by drugs in about 10–20% of cases. Skin manifestations include target-like lesions, maculopapular rashes, urticaria and vesicles. Lesions are typically symmetrical and frequently occur on the extensor surfaces of the limbs. In the most severe form of this reaction, known as Stevens-Johnson syndrome, there are mucosal and conjunctival lesions, and up to 10% of the epidermis may be lost. More than a hundred drugs have been implicated as causes of Stevens-Johnson syndrome, although infections or a combination of infection and drugs have also been implicated. The drugs associated with substantial relative increases in risk include the sulphonamide antibiotics, oxicam NSAIDs, antiepileptics, and allopurinol. Significant associations with many antibiotics and corticosteroids have also been reported (Roujeau et al., 1995). Fever and influenza like symptoms often precede the mucocutaneous lesions by one to three days. Visceral involvement may occur and is associated with a poor prognosis. Treatment is supportive and the early use of corticosteroids is recommended, as they appear to prevent visceral involvement and decrease both the duration and severity of clinical symptoms.

Anticonvulsant hypersensitivity syndrome (AHS)

Anticonvulsant hypersensitivity syndrome is a potentially fatal drug reaction that is estimated to occur in 1 in 1000 to 1 in 10 0000 patients treated with the antiepileptics phenytoin, carbamazepine, and phenobarbital sodium. The hallmark features of the syndrome are fever, rash and lymphadenopathy (Table 5.6). The rash is usually generalized and consists of irregular and ill-defined patches of macular erythema. It is usually pruritic and resolves with a desquamation reminiscent of that seen in scarlet fever. There is severe facial oedema, and periorbital oedema may be so severe as to prevent the patient's eyelids from opening. The mucous membranes are involved with erythema in the pharynx and oral mucosa (Stanley and Fallon-Pellicci, 1978). The reaction usually begins within one to three weeks of initiating antiepileptic therapy, but may develop after three months or more of treatment.

There is some debate as to the underlying mechanism of AHS. However, AHS probably results from an inherited deficiency of epoxide hydrolase. Phenytoin, carbamazepine and phenobarbital are all metabolized by cytochrome P450 to an arene oxide metabolite. This is normally detoxified by the enzyme epoxide hydrolase. If this enzyme is lacking or mutated then detoxification will be defective and the toxic metabolite can cause cell death, or contribute to the formation of an antibody that triggers an immune response (Vittorio and Muglia, 1995).

Treatment consists of immediate discontinuation of the drug. As the degree of hepatitis is related to the interval between the onset of the syndrome and withdrawal of the drug, it is clear that prompt diagnosis is imperative, especially as liver failure is the main cause of death. The patient should also be monitored closely and appropriate supportive therapy given, with careful attention to hydration and electrolyte balance. The skin rash responds well to topical corticosteroids, wet wraps and antihistamines. Seizures need to be controlled

Table 5.6 Clinical features of anticonvulsant hypersensitivity syndrome (Vittorio and Muglia, 1995)

Clinical feature	*Incidence (%)*
Fever (38–40 °C)	90–100
Rash	90
Lymphadenopathy	70
Multi organ system involvement	60
Hepatitis–anicteric or icteric	50–60
Leucocytosis, eosinophilia, leucopenia	50
Periorbital or facial oedema	25
Myalgia, arthralgia	21
Pharyngitis	10

using drugs that are non-arene oxide producing, for example valproic acid, gabapentin, lamotrigine, and vigabatrin.

Toxic epidermal necrolysis (Lyell syndrome)

This acute illness is usually drug-related and is characterized by fever, epidermal loss exceeding 30% of the body surface area, and visceral involvement with an associated mortality of 30–40%. It is sometimes difficult clinically to separate toxic epidermal necrolysis from Stevens-Johnson syndrome; it is associated with the same drugs. Treatment is supportive but corticosteroids are not recommended for toxic epidermal necrolysis.

Idiosyncratic effects

Idiosyncratic effects are inherited abnormal responses to drugs mediated by single genes. The response can be increased, decreased or bizarre (Table 5.7).

Glucose-6-phosphate dehydrogenase (G-6-PD)

Glucose-6-phosphate dehydrogenase is an enzyme that is involved in chemical reactions that are important in maintaining the integrity of red blood cells, which includes protecting them from oxidation. Consequently, people who are deficient in this enzyme may suffer acute haemolysis if they are exposed to oxidant substances, including a wide selection of drugs (Table 5.8).

The prevalence of the defect varies with race. It is rare amongst Caucasians, and occurs most commonly amongst those of Mediterranean, African or Southeast Asian origin. G-6-PD deficiency is an X-linked recessive trait, but its inheritance is complex. There are two main varieties of deficiency, namely the Black and the Mediterranean variety. In the former, G-6-PD production appears normal, but its degradation is accelerated, so that old red blood cells are affected. In this form, there is a self-limiting acute haemolytic episode two to three days after starting the drug; thereafter continued drug administration causes chronic, but mild, haemolysis. In the Mediterranean variety, the enzyme is abnormal and both young and old cells are affected. Consequently, in this form of G-6-PD deficiency severe haemolysis occurs on first administration of the responsible drug, and is maintained with continued administration.

Table 5.7 Examples of idiosyncratic responses (Schmidt, 1998)

Gene	*Drug Example*	*Response*
Apolipoprotein E	Tacrine	The ApoE4 form of this gene is associated with an increased risk of Alzheimer's and a poor response to tacrine
Butyrylcholinesterase	Suxamethonium	People who have a deficiency of the cholinesterase enzyme cannot rapidly inactivate suxamethonium, so it carries on working. See Chapter 2
Cholesterol ester transfer protein, lipoprotein lipase, and ß-fibrinogen	Pravastatin	Certain variants of these genes are associated with atherosclerosis progression as well as altered response to pravastatin
CYP2D6-part of the cytochrome P450 gene family	Desipramine	People with a CYP2D6 defect tend to metabolize drugs slowly and so suffer with toxicity effects
Glucose-6-phosphate dehydrogenase	Primaquine	Haemolysis
N-acetyltransferase	Isoniazid, procainamide	Individuals who are 'slow acetylators' are susceptible to toxic side-effects, as they cannot clear the drug from the body fast enough
Serotonin receptor subtype 5-HT_{2A}	Clozapine	People with 2 copies of the C102 form of this gene are less likely to respond to clozapine

Table 5.8 Examples of drugs that may precipitate haemolysis in people with G-6-PD deficiency (Grahame-Smith and Aronson, 1992)

- Analgesics, e.g. aspirin
- Antimalarials, e.g. chloroquine, mepacrine, quinidine, quinine
- Chloramphenicol
- Dapsone and other sulphones
- Doxorubicin
- Nalidixic acid
- Nitrofurantoin
- Primaquine
- Probenecid
- Sulphonamides, e.g. sulfamethoxazole (sulphamethoxazole), sulfasalazine (sulphasalazine)

People with G-6-PD deficiency are also susceptible to exposure to nitrates, anilines, and naphthalenes found in mothballs. Some individuals experience haemolysis after eating the broad bean *Vicia faba*, and hence the term 'favism'.

Malignant hyperthermia and neuroleptic malignant syndrome (NMS)

Malignant hyperthermia is a potentially lethal complication of an inherited muscular disorder (Beck, 1994). It is precipitated by the administration of volatile anaesthetics, e.g. halothane, and neuromuscular blocking agents, e.g. succinylcholine, with an incidence of 1:15000 for children and 1:100 000 for adults receiving anaesthesia, and a mortality of 10% (Beck, 1994). Other drugs such as diuretics, anti-epileptic drugs, analgesics, anti-arrhythmics and antibiotics can also trigger it (Cunha and Tu, 1988). The drugs, in some way that is not fully understood, trigger the release of calcium from the sarcoplasmic reticulum, where it is stored, into the cytoplasm of muscle cells (Donnelly, 1994). The increase in intracellular calcium results in continuous contracture of the skeletal muscle. The metabolism involved in the muscular contraction results in high oxygen consumption, production of lactic acid, carbon dioxide and heat. So much heat is generated that the patient's temperature rises dramatically, e.g. to 43°C within minutes. Other symptoms include tachycardia, cardiac dysrhythmias, tachypnoea, unstable blood pressure, muscle rigidity, cyanosis, and elevated levels of creatinine phosphokinase. Management of the condition involves discontinuing the triggering agent, hyperventilating the patient with 100% oxygen at high flow rates, and administering intravenous dantrolene, a skeletal muscle relaxant that inhibits the release of calcium from the sarcoplasmic reticulum.

Neuroleptic malignant syndrome (NMS) has many clinical similarities to malignant hyperthermia, but despite the similarities, most authorities believe them to be two different syndromes. NMS has an incidence of 0.5–1.4% (Byrd, 1993), and is a potentially fatal response to drugs used to treat psychosis, including the phenothiazines, butyrophenones, and thioxanthenes, as well as a variety of other drugs (Table 5.9). It most commonly occurs with the high potency neuroleptics such as haloperidol, and the long-acting agents such as fluphenazine. The exact pathophysiological mechanism of NMS is unclear, but it would appear that the syndrome is the result of dopamine blockade in the basal ganglia and hypothalamus. This is supported by the fact that NMS can also occur with the discontinuation of anti-parkinsonian drugs. The syndrome is characterized by hyperthermia of up to 41°C, muscular rigidity, akinesia, impaired consciousness and autonomic nervous system instability. The latter manifests itself with tachycardia, cardiac dysrhythmias, hypotension or hypertension, dyspnoea, sweating, pallor and incontinence. Due to the severe muscle rigidity, serum skeletal muscle creatinine phosphokinase levels are usually three times normal (Foley, 1993). The symptoms of NMS may develop in a few hours or several weeks after administration of the offending agent, and can develop after just one dose (Stewart, 1995). Rapid neuroleptization, high dosages, dehydration, malnutrition, anticholinergic agents, and restraints may increase the risk of NMS (Levenson, 1985).

Table 5.9 Non-neuroleptic drugs that can cause neuroleptic malignant syndrome (Blair and Dauner, 1993)

Drug group	*Examples*
Antiemetics	• Metoclopramide
	• Prochlorperazine
Mono-amine oxidase inhibitors	• Isocarboxazid
	• Phenelzine
	• Tranylcypromine
Tricyclic antidepressants	• Amitriptyline + perphenazine
	• Amoxapine
	• Desipramine
	• Doxepin
	• Imipramine
	• Nortriptyline
Others	• Fluoxetine
	• Lithium

The mortality statistics for NMS range from 0–76% with a current mean mortality rate of 11.6% (Foley, 1993). Because of this high mortality rate, patients should be managed in an intensive care setting. The treatment regimen consists of immediate discontinuation of the offending neuroleptic drug, although many patients are able to resume the drug at a later date with no ill effects (Byrd, 1993). If the NMS has been caused by the discontinuation of levodopa this should be reinstated. Supportive care should include hydration, nutrition, and control of hyperthermia with a cooling blanket and antipyretics. Because of the long half-lives of neuroleptic drugs and the extended effect of depot forms, time to response can take up to seven days. Use of a dopamine agonist, i.e. bromocriptine or amantadine, and use of the skeletal muscle relaxant dantrolene can decreases the response time to about a day.

N-acetyltransferase

During metabolism, many drugs undergo acetylation in Phase II conjugation. The enzyme that controls this reaction, N-acetyltransferase, occurs in several forms, i.e. it is polymorphic, and consequently individuals can be either slow or fast acetylators. About 50% of Caucasians are fast acetylators while in the Japanese the proportion is as high as 95% (Waller, 1993). Important drugs that are substrates for the acetylating enzyme N-acetyltransferase are the vasodilator hydralazine, the antiarrhythmic procainamide, the antituberculous drug isoniazid, and the antileprosy drug dapsone. Adverse effects can result in both slow and fast acetylators. For example, isoniazid may cause peripheral neuropathy in slow acetylators on standard doses, while acute hepatocellular necrosis is more common with fast acetylators, possibly because they more readily form a hepatotoxic metabolite. However, generally poor metabolizers show an enhanced therapeutic response and have a higher risk of developing drug-induced systemic lupus erythematosus.

References and further reading

Beck CF (1994) Malignant hyperthermia: are you prepared? AORN Journal 59: 367-90

Blair DT, Dauner A (1993) Neuroleptic malignant syndrome: liability in nursing practice. Journal of Psychosociological Nursing and the Mental Health Service 31: 5-35.

Byrd C (1993) Neuroleptic malignant syndrome: a dangerous complication of neuroleptic therapy. Journal of Neuroscience Nursing 25: 62-5

Campbell J (1997) Anaphylaxis. Professional Nurse 12: 429-32

Carr A (1997) Role of desensitisation for drug hypersensitivity in patients with HIV infection. Drug Safety 17: 119-26

Cunha B, Tu R (1988) Fever in the neurosurgical patient. Heart and Lung 17: 608-11

Department of Health (1996) Immunisation Against Infectious Diseases. London: HMSO

deShazo RD, Kemp SF (1997) Allergic reactions to drugs and biologic agents. Journal of the American Medical Association 278: 1895-906

Donnelly A (1994) Malignant hyperthermia: epidemiology, pathophysiology, treatment. AORN Journal 59: 393-405

Foley JJ (1993) Recognition and treatment of neuroleptic malignant syndrome. Journal of Emergency Nursing 19: 139-41

Grahame-Smith DG, Aronson JK (1992) Oxford Textbook of Clinical Pharmacology and Drug Therapy 2nd edn. Oxford: Oxford University Press

Khrais J, Ouellette S (1995) Mechanisms and management of allergic reactions in the surgical patient. Clinical Forum for Nurse Anesthetists 6: 146-58

Levenson JL (1985) Neuroleptic malignant syndrome. American Journal of Psychiatry 142: 1137-45

Mackowiak PA, LeMaistre CF (1987) Drug fever: a critical appraisal of conventional concepts. Annals of Internal Medicine 106: 728-33

Roujeau J, Kelly J, Naldi L, Rzany B, Stern RS, Anderson T, Auquier A, Bastuji-Garin S, Correia O, Locati F (1995) Medication use and the risk of Stevens-Johnson syndrome or toxic epidermal necrolysis. New England Journal of Medicine 333: 1600-7

Schmidt K (1998) Just for you. New Scientist 160: 32-6

Small DM, Allen JE (1995) Aspirin sensitivity. Journal of Pharmaceutical Care in Pain and Symptom Control 3: 57-64

Stewart KB (1995) What's wrong with this patient? RN 58: 45-8

Waller D (1993) How relevant is drug metabolism to prescribing? Prescriber 4: 53-7

Vittorio CC, Muglia JJ (1995) Anticonvulsant hypersensitivity syndrome. Archives of Internal Medicine 155: 2285-90

Youlten L (1996) Recognising and treating anaphylactic reactions. Prescriber 7: 89-93

Chapter 6
Client groups

Introduction

Developmental change occurs throughout an individual's life, and must be considered as a potential influence on drug action. As an individual passes from being a foetus to a neonate, through infancy to childhood, adolescence, maturity and old age major changes in anatomy and physiology occur, not to mention psychological and social changes. These changes are reflected in different abilities to handle and respond to drugs. Age, or more correctly state of development, must be considered when prescribing and administering drug treatments if adverse effects are to be avoided.

The foetus

For the first half of this century, it was believed that the placenta, which separates the blood vessels of the mother and the foetus, constituted a complete barrier to environmental teratogens. It was not until the thalidomide disaster in the early 1960s, when it was found that the use of this sedative during early pregnancy could lead to foetal abnormality, most notably malformation of the limbs, that this belief was seriously researched. It is now clear that despite the thickness of the placenta, and the tissue enzymes within it which inactivate some chemicals, e.g. catecholamines, the placenta does not afford the foetus complete protection. Lipid-soluble drugs can cross the placenta preferentially, but so can a large number of lipid insoluble drugs. Consequently many drugs intended to treat the mother may cross the placenta and exert a harmful effect on the developing foetus. Among the drugs most easily transported across the placenta are steroids, narcotics, anaesthetics and some antibiotics.

Drugs can have harmful effects on the foetus at any time during pregnancy, although the risks are greatest during the first trimester. Drugs taken during this time may produce congenital malformations (teratogenesis); the period of greatest risk is from the third to the eleventh week of pregnancy. During the second and third trimesters, drugs may still have adverse effects by affecting the growth and functional development of the foetus, or by having toxic effects on foetal tissue. Drugs given shortly before term or during labour may have adverse effects on labour or on the neonate after delivery. Drugs should thus be prescribed in pregnancy only if the expected health benefit to the mother is believed to be greater than the risk to the foetus. However, carrying out this cost-benefit analysis can be problematic. Firstly, identifying the degree of risk of a drug to the foetus is difficult as the data is very limited, and much of it is derived from animal studies and anecdotal material. Secondly, although the teratogenic effects of prescription drugs are low and are recognized to cause less than 1% of congenital abnormalities (Ruggiero, 1992), the public have lost confidence in the medical profession after the thalidomide disaster. Consequently, when drugs are of a positive benefit to a pregnant woman she may refuse to take them even if they are prescribed. This is supported by a study by Butters and Howie (1990) which identified that of 514 women on postnatal wards, 48% would not take a prescribed antibiotic.

Epidemiological studies have shown that pregnant women do still take substantial quantities of drugs, particularly social drugs such as alcohol, as well as over-the-counter medications. A study by Rubin et al. (1986) found that of 2765 women 13% were taking non-narcotic analgesics, 10% antacids, and 6% anti-emetics. However, the more recent study by Butters and Howie (1990) identified that the majority of women (85%) recognized that drugs were particularly harmful to the foetus during the first 3 months of pregnancy, and they demonstrated a generally high level of awareness of commonly used drugs. For example, 70% of respondents were aware that paracetamol-containing analgesics were preferable to aspirin in pregnancy. However, the authors also identified the need for continued health education.

Table 6.1 lists a selection of drugs that should be avoided in early pregnancy, whilst Table 6.2 identifies drugs that should be avoided during later pregnancy. However, it must be stressed that these tables are purely for interest. An up-to-date copy of Appendix 4 of the

British National Formulary, must be consulted when advising pregnant women about drugs, as clinical data on drugs in pregnancy is subject to continuous change.

Table 6.1 Drugs to avoid in early pregnancy (Gal and Sharpless 1984; Laudano et al., 1990; McManus Kuller, 1990; Ruggiero, 1992; Budd, 1995; Sundaram, 1995)

Drug	*Adverse Effect*
Alcohol	Foetal alcohol syndrome
Antiepileptics, particularly phenytoin	Foetal hydantoin syndrome
Carbimazole	Aplasia cutis
Cocaine	*In utero* cerebrovascular accident, bowel atresia, spontaneous abortion
Corticosteroids–high dose	Cleft palate
Diethylstilbestrol (stilboestrol)	Vaginal adenosis in female foetus; vaginal or cervical cancer 20+ years later
Fibrinolytic drugs, e.g. streptokinase	Separation of placenta
Sodium iodide	Partial or complete destruction of thyroid
Tetracyclines	Inhibition of bone growth, discoloration of teeth
Valproate	Neural tube defects
Vitamin A–high doses; including isotretinoin	Microtia, facial palsy, cardiac defects, limb reductions, gastrointestinal atresia
Warfarin	Foetal warfarin syndrome

Table 6.2 Drugs to avoid in the second and third trimester

Drug	*Adverse Effect*
Aminoglycosides	Eighth cranial nerve damage
Antithyroid drugs	Goitre and hypothyroidism
Antipsychotics	Extrapyramidal effects
Benzodiazepines	Floppy infant syndrome
Chloramphenicol	Grey baby syndrome
Disopyramide	May induce labour
Nitrofurantoin	Neonatal haemolysis if used at term
NSAIDs	Premature closure of ductus arteriosus in utero
Opioid analgesics	Respiratory depression, drug withdrawal symptoms if mother addicted
Primaquine	Neonatal haemolysis and methaemoglobinaemia
Sulphonylureas	Hypoglycaemia
Sulphonamides	Neonatal haemolysis
Thiazide diuretics	Thrombocytopenia

It should be noted that women suffering from epilepsy have a major difficulty when it comes to drug therapy during pregnancy. Studies have shown that both the disease process itself and the drugs used to treat it contribute to the incidence of congenital abnormalities that is two or three times higher than the average (McManus Kuller, 1990). During pregnancy, a single convulsion can lead to foetal mortality, or morbidity from hypoxia or a placental abruption. Conversely, as Table 6.1 shows the anti-epileptic drugs are harmful to the foetus. This dilemma needs to be discussed with the mother so that she is fully informed of the risks and is involved in the decision of choosing how to manage her epilepsy most effectively for herself and her baby. This usually means giving the lowest effective dose of the favoured antiepileptic, and monitoring blood levels of the drug throughout pregnancy.

Breastfeeding

It is true that most drugs can be detected in breast milk. However, the advantages of breastfeeding to both the mother and baby are too great for medications to be a reason to give up breastfeeding. Most drugs appear only in very small amounts in breast milk and there are few medications that are truly contraindicated for the breastfeeding mother (see Table 6.3 for examples and the British National

Table 6.3 Examples of drugs that are contraindicated during breastfeeding

Drug	*Rationale*
Androgens	May cause masculization of female infants or precocious development of male infants; high doses suppress lactation
Aspirin	Possible risk of Reye's syndrome
Benzodiazepines	Lethargy and weight loss
Bromocriptine	Suppresses lactation
Chloramphenicol	Bone marrow toxicity
Corticosteroids	Doses greater than 10 mg/day prednisolone may suppress infant's adrenal function
Ergotamine	Vomiting, diarrhoea, convulsions
Iodine	Concentrated in breast milk; neonatal hypothyroidism or goitre
Lithium	Intoxication–apathy, restlessness, vomiting, ataxia
Phenindione	Risk of haemorrhage, increased by vitamin K deficiency
Phenobarbital (phenobarbitone)	Inhibits sucking reflex
Sulphonamides	Small risk of kernicterus in jaundiced infants

Formulary Appendix 5 for a more detailed and up-to-date list). Instead, it is more useful to consider the factors that influence the passage of drugs into breast milk and to consider strategies to minimize infant exposure to drugs while breastfeeding (Table 6.4).

Table 6.4 Strategies for minimizing infant exposure and risk to drugs while breastfeeding (Committee on Drugs, 1994; Banta-Wright, 1997)

- Only take essential medication
- Consider delaying drug therapy until after breastfeeding is complete
- Avoid drugs new to the market, as their safety profile may not be complete
- Take drugs that do not pass easily into milk, e.g. take paracetamol rather than aspirin
- Consider the route of drug administration and utilize routes that minimize amount of drug passed into breast milk, e.g. inhaled steroids for asthma rather than oral
- Take drugs immediately after breastfeeding and in the case of once a day drugs take immediately before the baby's longest sleep period

Immediately after birth the spaces between the myoepithelial cells of the alveolae of the breast are large and allow the passage of large plasma proteins like IgA, as well as drugs, into breast milk. However, within a week of birth the spaces close, so that only drugs with a molecular weight of less than 200 kDa can pass into breast milk. Thus, drugs such as heparin and insulin are normally unable to cross the alveolar membrane. In addition, if drugs are highly protein bound, like phenytoin, they are confined to the plasma compartment and only transfer to breast milk in small amounts. Conversely, drugs that are highly lipid soluble transfer easily into breast milk, so drugs like diazepam can rapidly accumulate in milk. The pH of breast milk is 7.2, making it significantly lower than plasma at 7.4. Weak bases, such as erythromycin and antihistamines, are non-ionized in maternal plasma. This increases their lipid solubility and hence their passage into breast milk. At the lower pH of breast milk, weak bases may become ionized and hence trapped in the milk, achieving higher concentrations than might otherwise be expected.

Breast milk is manufactured whilst the infant is suckling, thus a drug taken immediately after breastfeeding has the maximum time to clear the maternal blood, before more milk is made. The amount of milk the baby is taking is relevant as the more milk the baby takes, the more drug it will consume. Not surprisingly, if the mother takes high doses of a drug, the breast milk will contain more of it. In addition, if the drug is given intravenously, its concentration is likely to be higher than if it is administered by an alternative route where the drug needs to be absorbed first. Drugs with a long-half life will be expected to accumulate in the mother, and consequently in her breast milk, and therefore in the infant.

The physiology of both mother and baby are important. If the mother has poor liver or kidney function, then the drug will not be metabolized and excreted, and so a greater quantity will accumulate in breast milk. In the case of the baby, its glomerular filtration rate is poor at birth, but by two to three days post delivery the glomerular filtration rates are three times those of the first day of delivery. Hepatic enzymes mature at varying rates. For example, phenytoin is metabolized at adult rates within one to two weeks of delivery. However, theophylline metabolism does not reach adult capacity until one year of age.

Neonates, infants and children

It is a truism to say that children are not miniature adults. They differ from adults in size, in the proportions and constituents of their bodies, and in the functioning of their physiological systems. Furthermore, as a group they are very diverse due to the major developmental changes that occur as they move from neonate, through infancy and childhood, to adolescence. With increasingly sophisticated technology younger and younger preterm infants are being cared for, adding to the developmental diversity to be catered for. It is important to allow for these differences when prescribing and administering drugs to young people, who contrary to popular belief receive substantial amounts of drugs. A study documenting prescription medication use in 222 paediatric patients, found that the average number of drug courses received was 8.5 during the first five years of life (Fosarelli et al., 1987). Another study estimated that a 1.5 kg preterm infant receives about 20 prescribed drugs between conception and discharge from hospital (Aranda et al., 1976).

When prescribing for children it is difficult to allow for the differences in pharmokinetic and pharmacodynamic parameters, because although these processes are well described for many drugs for the adult, such information is sparse for the child (Zenk, 1994). Furthermore, concern over the occurrence of severe adverse drug events in children has meant that practitioners focus on drug safety, sometimes at the expense of therapeutic efficacy, and consequently progress in paediatric research has been stifled (Gilman and Gal, 1992).

Calculating drug dosages can also be a problem in children. They may be calculated according to age, but this is highly inaccurate due to the vast variations in body mass of children of similar age (Ellis, 1995). The most commonly used method is by body weight up to 40 kg (Kanneh, 1998a), but adjustment according to body surface area (BSA) may be more appropriate as this is directly related to metabolic rate. It is obtained by calculating the body weight to the power of 0.7 (Laurence et al., 1997). For a five-year-old child, the BSA-based dose is 50% greater than the dose adjusted for body weight. The choice of weight or body surface area is often arbitrary and may be an important confounding variable when evaluating drugs over wide ranges of age in paediatric patients or comparing two drugs for which doses are not adjusted in a similar manner (Rodman, 1994).

Administration and absorption

Table 6.5 outlines the pharmokinetic differences between neonates, infants and children. Starting with absorption, the drug formulation needs to be considered first. At the younger end of the scale, tablets are not an option as babies and young children cannot swallow them. Thus, drugs have to be given by naso-gastric tube or parenterally. However, problems can arise, as many drugs are only available in solid dosage forms. Where liquid formulations are available, parents may object to them because of concern about the sugar content of the formulation and the risk of dental caries. However, it may not just be liquid formulations that cause tooth damage, as a recent study suggests that the powdered drugs used to treat asthma are so acidic that they may cause tooth erosion (O'Sullivan and Curzon, 1998). The dyes, particularly tartrazine and sunset yellow, which are used in some formulations to promote compliance, have been criticized as a cause of hyperkinesis in some children. A further problem for the very young is that medications are not available in concentrations suitable for neonatal administration (Skaer, 1991). Consequently, complex dilutions have to be carried out, which increases the risk of drug errors. In addition, suspensions of for example anti-epileptic drugs, are prone to variable errors in dosing because of inadequate mixing (McLeod and Evans, 1992).

Table 6.5 Pharmokinetic differences between neonates, infants and children

	Neonate (under 1 month old)	*Infant (1–12 months old)*	*Child (1–12 years old)*
Absorption			
Gastric acidity	Neutral from 10–30 days after birth.	Reaches adult levels at 1–2 years	
Gastric emptying	Prolonged, usually 6–8 hours. Irregular peristalsis.	Reaches adult levels at 6–8 months.	Same as adult
Gut motility	Highly variable. Influenced by presence of food		
Pancreatic enzyme activity	Decreased	Full activity achieved at variable times depending on enzyme	
Skin permeability	Thin stratum corneum. Increased surface area to volume ratio.	Thinner stratum corneum than adult	
Distribution			
Total body water Adipose content	75–85% 5–12%	55–60% 21–26%	Reaches adult levels of 50–70% by 12 years Adolescent boys lose fat (12%) whilst adolescent girls gain fat (25%)
Protein binding	Lower albumin levels (3–4 gm/dL). Lower binding affinity.	Plasma proteins reach adult levels by 1 year. Binding affinity reaches adult levels by 2–3 years	
Blood-brain barrier	Permeable.	Similar to adult	
Metabolism			
Liver metabolism	Decreased		Similar to adult
Microsomal enzymes	Low		Most enzyme systems mature by 2–4 years
Elimination			
Renal blood flow	12 mL/min	Reaches adult levels of 140 mL/min at 6–9 months	
Glomerular filtration	8–20 mL/min	Reaches adult levels of 120 mL/min at 3–6 months	
Tubular secretion	Decreased	Reaches adult levels after 9 months	Decrease in renal tubular clearance with onset of adolescence

Many factors alter the absorption of drugs in children. Most medications are absorbed in the intestines, but several are absorbed in the stomach. Drug absorption from the stomach is affected by gastric acidity, which varies in the child. From birth to ten days the gastric pH is between one and three, it is then neutral until the end of the first month (Niederhauser, 1997). Stomach pH returns to adult levels by two years of age. Because of the increase in gastric pH drugs such as aspirin, phenobarbital (phenobarbitone) and phenytoin are not effectively absorbed in the neonate. Also, the absorption of acidic drugs will decrease if they are given with milk or infant formula, due to the increase in pH. Conversely, some drugs are absorbed more effectively. Thus, there is 60% absorption of ampicillin in the neonate, compared with 30% in the adult. In addition, benzylpenicillin, which in later life cannot be given orally because it is inactivated by gastric acid, can be given orally to the neonate.

Gastric emptying time is prolonged in neonates and infants, and in conditions such as congenital heart disease and gastro-oesophageal reflux. This will increase absorption of acidic drugs like digoxin, but delay peak serum concentration of orally administered drugs that are absorbed best in the intestines. Also, intestinal transit time is variable in infancy, and this will alter the absorption of some drugs. Common illnesses and side-effects of drugs, such as vomiting and diarrhoea, will increase gastric motility and cause decreased absorption of drugs in infants and children. Pancreatic enzyme activity is decreased at birth and the age at which adult levels of activity develop is dependent on the specific enzyme. Any drugs that rely on a specific enzyme to aid in absorption may demonstrate a variable bioavailability. Reduced levels of bacterial flora increases the bioavailability of drugs such as digoxin, which is normally reduced by intestinal organisms (Wink, 1991).

During the neonatal period regional blood flow is quite variable, and may reduce intramuscular and subcutaneous absorption rates substantially. Moreover, absorption may be compromised in the neonate due to the reduced muscle mass and subcutaneous fat relative to that seen in the older child (Dionne and McManus, 1993). Reductions in absorption of intramuscular digoxin and gentamicin have been reported in neonates (Guyon, 1989).

Another route of drug administration is topically. Neonates, infants and children all have a thinner stratum corneum than the adult, and thus percutaneous absorption is increased 2.7-fold in the newborn and young infant, compared with the adult (Dionne and McManus, 1993). Premature neonates may have a greater absorption problem because the barrier function of the skin is not intact until 21 days. Furthermore, compared with older children neonates and infants have a larger surface to volume ratio. Consequently, drugs applied topically, including corticosteroids, may be absorbed excessively. The antiseptic hexachlorophene has been known to be absorbed sufficiently to cause neurotoxicity (Smith, 1995), while deafness has resulted from aminoglycoside/polymixin antibacterial sprays on burns (Grahame-Smith and Aronson, 1992). Such agents should only be applied sparingly and only when absolutely necessary. Absorption is further increased by the use of occlusive dressings, nappies and skin diseases.

Distribution

Infants have lower body fat and higher water content than adults. Consequently, infants receiving lipid-soluble drugs, such as diazepam, require smaller doses than adults. Conversely, infants receiving water-soluble drugs require larger doses than adults, and so weight-related priming doses of aminoglycosides, aminophylline, digoxin and furosemide (frusemide) are larger for neonates than for older children (Laurence et al., 1997). As Table 6.5 shows, changes in body fat are quite considerable throughout childhood, with major changes occurring at adolescence such that fat accounts for 12% of body weight in boys in late puberty, and 25% in girls.

Neonates and infants have significantly less ability to bind drugs to plasma proteins. This is because they have lower concentrations of serum albumin, there is decreased intermolecular attraction between the drug and plasma protein (Guyon, 1989), and there is competition between the drugs and endogenous substances for the binding sites. Less extensive binding of drugs to plasma proteins is generally without clinical importance unless the drugs are normally more than 80–90% bound. An example of this is phenytoin, which is normally 90% plasma-protein bound, but is only 70% bound in neonates, so that if the dose is not adjusted accordingly there is a high risk of toxic effects (Niederhauser, 1997). The other concern is that endogenous chemicals may be displaced by competition with drugs. There is a significant risk of elevation of plasma bilirubin in the neonate following its displacement from protein binding sites by sulphonamide antibiotics, vitamin K, X-ray contrast media or indometacin (indomethacin). Because the blood-brain barrier in the neonate is more permeable than the adult, there is a danger that the bilirubin will cross into the brain and cause kernicterus. The increased permeability of the brain also means that drugs like phenobarbital (phenobarbitone), morphine and chloral hydrate have an enhanced effect.

Metabolism

Enzyme systems are present at birth but they are immature, and so for about the first 15 days after birth there is reduced capacity to dispose of drugs. Thereafter the metabolic capacity of the liver increases rapidly, but at variable rates in the different enzyme systems. In the case of some enzyme systems, there is a period of enhanced drug metabolism, after which the enzymes gradually decrease and reach adult levels. The variability in the enzyme systems means that there are dangers in making global assumptions about drug handling ability in children, as the few examples below illustrate.

Hepatic oxidative metabolism and conjugation with glucuronic acid are deficient in the newborn (Laurence et al., 1997). Consequently, incomplete metabolism of drugs such as morphine, benzodiazepines, paracetamol and phenobarbital (phenobarbitone) will slow their renal clearance and extend their duration of action. A drug of particular concern here is chloramphenicol. In neonates who have a decreased capacity for glucuronidation, chloramphenicol doses more than 25–50 mg/kg per day have been associated with an increased incidence of grey baby syndrome (McLeod and Evans, 1992). In this syndrome, the neonate suffers with vomiting, abdominal distension and anorexia that may progress to respiratory distress, hypotension, shock and death. Although immature glucuronidation is the primary cause, decreased tubular secretion of the glucuronidated chloramphenicol metabolite may also contribute to this toxic event.

The enzyme system for sulphate conjugation is present at birth, and neonates have a greater capacity for sulphation than adults do (Skaer, 1991). Consequently, the decreased glucuronidation of paracetamol in neonates is compensated for to some extent by their enhanced sulphation capacity. Paracetamol is excreted predominately as sulphate conjugates in children and as glucuronide conjugates in adults. This may account for a lower incidence of liver damage from paracetamol overdose in children than in adults.

Phenytoin is normally metabolized by hydroxylation, and this is poor in neonates, giving the drug a half-life of 30–100 hours, compared with 15–30 hours in adults. However phenytoin, in common with some other drugs, e.g. phenobarbital (phenobarbitone), carbamazepine and some sulphonamides, has a shorter half-life in infants, i.e. 2–7 hours, than in neonates and adults, and dosages have to be adjusted accordingly (Grahame-Smith and Aronson, 1992). Similarly, cyclosporin clearance is largely determined by metabolism, and in a study of children between 1 and 18 years undergoing bone marrow transplantation, average clearances in the children were found to be 150–200% higher than those reported for adults (Rodman, 1994).

It must be remembered that the formulation of a drug contains more than the active medicine. Inactive ingredients are often added to improve stability or shelf life, and these agents may cause adverse reactions. Benzyl alcohol, a common preservative, was linked to the death of 16 neonates whose intravenous lines were frequently flushed with saline (Ramirez, 1989). These infants developed 'gasping syndrome' and suffered with severe metabolic acidosis, central nervous system depression, respiratory failure and cardiovascular collapse. It has been suggested that premature infants are unable to fully metabolize benzyl alcohol.

Excretion

Despite the fact that proportionally the neonatal kidney is two times larger than the adult kidney (Skacr, 1991), neonates have poor renal function and do not excrete drugs well. Renal blood flow is reduced, averaging 12 mL per minute at birth and increasing to 140 mL per minute by year one (Wingard et al., 1991). The glomerular filtration rate at birth is about 30–40% of the adult value, corrected for body surface (Aronson, 1993), and tubular reabsorption and secretion are reduced. Consequently, for those drugs that are dependent on renal excretion for termination of activity, e.g. aminoglycosides, digoxin, penicillins, salicylates, and thiazide diuretics, dosage modifications must be considered for young infants. Table 6.6 demonstrates how slower metabolism and excretion increases the half-life of drugs. By 6–9 months, renal function in children is equivalent to that in healthy adults.

Table 6.6 Comparison of drug half-lives in the neonate with those in the adult

Drug	*Half-life in the Neonate*	*Half-life in the Adult*
Diazepam	25–100 hours	20–30 hours
Digoxin	20–80 hours	25–50 hours
Gentamicin	3–12 hours	1.5–3 hours
Indometacin (indomethacin)	15–30 hours	4–10 hours
Morphine	5–14 hours	2–4 hours
Phenytoin	30–100 hours	15–30 hours
Vancomycin	6–12 hours	5–8 hours

Pharmacodynamic factors

Pharmacodynamic differences between children and adults can lead to some unexpected outcomes of drug therapy and adverse effects. For example, antihistamines and barbiturates generally sedate adults, but these drugs can cause many children to become hyperactive (Kanneh, 1998b). Conversely, amphetamines, which increase motor and behavioural activity in adults, are used to treat hyperactive children, as these drugs appear to increase attention span and decrease disruptive social behaviour. In paediatrics, some drugs are not used as they are recognized as harmful to children (Table 6.7).

The elderly

Before looking at adverse reactions in the elderly it is important to point out that although the term 'the elderly' suggests a homogeneous group, this is far from the case, especially in the case of drug therapy. The elderly are very variable in their handling of and responses to drugs, and as they get older the variability increases, as ageing occurs at different rates. Consequently, monitoring individual drug response is vital and an important role for the nurse.

Table 6.7 Examples of drugs to avoid in children

Drug	*Reason for Avoidance*
Aspirin	Rarely administered to children less than 12 years old because of the risk of Reye's syndrome
EMLA (Eutetic Mixture of Local Anaesthetics)	Not used routinely on children under three months due to the potential risk of methaemoglobinaemia
Glucocorticosteroids	Suppress growth in children of all ages
Alimemazine (trimeprazine)	Not licensed for use in children less than six months old as there have been suggestions that it may increase the incidence of cot death

Statistics

The elderly take proportionally more drugs than any other age group, i.e. they make up 20% of the population yet they take 50% of prescribed drugs (Rajaei-Dehkordi and McPherson, 1997). This is not surprising, as the elderly take medication for the treatment of acute conditions and commonly use maintenance medications for chronic age-related disorders. Thus the typical elderly person takes on average 4–5 prescription medications at a time (Moore and Beers, 1992), while drugs brought over-the-counter account for over a third of all drugs consumed by the elderly (Pelly, 1992). In the case of elderly people who are in institutions, the number of drugs taken daily escalates, such that one third of them receive between 8 and 16 medications at a time (White, 1995). The benefits of these drugs, used appropriately, are profound. They have dramatically decreased the morbidity and mortality from diseases such as hypertension, stroke and other cardiovascular diseases, and they have greatly increased quality of life, as demonstrated by hormone replacement therapy. However, because a condition is diagnosed for which a treatment is available, it does not follow that treatment will bring benefit, particularly in the context of multiple pathologies (Bowman, 1997).

The beneficial effects of drugs used to treat the elderly are associated with many adverse effects. Naturally, the more drugs a person takes, the greater their risk of side-effects from the drugs per se, but also the greater the risk of drug interactions and the adverse effects that they in turn may cause. However, in the elderly the problems of adverse effects are also exacerbated by

- inappropriate prescribing and the use of 'high risk' drugs, i.e. drugs with a narrow therapeutic index
- age-related changes in physiology which decrease the patient's ability to deal with drugs and alter their responses to them (see Table 6.8)
- chronic diseases such as liver and renal failure which affect the metabolism and excretion of drugs
- environmental factors, e.g. the elderly frequently receive care from a number of sources which can result in contradicting information and multiple prescriptions of the same drug
- poor compliance with dosing regimens as a result of poor comprehension or memory of instructions and complicated drug regimens; however it must be noted that the elderly are no more non-compliant than any other client group (Weintraub, 1981).

The error rate in taking drugs is about 60% in patients over the age of 60, and the error increases if more than three drugs are prescribed (Grahame-Smith and Aronson, 1992). As a result, adverse drug reactions are 2–3 times more common in the elderly than other client groups (Grahame-Smith and Aronson, 1992), and adverse reactions account for an estimated 5–31% of elderly hospitalizations (Cunningham et al., 1997; Kemle, 1997). However, the actual incidence of adverse reactions is likely to be far greater. This is due firstly to under reporting by the elderly person who does not recognize the adverse effect for what it is, and secondly because the prescriber attributes the problem to effects of ageing rather than to drugs (French, 1996).

Table 6.8 Physiological changes in the elderly that may lead to adverse drug effects

- Increased pH of gastric mucosa
- Decreased gastro-intestinal absorptive surface and motility
- Decreased perfusion of gastro-intestinal tract
- Decrease in lean body mass, decrease in total body water, and increase in total body fat
- Altered protein binding and decreased serum albumin
- Decreased hepatic mass, blood flow and enzyme activity
- Decreased renal blood flow, glomerular filtration rate, and tubular function

Administration and absorption

Before a drug can be absorbed, it must be administered. This can be quite problematic if the drugs are dispensed in child-resistant containers or blister packs, as a significant number of elderly people cannot extract the contents (Sexton and Gokani, 1997). If drugs are provided as tablets the elderly can have problems with swallowing them due to a decline in saliva production (xerostomia) and general degenerative disease. Some tablets and capsules may adhere to the oesophageal mucosa where they can dissolve and cause ulceration (Table 6.9). It is therefore important that drugs are taken with at least 60 mL of fluid, and in an upright position (Channer, 1985). If drugs are given as elixirs, the elderly can have problems measuring out the correct dose due to decreased visual acuity and tremor. Subcutaneous and intramuscular administration also have their problems as decreased tissue perfusion, especially in the case of congestive cardiac failure, can slow down drug absorption. The transdermal route is in many ways the ideal route of drug administration for the elderly as it omits the peaks and troughs in serum drug level seen with conventional therapy, and the possible toxic effects that the peaks can produce. However, transdermal drugs may not be absorbed effectively in the elderly due to age-damaged skin, which has increased keratin and decreased hydration.

The elderly tend to have a slower rate of absorption of drugs. In the case of oral medication this occurs because there is a decline in gastric acidity, motility and mixing, as well as atrophy of the

Table 6.9 Drugs reported to cause oesophageal ulceration

- Aminophylline
- Ampicillin
- Ascorbic acid
- Clomethiazole (chlormethiazole)
- Clindamycin
- Codeine compound analgesics, i.e. tablets containing paracetamol or aspirin with codeine phosphate
- Co-trimoxazole
- Doxycycline
- Ferrous salts
- Glibenclamide
- Indometacin (indomethacin)
- Naftidrofuryl
- Pivampicillin
- Potassium chloride
- Quinidine
- Tetracycline
- Thioridazine
- Tolmetin sodium

microvilli and diminished intestinal blood perfusion. This is not usually problematic except for those drugs, e.g. ketoconazole, ampicillin, and iron compounds, that require an acid pH to render them non-ionized so that they can pass easily across the lipid cell membranes that separate the gut lumen from the blood. Delays in gastric emptying can produce prolonged contact between the medication and the mucosal surfaces, resulting in higher risk of ulceration from direct toxic agents such as non-steroidal anti-inflammatory drugs (NSAIDs) and potassium chloride. Some drugs may further delay gastric emptying and act synergistically with the ageing process to increase this risk, e.g. antacids, anti-cholinergics, narcotics, lithium and isoniazid. The use of enteric-coated drugs may appear to be a solution by protecting the stomach mucosa from toxic drugs. However, they will only be effective if the patient does not take them at the same time as antacids, which are frequently used to self-medicate oesophageal reflux and heartburn. If the pH of the stomach is increased to that of the intestine then the enteric coating will dissolve in the stomach, rendering the coating useless.

Distribution

Drug distribution is affected by the changes in body composition associated with ageing, particularly the increase in adiposity, which rises from 18% and 36% in young men and women respectively, to 36% and 48% in elderly men and women respectively (Hudson and Boyter, 1997). As a result, lipid soluble drugs such as diazepam tend to accumulate with time, and this can lead to toxic effects. Anaesthetics are highly fat-soluble drugs and so are retained in fatty tissue, partially explaining why the elderly can take several days to recover fully from a general anaesthetic. The elderly also experience a decline in lean body mass, which together with the increase in fat, results in a decrease in total body water. Thus, there is a reduced volume of distribution for water-soluble drugs such as ethanol, cimetidine, digoxin, and lithium. This normal anatomical change may be exacerbated by the use of diuretics, which are frequently used to treat conditions such as congestive cardiac failure. As a result of the decrease in total body water, the concentration of water-soluble drugs will be greater, and if the dose is not adjusted accordingly, there is a chance of increased adverse effects.

The other major distribution problem that the elderly have is with plasma proteins. These decrease only slightly with age, but may fall markedly with acute diseases, e.g. pneumonia, myocardial infarction. As a result there are less binding sites for protein-bound drugs, and so there is an increase in free drug. This problem is increased when the patient uses more than one protein bound drug and there is competition between the drugs for the binding sites. Poor nutritional intake may also add to the problem.

Metabolism

Between the ages of 40 and 80 there is a decrease in hepatic blood flow of 40%, and consequently a decrease in first pass metabolism. There is also a decrease in hepatic mass of around 45% and enzyme activity leading to reduced metabolism of a variety of drugs, including propranolol, paracetamol and nifedipine. Consequently, the half-life of these drugs is prolonged, requiring alteration in dosage regimes in order to minimize the development of toxicity. The problem is increased if liver disease is present.

Not all enzyme systems are affected equally by ageing. There is a decline in the P450 cytochrome system, which is responsible for the oxidative phase of metabolism, however the transamination phase is unchanged by the ageing process. Thus agents metabolized by the transamination route, e.g. lorazepam and temazepam, are preferable to those metabolized by the oxidative route, e.g. diazepam and chlordiazepoxide. Another aspect of metabolism that is changed is the capacity for liver enzyme induction.

Excretion

By the age of 80, the glomerular filtration rate has on average dropped from 125 mL per minute in the young adult to 60–70 mL per minute. This combined with a decrease in renal size, number of functional glomeruli, and renal blood flow, can result in decreased renal clearance. With chronic diseases such as hypertension and diabetes, renal function may be reduced further. The decrease in clearance is particularly problematic with drugs that are excreted in their active state or as active metabolites, and which have a narrow therapeutic index, e.g. allopurinol, aminoglycosides, chlorpropamide, and digoxin. The usual method of measuring renal function is to measure creatinine clearance. However, because muscles produce serum creatinine, and the decline of lean muscle mass in the aged corresponds with reduced renal function, creatinine levels may be normal even with markedly reduced renal function. Thus in the elderly serum creatinine clearance becomes a less reliable sign of renal function, making it more difficult to predict the patient's ability to excrete drugs effectively.

Pharmacodynamic factors

For a variety of reasons, that are not fully understood, the elderly have increased sensitivity to some drugs, independent of pharmacokinetics. One reason for this altered sensitivity is a change in homeostatic mechanisms due to age (Dunbar, 1996). These mechanisms assist the body to adjust to or counteract stressors, including drug effects. Among the changes that may occur in the elderly are a decreased autonomic nervous system response to positional changes resulting in postural hypotension, autonomic mediated changes in bladder and bowel function, impairment in thermoregulation, reduction of cognitive function, impairment of postural neuromuscular stability, glucose intolerance, and reduced immune response (Planchock and Slay, 1996). Thus falls, urinary retention, and confusion can result from indiscrete drug prescribing.

As well as homeostatic changes, altered drug response can also result from an increased sensitivity of the drug-binding site, as illustrated by digoxin. This drug inhibits the sodium-potassium pump (Na^+-K^+-ATPase) found in the cardiac cell membrane, and as a consequence leads to an increase in intracellular calcium and hence improved myocardial contraction. In the elderly, the sensitivity of the pump to digoxin increases, which means that digoxin dosage must be monitored very carefully. As digoxin and potassium ions compete for a binding site on the Na^+-K^+-ATPase, the effects of digoxin can be dangerously increased if hypokalaemia develops through the use of diuretics, which are commonly taken by the elderly.

Other drugs where there is increased sensitivity are aminophylline, warfarin, diuretics, hypnotics, sedatives, tranquillizers, antidepressants, neuroleptics and opiates. Part of the reason for the increased sensitivity to drugs acting on the central nervous system is the age-related depletion of the neurotransmitters acetylcholine, dopamine, and serotonin level (French, 1996). However, increased sensitivity is not the rule and occasionally there is decreased sensitivity as in the case of ß-adrenoceptors resulting in diminished pharmacological response to ß-blockers and ß-agonists. Common sense and a few simple strategies (see Table 6.10) can help to minimize adverse drug effects in the elderly.

Table 6.10 Strategies to minimize adverse effects in the elderly

- Always consider non-pharmacological treatments first
- Assess the need for the drug weighing up risks and benefits
- Assess what drugs the patient is currently taking, including over-the-counter medications
- Select drugs with least adverse effects and avoid, where possible, drugs in Table 6.11
- Use the lowest possible dose to achieve the desired therapeutic effect
- Keep the number of drugs to a minimum and the regimen as simple as possible
- Ensure that the patient understands the regimen and the adverse effects to monitor for
- Frequently review medication regimens in the elderly
- Discontinue medications as soon as they are no longer needed
- If an elderly person's condition deteriorates or a new symptom appears, always consider that a drug may be the cause
- Advanced patient age, in itself should never be considered a contraindication to potentially beneficial therapy

Table 6.11 Common drugs with a high potential for adverse drug reactions in the elderly (Planchock and Slay, 1996)

Drug	*Rationale*
Angiotensin-converting enzyme inhibitors, e.g. captopril	May cause profound first dose hypotension, especially in those with mild to moderate heart failure. Reduced baroreceptor function in the elderly that can lead to hypotension after any antihypertensives
Aminoglycosides, e.g. gentamicin	Dependent on renal clearance, which is decreased in the elderly
Anticoagulants, e.g. warfarin	Increased sensitivity to anticoagulant effects
Antidepressants, e.g. amitriptyline	Excess anticholinergic effects. Orthostatic hypotension
ß-adrenergic blockers, e.g. propranolol	Decreased sensitivity of ß-adrenoceptors, especially in the heart, which reduces pharmacological effect of ß-adrenoceptor agonists and antagonists

Table 6.11 (contd)

Drug	*Rationale*
Calcium channel blockers, e.g. nifedipine	Should be avoided in heart failure, a common problem of the elderly, as they may further depress cardiac function. Reduced metabolism of nifedipine leads to a prolonged half-life
Digoxin	Increased receptor sensitivity which is increased by concomitant use of diuretics and calcium channel blockers; delayed clearance secondary to renal insufficiency
Diuretics, e.g. furosemide (frusemide)	Elderly patients particularly susceptible to diuretic induced hypokalaemia; a brisk diuresis in a man with prostatic enlargement can cause urinary retention; in the case of women, incontinence may ensue; gout may be precipitated. Reduced tubular secretion of furosemide (frusemide)
Histamine blockers, e.g. cimetidine	Can cause confusion, psychosis and hallucinations
Hypnotics, e.g. diazepam	Central nervous system very susceptible to effects leading to daytime drowsiness and increased risk of falls. Half-life of benzodiazepines can be prolonged threefold in the elderly
Narcotics	Elderly more sensitive, leading to excessive sedation, falls, delirium and constipation
Neuroleptics, e.g. chlorpromazine, haloperidol	May precipitate severe parkinsonism to which the elderly are prone
Non-steroidal anti-inflammatory drugs, e.g. indometacin (indomethacin)	Decreased mucosal protection and delayed gastric emptying leads to gastric bleeding and ulceration; increased risk of renal toxicity where there is dehydration
Oral hypoglycaemics, e.g. chlorpropamide	Long half-life
Theophylline	Metabolism reduced, leading to a prolonged half-life

References and further reading

Aranda JV, Cohen S, Neims AH (1976) Drug utilization in a newborn intensive care unit. Journal of Pediatrics 89: 315-17

Aronson J (1993) Drug excretion: what the prescriber should know. Prescriber 4: 31-4

Banta-Wright SA (1997) Minimizing infant exposure to and risks from medications while breastfeeding. Journal of Perinatal and Neonatal Nursing 11: 71-84

Bowman C (1997) Challenge of prescribing for elderly patients. Prescriber 8: 19-23

Budd KW (1995) Perinatal substance use: promoting abstinence in acute care settings. AACN Clinical Issues 6: 70-8

Butters L, Howie CA (1990) Awareness among pregnant women of the effect on the fetus of commonly used drugs. Midwifery 6: 146-54

Channer K (1985) Stand up and take your medicine. Nursing Times 81(28): 41-2

Committee on Drugs (1994) The transfer of drugs and other chemicals into human milk. Pediatrics 93: 137-50

Cunningham G, Dodd TRP, Grant DJ, McMurdo MET, Richards RME (1997) Drug-related problems in elderly patients admitted to Tayside hospitals, methods for prevention and subsequent reassessment. Age & Ageing 26: 375-82

Dionne R, McManus C (1993) Pediatric critical care pharmacodynamics. Critical Care Nursing Clinics of North America 5: 367-75

Dunbar A (1996) Altered presentation of illness in old age. Nursing Standard 10: 49-52

Ellis J (1995) Administering drugs. Paediatric Nursing 7: 29-39

Fosarelli P, Wilson M, DeAngelis C (1987) Prescription medications in infants and early childhood. American Journal of Diseases of Children 141: 772-5

French DG (1996) Avoiding adverse drug reactions in the elderly patient: issues and strategies. Nurse Practitioner 21: 90-105

Gilman J, Gal P (1992) Pharmacokinetics and pharmacodynamic data collection in children and neonates. Clinical Pharmokinetics 23: 1-9

Gal P, Sharpless MK (1984) Fetal drug exposure—behavioural teratogenesis. Drug Intelligence and Clinical Pharmacy 18: 187-201

Grahame-Smith DG, Aronson JK (1992). Oxford Textbook of Clinical Pharmacology and Drug Therapy 2nd edn. Oxford: Oxford University Press.

Guyon G (1989) Pharmacokinetic considerations in neonatal drug therapy. Neonatal Network 7: 9-12

Hudson SA, Boyter AC (1997) Pharmaceutical care in the elderly. The Pharmaceutical Journal 259: 686-8

Kanneh A (1998a) Pharmacological principles applied to children: Part 2. Paediatric Nursing 10: 24-7

Kanneh A (1998b) Pharmacological principles applied to children. Paediatric Nursing 10: 17-20

Kemle K (1997) Drug therapy in the elderly. Physician Assistant 21: 34-65

Laudano JB, Leach EE, Armstrong RB (1990) Acne: therapeutic perspective with an emphasis on the role of isotretinoin. Dermatology Nursing 2: 328-37

Laurence DR, Bennett PN, Brown MJ (1997) Clinical pharmacology. 8th edn. Edinburgh: Churchill Livingstone

McLeod HL, Evans WE (1992) Pediatric pharmacokinetics and therapeutic drug monitoring. Pediatrics in Review 13(11): 413-21

McManus Kuller J (1990) Effects on the fetus and newborn of medications commonly used during pregnancy. Journal of Perinatal Neonatal Nursing 3: 73-87

Moore A, Beers M (1992) Drug interactions in the elderly. Hospital Medicine 117: 684-9

Niederhauser VP (1997) Prescribing for children: issues in pediatric pharmacology. The Nurse Practitioner 22: 16-30

O'Sullivan EA, Curzon MEJ (1998) Drug treatments for asthma may cause erosive tooth damage. British Medical Journal 317(7161): 820

Pelly M (1992) Polypharmacy: too much of a good thing? Prescriber 3(16): 28-31

Planchock NY, Slay LE (1996) Pharmacokinetic and pharmacodynamic monitoring of the elderly in critical care. Critical Care Nursing Clinics of North America 8: 79-89

Rajaei-Dehkordi Z, McPherson G (1997) The effects of multiple medication in the elderly. Nursing Times 93(27): 56-8

Ramirez A (1989) the neonate's unique response to drugs: unravelling the causes of drug iatrogenesis. Neonatal Network 7: 45-9

Rodman JH (1994) Pharmokinetic variability in the adolescent: implications for body size and organ function for dosage regimen design. Journal of Adolescent Health 15: 654-62

Rubin PC, Craig GF, Gavin K, Sumner D (1986) Prospective survey of use of therapeutic drugs, alcohol and cigarette during pregnancy. British Medical Journal 292: 81-3

Ruggiero RJ (1992) Drugs in pregnancy. Neonatal Pharmacology Quarterly 1: 25-32

Sexton J, Gokani R (1997) Pharmaceutical packaging and the elderly. The Pharmaceutical Journal 259: 697-700

Skaer TL (1991) Dosing considerations in the paediatric patient. Clinical Therapeutics 13: 526-44

Sundaram B (1995) Tackling the aftermath faced by the daughters of DES. Nursing Times 91: 34-5

Smith S (1985) How drugs act. Six Drugs at different ages. Nursing Times 81: 37-9

Weintraub M (1981) Intelligent non-compliance with special emphasis on the elderly. Contemporary Pharmacy Practice 4: 8-11

White P (1995) Polypharmacy and the older patient. Journal of the American Academy of Nursing Practitioners 7: 545-8

Wingard LB, Brody TM, Larner J, Schwartz A (1991) Human Pharmacology Molecular-to-Clinical. St Louis: Mosby p848

Wink DM (1991) Giving infants and children drugs: precision + caution = safety. American Journal of Maternal and Child Nursing 16: 317-21

Zenk KE 1994) Challenges in providing pharmaceutical care to pediatric patents. American Journal of Hospital Pharmacology 51: 688-94

Chapter 7
Gastro-intestinal and hepatic effects

Introduction

Almost every drug has possible gastrointestinal side-effects associated with it (Everette, 1995). These can range from mild indigestion through to life-threatening gastro-intestinal haemorrhage, with the most commonly reported being nausea, vomiting, constipation or diarrhoea. In 1996, the GI tract was involved in 17.5% of the yellow card reports made to the Committee on the Safety of Medicines (Lee and Morris, 1997).

The mouth

Perhaps surprisingly, drugs can have a variety of adverse effects on the mouth (Table 7.1).

Table 7.1 Examples of drugs with adverse effects on the mouth

Adverse effect	*Causative drug*
Dry mouth (xerostomia)	Anticholinergics, antihistamines, phenothiazines, tricyclic antidepressants
Contact stomatitis	Antiseptic lozenges, mouthwashes
Erythema multiforme (see Chapter 5)	Penicillins, phenytoin, sulphonamides
Gum hyperplasia	Calcium channel blockers, cyclosporin, phenytoin
Lichen planus	ß-blockers, chloroquine, quinidine, thiazide diuretics
Mouth ulcers	Cocaine, cytotoxics, gold salts, isoprenaline, NSAIDs, sulfasalazine (sulphasalazine)
Taste disturbances	Acetazolamide, ACE inhibitors, systemic griseofulvin, metronidazole, penicillamine, terbinafine

Many drugs can affect the sensation of taste, although the mechanism by which they do so is not clear. Taste may be blunted (hypogeusia), distorted (dysgeusia) or lost completely (ageusia). Penicillamine, which chelates copper, and the ACE-inhibitor captopril commonly lead to taste disturbances, while drugs like gold, levodopa, metronidazole and metformin can produce a metallic taste. Alteration in taste may seem a minor adverse effect, but it can lead to drug non-compliance as well as loss of appetite and weight loss. Taste problems usually resolve when the drug is discontinued, but it can take some months.

Dry mouth or xerostomia occurs when production of saliva is inhibited. The release of saliva is controlled by the autonomic nervous system, and so drugs that antagonize acetylcholine at parasympathetic junctions are the main cause of xerostomia. Those most commonly implicated include anticholinergic drugs such as atropine, tricyclic antidepressants, and phenothiazines. If saliva production is inhibited for a long time dental caries can result as saliva plays an important role in reducing mouth infections. Patients should be warned about the need for good oral hygiene, and advised to use mouthwashes, sugar free gum and saliva substitutes in order to relieve the problem.

The pathogenesis of gum hyperplasia, or gingival overgrowth, is not fully understood although it has been suggested that the drug, or its metabolite, stimulate gingival fibroblasts to produce too much collagen. The problem occurs after about three months of taking the drug, and prevalence studies suggest that 50% of patients taking phenytoin, 30% of those taking cyclosporin and 10% of those taking dihydropyridine calcium antagonists, such as nifedipine, experience gingival hyperplasia (Seymour, 1994). Symptoms include pain, tenderness and bleeding gums. Management is either to withdraw the drug, or where that is not possible, to encourage good oral hygiene as poor hygiene makes the hyperplasia worse. In some cases, extensive oral surgery is required, which may have to be repeated.

Contact stomatitis is a hypersensitivity reaction of the oral mucosa to repeated contact with an allergen. Common causes are not usually drugs but hygiene products such as toothpaste, mouthwash, and chewing gum, although antiseptic lozenges may be a cause.

Lichen planus is a dermatological condition that manifests in the mouth as areas of desquamation which can develop into ulcers. The surrounding mucosa is often covered with white striae, which gives a characteristic lace pattern (Seymour, 1994). Drugs that can induce this condition include ß-blockers, chloroquine, lithium, phenothiazines and thiazide diuretics. Unlike true lichen planus, the drug-induced eruptions disappear when the drug is withdrawn.

Mouth ulcers can result from topical application of various drugs that act as irritants to the oral mucosa. Drugs associated with this problem are aspirin (when applied against a painful tooth), potassium chloride, and isoprenaline. Topical application of cocaine by drug abusers can result in ulceration due to the intense vasoconstrictive properties of the drug. Discontinuation of the offending drug allows the ulcers to heal. The second main cause of mouth ulcers is drug-induced neutropenia. This commonly occurs with cytotoxic drugs, when the ulceration can be severe, making eating a very painful experience. The ulcers may also become infected with oral candidiasis, adding to the patient's problems. Other drugs that cause ulceration are gold compounds, proguanil, and sulfasalazine (sulphasalazine). Oral candidiasis may also occur as an opportunistic infection following the use of broad-spectrum antibiotics, oral steroids and hydrogen peroxide mouthwashes (Campbell, 1995).

Oesophagus

Adverse drug reactions in the oesophagus are uncommon. When they do occur they take the form of oesophageal reflux, oesophagitis, ulceration and stricture. Drugs like anticholinergic drugs, calcium-channel blockers, and opioids relax the cardiac sphincter and allow acid reflux with consequent heartburn. Tetracycline and doxycycline have been implicated in several case reports of oesophageal ulcer, and more recently a new bisphosphonate, alendronate, has been recognized as an important cause. In order to minimize the risk the patient prescribed alendronate should be advised that the drug must be taken with at least 200 mL of water. The patient must not lie down for at least 30 minutes after taking the drug, and not until after eating, which should be at least 30 minutes after taking the drug (Lee and Morris, 1997). Alendronate should not be taken at bedtime, and concurrent use with NSAIDs or aspirin should be avoided.

NSAIDs are a major cause of oesophagitis and stricture. One study (Hirschowitz 1997) found that 60% of 55 patients with oesophagitis and 80% of 30 patients with oesophageal stricture used NSAIDs (especially aspirin). It is believed that the NSAIDs initiate oesophageal damage by compromising the integrity of the mucosa and rendering it susceptible to acid and pepsin. NSAIDs can also cause direct ulceration if the tablets are stalled, even transiently, in the oesophagus (pill oesophagitis).

Stomach and duodenum

The NSAIDs are the main cause of adverse effects in the stomach and duodenum. Problems range from symptoms of pain, dyspepsia, and nausea to ulceration, bleeding, and perforation. Twenty to thirty percent of patients taking therapeutic doses of NSAIDs chronically experience dyspepsia, nausea or abdominal pain, and 10–30% develop chronic gastric and duodenal ulcers (Hirschowitz, 1997). NSAIDs cause these gastro-intestinal side-effects because they inhibit the enzyme cyclooxygenase, which is required for prostaglandin synthesis. Prostaglandins produce the symptoms of pain, inflammation, and pyrexia, and it is for this reason that NSAIDs are taken. However, in the gastro-duodenal mucosa prostaglandins also appear to function as paracrine signals coordinating a variety of defences against gastric acid and pepsin attack (Table 7.2).

Table 7.2 Gastric protective effects of prostaglandins

In response to prostaglandins:
• The gastric and duodenal epithelial cells increase their secretion of mucus and bicarbonate ions, which buffer hydrogen ions
• The gastric and duodenal cells increase their secretion of mucopolysaccharide which traps hydrogen ions
• The mucosal blood flow increases delivering oxygen, nutrients and bicarbonates and removing harmful metabolites
• The gastric mucosa increases its self-renewal
• The tight intracellular junctions are strengthened and keep hydrogen ions from penetrating the epithelium
• The secretion of gastric acid is suppressed

NSAIDs do not only inhibit the protective effects of prostaglandins, they also damage the gut mucosa directly because they are highly acidic. Due to their acidic nature, NSAIDs only dissociate slightly in the highly acid gastric lumen, but at the more alkaline pH of the mucous gel, which lies over the gastric epithelium, they release harmful hydrogen ions, that diffuse into the epithelium of the gut wall and damage it (Wolfe, 1996). Everette (1995) suggests that when the stomach pH is less than 3.5 the non-ionized drug is lipid soluble and so is absorbed directly into the gastric mucosa, where it destroys the mucosal cells, exposing the gastric capillaries to direct vascular injury.

Strategies for the prevention of gastro-intestinal symptoms produced by NSAIDs include dosage reduction, discontinuation of therapy, the use of low risk NSAIDs, giving an antacid, an H_2-histamine receptor antagonist, or misoprostol (Gabriel, 1997). Ibuprofen is associated with the lowest risk, diclofenac, naproxen and indometacin (indomethacin) are intermediate risk, ketoprofen and piroxicam have a greater risk, and azapropazone has the highest risk (Lee and Morris, 1997). Newer NSAIDs, for example nabumetone and meloxicam, which have less effect on COX-1, the form of cyclooxygenase that is important in the synthesis of protective prostaglandins, may be less toxic, but this requires confirmation (Needleman and Isakson, 1998). Many NSAIDs are available as a pro-drug, suppository or enteric-coated formulation, which may reduce any direct action on the mucosa. However, the active agent nevertheless reaches the gut via the vascular system and may still result in ulceration (Reardon and Holman, 1995).

NSAIDs are known to impair the ability of H_2-antagonists, such as cimetidine, to heal NSAID-related ulcers, unlike proton pump inhibitors such as omeprazole which have been found to be effective (Wolfe, 1996). As far as prophylaxis is concerned mucosal protectives, like sucralfate, have been shown to be ineffective as have the H_2-histamine receptor antagonists (Wolfe, 1996). Exogenous prostaglandins like misoprostol, however, are effective. At any dosage prostaglandins promote mucosal protection, but only at high doses do they inhibit gastric acid secretion and demonstrate a clinical capacity to prevent NSAID-related ulceration. At this dosage, they cause diarrhoea, which considerably decreases patient compliance. Risk factors for NSAID-induced ulceration are age over 75 years, a previous peptic ulcer, previous gastro-intestinal bleeding, and a history of cardiovascular disease. Patients with all four risk factors have a 9% risk of major complication over a six-month period (Wolfe, 1996) and thus would appear to be particularly in need of prophylaxis.

Glucocorticoid therapy has been associated with an increased incidence of gastric or duodenal ulceration. However, Baxter (1992) maintains that the overall incidence of gastrointestinal haemorrhage linked to glucocorticoid therapy is so low that in general it should not be a major problem. He maintains that much of the ulcer disease seen in patients taking glucocorticoids results from the NSAIDs that are being taken simultaneously.

Nausea and vomiting

Many drugs have the potential to cause nausea and vomiting. They do this either by stimulating the chemoreceptor trigger zone in the brain, or by causing gastric irritation as occurs with iron salts and potassium. It is important is to be aware of those drugs which invariably cause nausea and vomiting, i.e. most cytotoxics, levodopa and opioids. Symptoms will often resolve with continued use of the drug, as occurs with opioids (Walsh, 1990) otherwise concurrent antiemetics may be required.

Surgery is associated with postoperative nausea and vomiting. The incidence varies from 13% in ophthalmic surgery to 42% in gynaecological surgery (Rowbotham, 1995). Numerous anaesthetic agents have been implicated as the primary cause, for example etomidate, ketamine, nitrous oxide, ketorlac (Mann, 1998). However, a variety of factors contribute to postoperative nausea and vomiting as indicated in Table 7.3.

No matter what the cause, postoperative nausea and vomiting is a serious complication as it can result in patient distress and anxiety, dehydration and electrolyte imbalance, aspiration pneumonia, wound dehiscence, Mallory-Weiss tears, and even rib fractures. Consequently, it is important that those at risk are identified by good preoperative assessment so that measures can be taken to minimize the effects. These may include reducing the period of preoperative fluid restriction (Smith et al., 1997), using newer anaesthetic agents such as propofol that are less emetogenic (Mathias, 1995), using antiemetics (Tate and Cook, 1996), and complimentary therapies

Table 7.3 Risk factors for post-operative nausea and vomiting

Risk factors	*Comments*
Age	Low risk under 3 and over 70 years old; high risk 3–15 years old
Drugs	Opioids in premedication and post-operative pain relief. Induction agents, e.g. thiopental (thiopentone). Inhaled anaesthetics, e.g. nitrous oxide. Prostaglandins used in gynaecological and obstetric surgery
Gender	Women, particularly during the second half of the menstrual cycle
History	Motion sickness, migraine or previous post-operative nausea and vomiting
Movement	Excessive movement in the immediate post-operative period, particularly sitting up before blood pressure has stabilized
Obesity	Fat takes up anaesthetic and acts as a reservoir
Starvation	Prolonged pre- and post-operative starvation increases risk Eating and drinking in the first 2–3 hours post-operatively increases risk
Surgical procedure	Gall bladder surgery, laparoscopy, middle ear procedures

such as ginger root (Bone et al., 1990) and acupressure (Jackson, 1995).

Chemotherapy-induced nausea and vomiting is a major disrupter of quality of life in many patients who receive chemotherapy, and it can be so severe that the patient refuses potentially curative treatment (Wickham, 1989). The risk of nausea and vomiting depends on the agent used (Table 7.4). Generally, agents associated with a high risk of emesis also induce the most severe vomiting. It has also been suggested that there is a correlation between the emetic potential of a chemotherapeutic agent and the onset of emesis (Tortorice and O'Connell, 1990). Thus highly emetogenic agents like cisplatin and dacarbazine can cause an emetic response within one to two hours of infusion. Vomiting usually occurs within six hours when the agent has moderate emetogenic potential, and can be delayed for up to 12 hours in agents with moderately low emetogenicity. Cyclophosphamide is metabolized in the liver to its active form before it exerts cytotoxic or emetic effects. Thus, patients who receive cyclophosphamide require antiemetic coverage for at least 18–24 hours following drug administration. Furthermore, it must be remembered that when cytotoxics are used in combination the emetogenic potential of each agent is additive (Veyrat-Follet, 1997).

Table 7.4 The potential of some cytotoxic drugs to cause nausea and vomiting (adapted from Goodman, 1997)

Low risk	*Moderate Risk*	*High Risk*
• Bleomycin	• Asparaginase	• Actinomycin D
• Chlorambucil	• Azacytidine	• Carmustine> 200 mg/m^2
• Etoposide	• Daunorubicin	• Cisplatin
• Paclitaxel	• Fluorouracil	• Cyclophosphamide> 600 mg/m^2
• Pentostatin	• Idarubicin	• Dacarbazine
• Thiotepa	• Mitomycin	• Doxorubicin > 50 mg/m^2
• Vinblastine	• Procarbazine	• Methotrexate > 250 mg/m^2
• Vincristine	• Topotecan	• Melphalan > 100 mg/m^2

In the case of cytotoxics, it is necessary to prevent rather than just treat nausea and vomiting, because once it is allowed to occur the patient may develop anticipatory nausea and vomiting, so they only need to smell the hospital or see the nurse to start vomiting. For highly emetogenic chemotherapy regimens, the combination of 5-HT_3 serotonin receptor antagonists, such as ondansetron, and dexamethasone appear to be superior to single agents or combinations in preventing nausea and vomiting (Goodman, 1997). For some drugs, for example digoxin and theophylline, nausea and vomiting may be a sign of toxicity.

Small intestine

The main adverse drug effects suffered by the small intestine are ulceration and perforation, malabsorption, and paralytic ileus and pseudo-obstruction. The stomach and duodenum are usually associated with NSAID-induced ulceration, but the small and large bowel can also be affected. Small bowel ulceration and perforation have also been described with slow-release potassium preparations (Lee and Morris, 1997).

Drug-induced malabsorption usually occurs as a result of an interaction between drugs and certain nutrients. The anion-exchange resins colestyramine (cholestyramine) and colestipol, and the faecal softener liquid paraffin can interfere with the absorption of the fat-soluble vitamins, i.e. A, D, E and K. Metformin can interfere with the absorption of vitamin B_{12} and a third of patients who have been on the drug for four to five years have B_{12} malabsorption (Callaghan et al., 1980). In some cases, this can be severe enough for megaloblastic anaemia to result, and so vitamin B_{12} levels should consequently be checked annually in patients taking this drug.

Drugs can induce reduction in the activity of the small bowel severe enough to cause paralytic ileus and obstruction, which can progress to necrotizing enterocolitis with extensive necrosis of the intestinal mucosa. Loperamide has been implicated in causing this severe reaction, and so it should be avoided where there is ileus or abdominal distension, or in patients with acute pseudomembranous colitis associated with broad-spectrum antibiotics. Pseudo-obstruction has also been reported with opioid addicts, phenothiazines, tricyclic antidepressants and vincristine.

Pancreas

The main adverse effect of drugs on the pancreas is drug-induced pancreatitis, which accounts for about 2% of cases of the disease (Lee and Morris, 1997). Most cases of drug-induced pancreatitis are mild. Treatment consists of immediate removal of the suspected drug, and the commencement of standard supportive management of pancreatitis. Drugs that have consistently been associated with pancreatitis include aminosalicylates, didanosine, oestrogen and sodium valproate (Lee and Morris, 1997). In the case of sodium valproate, most cases occur within a year of starting treatment. There is no obvious relationship to dose or serum concentration, suggesting that this is an idiosyncratic reaction. Other drugs which may cause pancreatitis, but which have not been proven to do so, are ACE inhibitors, clozapine, corticosteroids and thiazide diuretics.

Large intestine

Other than constipation and diarrhoea (see below), the large intestine is rarely affected by adverse drug reactions. The main adverse effect is ischaemic colitis, which commonly presents with sudden onset of abdominal pain, passage of blood, nausea and vomiting, and diarrhoea, tachycardia, raised white blood count and pyrexia. Drugs that cause this reaction include amphetamines, cocaine, digoxin, ergotamine and oestrogens (Lee and Morris, 1997), and need to be withdrawn if ischaemic colitis arises.

Rectal necrosis is a rare but serious injury sustained during administration of phosphate enema. Samadian (1990) describes a case in which an 84-year-old gentleman was given two 130 mL disposable phosphate enemas, and eight days later developed ulceration of the rectal and perianal tissues which developed into a deep cavity extending into the perineum. It is believed that the necrosis results from injury to the rectum caused by the tip of the enema. The enema fluid is then injected through the injury causing an inflammatory reaction, which may be worsened by bacterial invasion. It is therefore advisable that enemas are only given by those who understand the possible hazards of the procedure.

Constipation

Medication has been found to be a factor in more than 50% of constipated patients admitted to hospital (Ross, 1998), and a wide variety of drugs have been found to be involved (Table 7.5). Many older people have grown up in a culture where daily bowel movement was seen as desirable, and they may have come to depend on daily laxatives to achieve this. Long-term use of stimulant laxatives may result in cathartic damage to the colon and will cause the natural defecation reflex to weaken and colonic muscle tone to deteriorate. Bulk forming laxatives can result in the bowel filling with soft faeces that are difficult to expel, resulting in thickening and hypertrophy of the bowel wall and muscle atrophy (Nazarko, 1996).

Constipation is regarded by many physicians as a trivial problem, and hence often receives little attention (Cameron, 1992). However, for patients it can be a very unpleasant problem with symptoms as diverse as headache, nausea, abdominal and rectal pain, confusion, faecal incontinence and overflow diarrhoea. Action must be taken to minimize these adverse effect by encouraging the patient to drink plenty of fluids, have a high fibre intake and to exercise gently. If withdrawal of the causative drug is not feasible, as when treating intractable pain with an opioid, constipation should be anticipated and a laxative prescribed simultaneously. Walsh (1990) suggests the combination of a stool softener, such as docusate sodium, and an osmotic laxative, such as lactulose. The dosage should be titrated to the comfort of defecation and the nature of the stools passed. Where possible codeine-based drugs should be avoided due to their propensity to cause constipation.

Table 7.5 Drugs that commonly give rise to constipation

Drug	*Mode of action*
Anion-exchange resins, e.g. colestyramine (cholestyramine)	Bind unabsorbed bile salts, which stimulate defecation
Antimuscarinics, e.g. atropine	Reduce intestinal motility by antagonizing acetylcholine on gut smooth muscle
Antacids containing aluminium salts	Aluminium salts relax the smooth muscle of the stomach and delay gastric emptying as well as decreasing intestinal motility
Antihistamines, e.g. promethazine	Act as peripheral antimuscarinics
Calcium channel blockers, e.g. nifedipine, verapamil	Prevent the influx of calcium ions required for smooth muscle cells to contract during peristalsis
Diuretics, e.g. furosemide (frusemide)	May cause dehydration and hard stools
Iron, e.g. ferrous sulphate	Has an irritant effect on the bowel which results in altered bowel habit, i.e. constipation or diarrhoea; oral preparations, particularly in the elderly have a constipating effect and may cause faecal impaction
Mono-amine oxidase inhibitors	Act as peripheral antimuscarinics
Opioids, e.g. morphine	Agonistic action on opioid receptors on bowel wall. Results in an increase in segmentation but decrease in propulsive movements, so that faecal material is repeatedly brought in contact with the intestinal mucosa but is not propelled forward; this results in dried impacted faeces
Phenothiazines, e.g. prochlorperazine	Have antimuscarinic effects
Tricyclic antidepressants, e.g. amitriptyline	Have antimuscarinic effects
Vinca alkaloids, e.g. vincristine	Neurotoxic to peripheral nerves including autonomic nerves of bowel, leading to decreased peristalsis

Diarrhoea

As Table 7.6 indicates, many drugs can lead to diarrhoea as an adverse effect. The main offenders are antibiotics, with as many as 20% of patients who take them developing diarrhoea. Occasionally the diarrhoea is accompanied by colitis, or more seriously by life-threatening pseudomembranous colitis (Rowland, 1989). Nearly any antibiotic can cause diarrhoea, but it is more likely to occur with oral or multiple antibiotic therapy. The most common culprits are clindamycin, ampicillin, and the cephalosporins, which account for over 80% of cases seen (Everette, 1995). Antibiotics cause diarrhoea in some cases by stimulating bowel motility, e.g. erythromycin. However, their main effect seems to be to kill protective anaerobes found in the gut (Hamilton, 1999), allowing the overgrowth of harmful bacteria such as *Clostridium difficile*, *Shigella* and *Salmonella*.

Table 7.6 Drugs that commonly give rise to diarrhoea

Drug	*Mode of action*
Antacids containing magnesium	Osmotic suction of fluid into colon
Antibiotics, e.g. ampicillin, cephalosporins, clindamycin	Alteration of endogenous bowel flora
Anti-neoplastics	Destroy rapidly dividing cells, including those of the gut leading to increased motility and decreased absorption of fluids
Colchicine	Increase bowel motility
Digoxin	Increases vagal activity and thus peristalsis
Laxative abuse	Depends on the laxative being abused
NSAIDs, e.g. mefenamic acid	Inhibition of prostaglandin synthesis prevents damaged gut cells from repairing themselves and maintaining their integrity, resulting in increased permeability and fluid loss
Prostaglandin E analogues, e.g. misoprostol	Cause contraction of gut smooth muscle and so increase bowel motility
Sorbitol	Osmotic suction of fluid into colon

Minimizing the use of antibiotics will cut down on this problem, but where antibiotics are absolutely necessary it has been suggested that the use of the non-pathogenic yeast *Saccharomyces boulardii* may have some prophylactic value, while eating yoghurt or other products containing live lactobacilli also helps some people (Rowland, 1989).

Overgrowth of *Clostridium difficile* is responsible for about 20% of cases of antibiotic induced diarrhoea. The bacteria release toxins that cause mucosal damage and inflammation of the colon, leading to diarrhoea. Onset of diarrhoea usually occurs between five and ten days after starting the antibiotic (Robinson, 1993). It tends to be explosive, watery and foul smelling and can be particularly debilitating to the elderly. Antibiotic therapy should be stopped as soon as possible in a patient who develops diarrhoea. Patients with proven or suspected *C. difficile* may require treatment with oral metronidazole or vancomycin. If it is necessary to continue an antibiotic for the primary infection, one that is less likely to cause diarrhoea, e.g. a quinolone or a parenteral aminoglycoside should be used.

Liver

Drug-induced liver damage has been associated with more than 800 different drugs and accounts for 2–3% of all hospitalizations due to adverse drug reactions (Dossing and Sonne, 1993). This is perhaps not surprising when it is remembered that the liver plays a major role in the metabolism of most foreign chemicals. Some drugs are converted to toxic intermediates and although they are usually rapidly detoxified in some cases, detoxification does not occur. This can transpire for two reasons. Either, it can be the result of a drug overdose when the capacity of the liver to detoxify the hepatotoxin is overwhelmed, or alternatively it can be an unpredictable reaction to a therapeutic dose leading to the over production of reactive metabolites (Magee and Beeley, 1992). The latter may occur because of genetically or environmentally induced variations in hepatic enzyme activity.

Recognizing drug-induced liver disease can be difficult, as the clinical symptoms may be minimal and vague. Furthermore, the duration of treatment until the appearance of liver injury (the latency period) may range from days even to years in the case of oral contraceptives, androgens and anabolic steroids. Symptoms of drug-induced liver disease include fever, general malaise, anorexia, nausea, and abdominal discomfort. The presence of dark urine, pale stools and jaundice help to identify liver disease, and if these symptoms are associated with pruritus, obstruction of the common bile duct should be suspected. The presence of a rash together with eosinophilia may suggest a hypersensitivity reaction. Confirmation of diagnosis is based on drug history, exclusion of other causes of liver disease, liver function tests and biopsy results. As most cases of drug-induced liver disorders are probably reversible until a certain point, early diagnosis is essential (Dossing and Sonne, 1993). Table 7.7 lists some of the common hepatotoxic drugs.

Some patients are more prone to drug-induced liver disease than others. The presence of pre-existing liver disease means that drugs cannot be detoxified as efficiently as normal and that the patient is at increased risk of adverse effects on all bodily systems, including the liver. Patients who have ascites, cirrhosis, or encephalopathy may require reduced doses of many drugs (Ward et al., 1997). Women

Table 7.7 Examples of drugs that may affect the liver

Disorder	*Associated drugs*
Acute dose-dependent hepatotoxicity	
Hepatotoxicity	Azathioprine, chlorambucil, cyclophosphamide, mercaptopurine, methotrexate, paracetamol, large IV doses of tetracycline
Dose-independent hepatotoxicity	
Acute hepatitis	Allopurinol, ACE inhibitors, co-trimoxazole, dantrolene, methyldopa, isoniazid, minocycline (Gough et al., 1996), monoamine oxidase inhibitors, nifedipine, phenytoin, rifampicin, verapamil
Acute hepatocellular necrosis	Allopurinol, aspirin, cocaine, dantrolene, ecstasy, halothane, isoniazid, NSAIDs e.g. diclofenac (Helfgott et al., 1990), paracetamol
Cholestasis without hepatitis	Cyclosporin, oral contraceptives, glibenclamide, griseofulvin, tamoxifen, warfarin
Cholestasis with hepatitis	Azathioprine, cimetidine, chlorpromazine, erythromycin, gold salts, imipramine, NSAIDs, nitrofurantoin, sulphonylureas
Fatty liver	Sodium valproate, steroids, tetracycline,
Fibrosis and cirrhosis	Dantrolene, isoniazid, methotrexate, methyldopa, nitrofurantoin, vitamin A in mega doses
Granulomatous hepatitis	Allopurinol, carbamazepine, methyldopa, quinidine, sulphonamides, sulphonylureas
Hepatic tumours	Oral contraceptives, danazol, anabolic steroids
Vascular disorders	Azathioprine, dacarbazine

appear to be twice as susceptible to drug-induced liver disease as are men (Cadman, 1996), and older patients have a higher incidence, with the drug-induced reaction tending to be more severe. Children rarely suffer drug-induced liver disease, but for two exceptions. Children under the age of two on multiple enzyme-inducing antiepileptics and with a developmental delay seem to be particularly susceptible to idiosyncratic hepatotoxicity with sodium valproate. The other exception is aspirin. The use of salicylates in children with a mild viral infection risks development of Reye's syndrome. This is a life-threatening illness associated with hypoglycaemia, liver failure, seizures and coma.

Other risk factors for the development of drug-induced liver disease are genetic factors which determine the cytochrome P450 isoenzymes found in the liver, and hence the ability to metabolize drugs. The use of other drugs, including alcohol, also play an important role, and the risk increases in patients on multi-drug regimens. Other factors, including renal disease, pregnancy, cigarette smoking and poor nutrition may all affect the capacity of the liver to metabolize drugs efficiently and put the patient at increased risk.

Liver damage caused by drugs can range from minor changes to massive hepatic necrosis. Many drugs can cause elevation of liver function tests without any clinical significance to the individual, and the enzymes return to normal levels on stopping the drug. Drug-induced disease can be classified according to the mechanism by which the injury is induced, or using clinicopathological criteria (Cadman, 1996), as is done here.

Acute dose-dependent hepatotoxicity

Drugs can have a direct toxic effect on the liver in a dose-dependent manner. The classical example of this is paracetamol overdose, which is the most common cause of drug-induced liver disease, leading to about 200 deaths each year in the UK (Ward et al., 1997). At normal therapeutic doses, paracetamol is rapidly metabolized in the liver to its glucuronide and sulphate conjugates, ready for excretion by the kidneys. As the dose of the paracetamol increases, the proportion of drug excreted as the sulphate conjugate falls due to saturation of the metabolic pathway. The paracetamol is oxidized instead to form toxic intermediates. These are normally rapidly inactivated by conjugation to glutathione and excreted. However, if the levels of glutathione are depleted, due to excessive paracetamol consumption or malnutrition, the toxic intermediates cannot be inactivated and so they accumulate, causing necrosis.

Most patients have no symptoms after paracetamol overdose, although nausea and vomiting may occur within the first few hours, followed by a period of apparent recovery until the signs of hepatic necrosis occur 48–72 hours after ingestion. These symptoms include abdominal pain, hypoglycaemia, jaundice, oliguria, ascites, haematuria, and haemorrhage. The lack of symptoms for 48 hours can lead to a delay in seeking medical advice, and thus increase the risk of fatal liver failure. Patients who present 12 or more hours after ingestion of paracetamol are at greater risk of serious liver damage because the antidotes are less effective after this time. Treatment of the overdose consists of gastric lavage and oral administration of activated charcoal (Davis, 1991), together with acetylcysteine, which is administered intravenously. Acetylcysteine enhances glutathione synthesis and reduces free radical damage of the liver (Budden and Vink, 1996).

The dose of paracetamol required to cause a significant risk of developing hepatic cell damage is 150 mg/kg, which equates to the ingestion of 10 g in a 70 kg adult (Budden and Vink, 1996). There is evidence that the public has a poor knowledge of paracetamol's toxicity in overdose, and accidental deaths have occurred after self-medication with multiple paracetamol preparations at the same time. Patients need more education in this matter and must be advised on the importance of not exceeding the maximum daily dose of 4 g.

The majority of hepatic drug reactions are dose-independent, idiosyncratic and unpredictable (Lee, 1995) and these are discussed below.

Acute dose-independent hepatocellular necrosis

This form of liver damage occurs in patients who have altered enzyme activity or immunoallergic mechanisms. For example, isoniazid induced liver necrosis seems to occur in those patients who are fast acetylators in whom some of the drug may be converted to a hepatotoxic metabolite.

Halothane also produces severe necrosis in a dose independent manner, although only after repeated administration. A metabolite of halothane alters liver cells to make them antigenic, with the result that antibodies are produced against them. As repeated administration of halothane has been abandoned this should no longer be a problem.

Granulomatous hepatitis

As its name suggests, granulomatous hepatitis is the infiltration of the liver by granulation tissue. This tissue is normally associated with wound healing, and consists of numerous capillaries together with collagen fibres. The reaction may be drug-induced and can be accompanied by a generalized granulomatous reaction throughout the body. As there are no specific features of drug-induced disease, diagnosis depends on the exclusion of other causes together with identification of a possible drug culprit.

Cholestasis

Cholestasis occurs when there is partial or complete obstruction of the common bile duct, resulting in the retention of bile acids. This may occur with or without associated hepatitis and bile duct injury or destruction. Clinical features are jaundice, pruritus, dark urine and pale stools. Malabsorption of the fat-soluble vitamin K can lead to bruising and there may be cutaneous deposits of cholesterol. Chlorpromazine is a common cause of cholestasis with an estimated incidence of 0.5–1% in patients taking the drug for more than two weeks (Ward et al., 1997). Symptoms usually resolve within four weeks of discontinuing the drug.

Acute hepatitis

Acute hepatitis usually occurs as a result of a viral infection, but it can also be drug-induced, and is independent of dose. A large number of drugs have been implicated in this type of hepatotoxicity, but the incidence of clinical disease is low. For example, 15–20% of patients receiving isoniazid as a single agent for prophylaxis against tuberculosis may have increased enzyme levels. However, only 1% have hepatic necrosis severe enough to require withdrawal of the drug (Lee, 1995) and the rate of fatal isoniazid-induced hepatitis is estimated to be less than seven per 100000 (Anon, 1997). In order to prevent fatal hepatitis patients receiving isoniazid should have monthly liver function tests.

Fatty liver

Both hepatic and cholestatic drug-induced lesions will be associated with some degree of lipid accumulation within liver cells. For some drugs, such as the corticosteroids and tetracycline, fatty infiltration is the primary feature of their toxicity.

Fibrosis and cirrhosis

Chronic liver disease is associated with fibrosis and cirrhosis, and may result from prolonged drug treatment. Fibrosis may occur without the development of cirrhosis and is partially reversible, whereas cirrhosis is characterized by the presence of dense fibrosis and hepatocellular degeneration that is irreversible. For example, up to 50% of patients receiving long-term methotrexate for psoriasis develop hepatic fibrosis, which in some cases can progress to cirrhosis (Magee and Beeley, 1992). To reduce the risk of liver damage, methotrexate is usually given in small, once-weekly doses.

Vascular disorders

Budd-Chiari syndrome is characterized by obstruction of large hepatic veins, usually by a thrombus. The clinical presentation varies from a severe acute illness to a mild chronic form, with or without jaundice. Drugs known to induce this condition include oral contraceptives and cytotoxics.

Veno-occlusive disease can mimic Budd-Chiari syndrome, except that narrowing of the small centrilobular veins, rather than thrombosis, causes it. Offending drugs include cytotoxics and herbal remedies, such as comfrey, which contain pyrrolizidine alkaloids.

Hepatic tumours

The relationship between a drug and malignancy is difficult to prove because the reaction is delayed and large scale monitoring is required. However, there does appear to be a causal relationship between the use of oral contraceptives and anabolic steroids and the development of hepatic adenoma and carcinoma (Magee and Beeley, 1992). Danazol has been implicated as a cause of hepatocellular carcinoma.

Drug therapy in liver disease

The central role of the liver in drug metabolism poses obvious problems for drug therapy in patients with liver disease. Predicting which drugs to avoid is not easy as studies have shown that the rate of metabolism of individual drugs varies considerably in patients with chronic liver disease (Finlayson, 1994). Patients with liver disease should not be deprived of drug therapy because of excessive fear of side-effects, but instead care needs to be taken with prescribing (Table 7.8).

Table 7.8 Drug therapy in patients with liver disease

- Pain is best treated with paracetamol or codeine, either alone or in combination. Powerful analgesics should only be used under close supervision, and pethidine is preferable to morphine
- Aspirin and NSAIDs should be avoided in patients with oesophageal varices due to their erosive properties
- NSAIDs should also be avoided in patients with ascites as they reduce sodium excretion and so increase the ascites
- If sedatives are required, benzodiazepines with a short half-life should be used, e.g. temazepam, while the preferred anxiolytics are lorazepam and oxazepam
- Tricyclic drugs given in the minimum effective dose are best for depression
- Responsiveness to loop diuretics may be impaired and excessive potassium loss may occur
- ACE-inhibitors should be avoided as they can cause serious hypotension
- Care must be taken with antacids. Those that contain sodium may cause fluid retention, whilst those that contain aluminium and calcium may cause constipation, which predisposes to encephalopathy as there is greater opportunity for absorption of toxic substances from the gut
- Antibiotics which are known to be hepatotoxic should be avoided e.g. isoniazid, erythromycin, rifampicin, tetracyclines. Ketoconazole is contraindicated unless there is no alternative
- Combined oral contraceptives should be avoided, especially in cholestatic liver disease
- Chlorpropamide and tolbutamide are more likely to induce hypoglycaemia so their use must be carefully monitored
- Where blood flow through the liver is reduced, drugs that have a high first-pass metabolism should be given at reduced dosage or frequency, e.g. ß-blockers, clomethiazole (chlormethiazole), diltiazem, and verapamil

References and further reading

Anon (1997) Isoniazid-associated fatal hepatitis. Nurses Drug Alert 21(8): 8
Baxter JD (1992) The effects of glucocorticoid therapy. Hospital Practice 27(9): 111–34
Bone ME, Wilkinson DJ, Young JR, McNeil J, Charlton S (1990) Ginger root – a new antiemetic. The effect of ginger root on post-operative nausea and vomiting after major gynaecological surgery. Anaesthesia 45(8): 669-71
Budden L, Vink R (1996) Paracetamol overdose: pathophysiology and nursing management. British Journal of Nursing 5(3): 145-52
Cadman B (1996) Drug induced liver disease. The Hospital Pharmacist 3(2): 31-5
Callaghan TS, Hadden DR, Tompkin GH (1980) Megaloblastic anaemia due to vitamin B12 malabsorption associated with long-term metformin treatment. British Medical Journal 280: 1214-15
Cameron JC (1992) Constipation related to narcotic therapy. A protocol for nurses and patients. Cancer Nursing 15: 372-7
Campbell S (1995) Treating oral candidiasis. Community Nurse (Nurse Prescriber) 1:12-13
Davis JE (1991) A consideration not to be overlooked. Activated charcoal in acute drug overdoses. Professional Nurse 6: 710-14
Dossing M, Sonne J (1993) Drug-induced hepatic disorders. Incidence, management and avoidance. Drug Safety 96: 441-9
Everette SS (1995) GI distress: clues in the patient's medications. Gastroenterology Nursing 18: 219-23
Finlayson NDC (1994) Drugs and the liver. Medicine International 22: 455-9
Veyrat-Follet C, Farinotti R, Palmer JL (1997) Physiology of chemotherapy-induced emesis and antiemetic therapy. Predictive models for evaluation of new compounds. Drugs 53: 206-34
Gabriel SN (1997) NSAIDs: knowing the risks promotes safer use. The Journal of Musculoskeletal Medicine 14: 39-48
Goodman M (1997) Risk factors and antiemetic management of chemotherapy-induced nausea and vomiting. Oncology Nursing Forum 24: 20-33
Gough A, Chapman S, Wagstaff K, Emery P, Elias E (1996) Minocycline induced autoimmune hepatitis and systemic lupus erythematosus syndrome. British Medical Journal 312: 169-72
Hamilton G (1999) Insider trading. New Scientist 162: 43-6
Helfgott SM, Sandberg-Cook J, Zakim D, Nestler J (1990) Diclofenac-associated hepatotoxicity. Journal of the American Medical Association 264: 2660-2
Hirschowitz BI (1997) NSAIDs and the gut: understanding and preventing problems. The Journal of Musculoskeletal Medicine 14: 38-46
Jackson A (1995) Acupressure for post-operative nausea. Nursing Times 91: 58
Lee A, Morris J (1997) Adverse drug reactions (2). Drug-induced gastro-intestinal disorders. The Pharmaceutical Journal 258: 742-6
Lee WM (1995) Drug-induced hepatotoxicity. The New England Journal of Medicine 333: 1118-26
Magee P, Beeley L (1992) Drug-induced liver disease. The Pharmaceutical Journal 248:188-90
Mann A (1998) A continuing postoperative complication: nausea and vomiting – who is affected, why, and what are the contributing factors? A review. CRNA: The Clinical Forum for Nurse Anesthetists 9: 19-29

Mathias JM (1995) New anaesthetics have fewer side-effects. Operating Room Manager 11: 16-19

Nazarko L (1996) Preventing constipation in older people. Professional Nurse 11: 816-18

Needleman P, Isakson PC (1998) Selective inhibition of cyclooxygenase 2. Science and Medicine 5: 26-35

Reardon M, Holman R (1995) Are all NSAIDs the same? Geriatric Medicine 25: 47-50

Robinson B (1993) Be alert to an avoidable problem. Management and prevention of antibiotic-acquired diarrhoea. Professional Nurse 8: 510-12

Ross H (1998) Constipation: cause and control in an acute hospital setting. British Journal of Nursing 7: 907-13

Rowbotham D (1995) Recognising risk factors. Nursing Times 91: 44-6

Rowland MA (1989) When drug therapy causes diarrhoea. RN 52: 32-5

Samadian S (1990) Rectal necrosis due to phosphate enema. Care of the Elderly 2: 291

Seymour R (194) Identifying and treating ADRs of the mouth. Prescriber 5: 63-8

Smith AF, Vallance H, Slater RM (1997) Shorter preoperative fluid fasts reduce postoperative emesis. British Medical Journal 314: 1486

Tate S, Cook H (1996) Postoperative nausea and vomiting 2: management and treatment. British Journal of Nursing 5: 1032-9

Tortorice PV, O'Connell MB (1990) Management of chemotherapy-induced nausea and vomiting. Pharmacotherapy 10: 129-45

Walsh TD (1990) Prevention of opioid side effects. Journal of Pain and Symptom Management 5: 362-3

Ward FM, Daly MJ, Lee A (1997) Adverse drug reactions (3). Drug-induced hepatic disorders. The Pharmaceutical Journal 258: 863-7

Wickham R (1989) Managing chemotherapy-related nausea and vomiting: the state of the art. Oncology Nursing Forum 6: 563-74.

Wolfe MM (1996) NSAIDs and the gastrointestinal mucosa. Hospital Practice 31:37-48

Chapter 8
Renal effects

The kidneys play a major role in the formation of urine, excretion of waste products (including drugs), regulation of fluid, electrolyte and pH balance, maintenance of blood pressure, formation and release of renin and erythropoietin, and vitamin D synthesis. The role of the kidneys in maintaining health is so important that if drugs have detrimental effects on them the results can be far reaching. Unfortunately, the kidneys appear to be more sensitive to drug toxicity than most other organs of the body (Finley, 1992). The kidneys are particularly at risk of adverse effects because delivery of blood-borne toxic substances to the kidneys is high as they receive about 25% of the cardiac output. Furthermore, their functions include filtering, concentrating and eliminating toxins. As water is reabsorbed, the concentration of chemicals in the nephron can increase to toxic levels, and in some cases, the concentration may exceed the solubility of the chemical, resulting in precipitation of the chemical and obstruction of the affected area. As the medulla of the kidney is very hypertonic and is the site where drugs are concentrated, it is particularly at risk of sustaining damage from toxicity effects. Similarly, there are high drug concentrations in the tubular cells of the nephron caused by their uptake and active secretion of many drugs.

As well as excreting drugs, the kidney also metabolizes some drugs, using the cytochrome P450 enzyme system located in the proximal convoluted tubule. This explains why this region is particularly susceptibility to chemical injury by for example, chloroform and paracetamol, which are converted by the cytochrome P450 to toxic metabolites in the proximal tubule.

As indicated in Chapter 2 the kidney is important in excreting drugs that are not metabolized to an inactive state by the liver. Thus if kidney function is impaired, through old age or disease, then active drugs will accumulate, leading to toxicity effects throughout the whole body, including the kidney. Furthermore, in renal failure the rate of metabolism of drugs is often slower anyway due to the resulting inhibition of hepatic enzymes (Evans, 1980).

The incidence of drug-induced renal disease is uncertain, but Cove-Smith (1995) suggests that 5–20% of cases of acute renal failure can be directly attributed to drugs and chemicals, but minor damage may pass undetected. Chronic damage may occur insidiously and the role of drugs may not be recognized. Drugs can exert their adverse effects by interacting with kidney function, or alternatively by acting as nephrotoxins, and these will be looked at in turn. It should be noted that some drugs, in particular NSAIDs, affect the kidney through several different mechanisms (Table 8.1).

Fluid and electrolyte balance

The most obvious drugs to affect renal function are the diuretics; the most commonly used being the thiazides. These promote the excretion of sodium, chloride and water by inhibiting their re-absorption in the early part of the distal convoluted tubule. Consequently, when the increased sodium load is delivered to the distal tubule there is a corresponding increase in potassium excretion. Furthermore, the decrease in circulating blood volume – due to the fluid loss promoted by the diuretic – stimulates aldosterone production. This leads to

Table 8.1 Effects of NSAIDs on kidney function

NSAIDs have both acute and chronic effects:

1. They inhibit the formation of renal prostaglandins which help to maintain
    - Fluid and electrolyte homeostasis by:
        - Inhibiting tubular reabsorption of sodium and chloride
        - Inhibiting tubular responsiveness to antidiuretic hormone
    - Renin release
    - Renal blood flow by producing vasodilation of the afferent arteriole
2. They can stimulate a hypersensitivity reaction
3. They are cytotoxic

further potassium loss, and possible hypokalaemia (Mendyka, 1992). Hyperuricaemia can also occur because thiazide diuretics decrease tubular secretion of uric acid, which can precipitate gout in susceptible people. When serum uric acid becomes too high, uric acid can crystallize in the glomeruli causing renal damage.

Antihypertensive drugs work through a variety of different mechanisms, but all reduce peripheral resistance directly or indirectly. Reduction of blood pressure can decrease renal blood flow with a concomitant decrease in glomerular filtration rate due to the reduction of filtrate pressure. This can trigger sodium and water retention causing oedema and weight gain (Knox and Martof, 1995).

In recent years, oestrogen usage has increased in an attempt to prevent osteoporosis and alleviate the symptoms of the menopause. This hormone increases levels of renin, which results in the production of angiotensin II. This is a powerful vasoconstrictor and it also acts as a trigger for the release of aldosterone from the adrenal cortex, which in turn causes sodium and water retention, resulting in oedema.

Renal prostaglandins are important in helping to maintain fluid and electrolyte homeostasis by inhibiting tubular reabsorption of sodium and chloride ions, and by inhibiting tubular responsiveness to anti-diuretic hormone. When this function is blocked by NSAIDs, sodium and water retention can occur, leading to or exacerbating hypertension and heart failure. The inhibition of prostaglandin synthesis by NSAIDs also decreases secretion of potassium by limiting the amount of sodium delivered, and hence available for exchange, to the distal convoluted tubule. The resulting hyperkalaemia is made worse because renal prostaglandins are also involved in the release of renin. By blunting the activity of renin, NSAIDs lead to decreased aldosterone production, so contributing to the hyperkalaemia.

Nephrotoxicity

Drug-induced nephrotoxicity is a common clinical problem, and NSAIDs and angiotensin converting enzyme inhibitors are currently amongst the commonest causes of acute renal failure (Rang et al., 1995). A variety of drugs can cause nephrotoxicity (Table 8.2), but fortunately most drug-induced renal damage is reversible, provided action is taken to limit the damage. In order to examine the drugs

Table 8.2 Nephrotoxic drugs

- Aciclovir– parenteral
- Allopurinol
- Aminoglycosides, e.g. gentamicin
- Amphotericin B–parenteral
- Capreomycin
- Captopril
- Cisplatin
- Cyclosporin
- Demeclocycline
- Enalapril
- Gold compounds
- Interleukin-2
- Lithium
- Methotrexate–high doses
- Neomycin–oral
- NSAIDs
- Penicillamine
- Pentamidine
- Plicamycin
- Radiographic contrast media
- Rifampicin
- Streptozotocin
- Sulphonamides–systemic
- Tetracyclines (except doxycycline and minocycline)
- Vancomycin–parenteral

that cause nephrotoxicity it is necessary to have some insight into kidney function and disease. The functional part of the kidney is the nephron, which consists of two parts, the glomerulus and the tubule. Functionally the activity of the glomerulus is mainly determined by the integrity of its structure, and therefore adverse drug effects will result from interfering with that structure. Conversely, the activity of the renal tubule is mainly determined by the metabolic activity of its epithelial cells, and so adverse drug effects will result from interfering with metabolic activity. Both glomerular and tubular function are heavily dependent on adequate perfusion with blood, and if this is disrupted, both functions are impaired (Stevens and Lowe, 1995).

Damage to the kidney can result in partial or total renal failure. Partial renal failure may be classified as nephritic if there is a disturbance of glomerular structure that involves reactive cellular proliferation. This causes reduced glomerular blood flow. Consequently, there is reduced urine output, leakage of red blood cells from the damaged glomeruli leading to haematuria, and retention of waste products and uraemia. Conversely, if the glomerular basement membrane is damaged, the glomerulus loses its ability for selective retention of proteins in the blood. Consequently, large amounts of protein are lost in the urine, leading to hypoalbuminaemia and oedema. This is termed the nephrotic syndrome.

Total renal failure can be acute or chronic. The kidney may recover from acute renal failure if the damaging stimulus is removed, whilst chronic renal failure is irreversible as it is caused by permanent destruction of nephrons.

Disruption of blood flow

The blood flow to the nephron can be affected in several ways by drugs. At its simplest, there may be volume depletion secondary to excessive use of diuretics or laxatives. Moreover, this may precipitate acute renal failure. Patients who are especially at risk include the elderly, those with renal impairment, and those receiving other nephrotoxic agents.

The glomerular filtration rate is largely controlled by the relative tone of the afferent and efferent arterioles. In the afferent arterioles, tone is mainly mediated by vasodilatory prostaglandin, while in the efferent arteriole the renin-angiotensin-aldosterone system is mainly involved. Non-steroidal anti-inflammatory drugs inhibit prostaglandin synthesis. In the kidney prostaglandins, in particular PGE_2 and PGI_2, are vital for maintaining renal blood flow. PGE_2 is particularly important in bringing about compensatory vasodilatation of the blood vessels supplying the kidney in response to the general vasoconstriction brought about by noradrenaline (norepinephrine) and angiotensin II (Spilman and Whelton, 1992). Consequently, use of NSAIDs can result in vasoconstriction, leading to a decrease in renal blood flow, and therefore glomerular filtration rate (Knox and Martof, 1995). In severe cases, this can result in acute ischaemic renal failure (Rang et al., 1995).

ACE inhibitors prevent the conversion of angiotensin I to angiotensin II. Angiotensin II is a potent vasoconstrictor of the systemic and the renal vascular bed. Consequently, ACE inhibitors produce systemic and renal vasodilation, resulting in decreased blood pressure and increased renal blood flow. As renal vasodilation is mediated mainly by the efferent arteriole, filtration pressure is reduced by ACE inhibition. The lower filtration pressure does not automatically lead to a reduction in glomerular filtration rate, but this may occur in some situations. Patients at risk include those with renal artery stenosis, particularly those with bilateral stenoses, those with severe cardiac failure, and those receiving NSAIDs or diuretics.

The overall incidence of acute renal failure in patients taking ACE inhibitors is less than 1%. However, it increases to 25% in those with bilateral renal disease (Hems and Lee, 1997). It is therefore vital to monitor renal function regularly throughout treatment in these at risk groups.

Glomerulonephritis

Glomerulonephritis is used to describe those diseases in which the primary pathology is structural damage to the glomerulus. There are several forms of glomerulonephritis, including minimal change glomerulonephritis, membranous glomerulonephritis, and lupus nephritis. Drugs can cause these glomerular diseases by acting as antigens and stimulating antibody production. The drug antigens and antibodies combine to form immune complexes (see Chapter 5) and it is these that do the damage. Drug-induced glomerulonephritis may present as proteinuria, or if sufficiently severe, it may result in the nephrotic syndrome, with symptoms of hypoalbuminaemia, oedema, hyperlipidaemia and hypercoagulability.

In minimal change glomerulonephritis, light microscopy shows normal glomeruli – hence the name – but electron microscopy reveals that the epithelial cells are abnormal. It is most commonly observed with NSAIDs, especially in elderly patients, those with renal failure, and those on diuretics. Nephrotic syndrome develops after two weeks to two years of therapy, and usually disappears after drug withdrawal. Steroids may assist recovery, but progression to chronic renal failure may occur despite their administration.

In membranous glomerulopathy, the antigen-antibody complexes deposited in the kidney produce thickening of the capillary basement membrane. It is associated with drugs such as antiepileptics, captopril, gold, NSAIDs, penicillamine and probenecid. Genetic factors appear to be important in conferring susceptibility.

More than 50 drugs have been associated with lupus nephritis, a syndrome resembling the autoimmune disease systemic lupus erythematosus (SLE). The drugs most commonly implicated in lupus nephritis are hydralazine, isoniazid and procainamide (Hems and Lee, 1997). Symptoms include fever, arthralgia, pleurisy and pericarditis. The disease usually resolves when the drug is withdrawn.

Tubular toxicity

Renal tubular damage may be minor or major, and may affect the proximal or distal convoluted tubule. The clinical features of minor proximal tubular toxicity include microscopic haematuria, tubular epithelial cells in the urine and the presence of granular and cellular casts. The signs of moderate damage include aminoaciduria, glycosuria and hyperphosphaturia. The most severe damage is acute tubular necrosis, which is the most common cause of acute renal failure, accounting for 75–90% of cases (Douglas, 1992). Acute tubular necrosis is the commonest drug-induced renal disease, the most important causes of which are aminoglycosides, cisplatin, cyclosporin and radiographic contrast media (Hems and Lee, 1997). These drugs produce a direct toxic effect on the tubule resulting in necrosis of the tubular cells and non-oliguric acute renal failure.

The main group of drugs responsible for precipitating acute tubular necrosis is the aminoglycosides. The exact mechanism of their toxicity is unclear, but the lysosomes in the tubular cells become full of drug and phospholipids, until the lysosomes rupture releasing toxic enzymes and high concentrations of drug into the cell cytoplasm, disrupting its function. Between 6 and 26% of recipients of gentamicin, develop renal impairment within ten days of treatment (Hems and Lee, 1997). Development of renal failure is dependent on the dose and duration of the therapy as well as intravascular volume depletion, diuretic use, renal or hepatic disease, or concurrent use of other nephrotoxic drugs. Renal function usually recovers once the aminoglycoside is withdrawn, but may take several weeks. Dosing with aminoglycosides has altered recently, so that larger doses are now given less frequently. It is hoped that once daily dosing will lead to reduced tissue accumulation of the drug and hence to reduced toxicity.

One of the main causes of nephrotoxic damage to the distal tubule and the ascending loop of Henle is intravenous amphotericin. It is estimated to cause renal toxicity in 80–90% of patients receiving it, with an increased risk amongst the elderly, the volume-depleted and those at the higher end of the 0.25–1.0 mg/kg daily dose range (Miano-Mason, 1997). Renal injury from amphotericin therapy may result in fluid and electrolyte disturbances and acute tubular necrosis. Normally, the intrarenal regulatory mechanism monitors sodium concentration and reduces glomerular filtration to conserve sodium and to maintain volume. Amphotericin appears to activate this tubular glomerular feedback, leading to a functional reduction of glomerular filtration of around 40%. Amphotericin also directly induces tubular acidosis, calcification of the tubular lining and interstitium, and nephrogenic diabetes insipidus. Renal function may return to pre-treatment levels in some patients while irreversible damage may be expected with large doses (4–5 g) and when combined with other nephrotoxic drugs. Suggestions for minimizing the nephrotoxic effects of amphotericin are shown in figure Table 8.3. The use of a lipid formulation of amphotericin would appear to be particularly beneficial as studies suggest that this formulation reduces the risk of nephrotoxicity, with only 12–20% of patients experiencing some degree of nephrotoxicity (Rust and Jameson, 1998).

Table 8.3 Recommendations for minimizing the toxic effects of amphotericin (Miano-Mason, 1997)

- Keep patient well hydrated
- Promote potassium rich diet
- Sodium loading of 90 mEq each day of intravenous amphotericin
- Avoid use of other nephrotoxic drugs
- Supplementation with magnesium oxide may be necessary
- Decrease dose or discontinue therapy when serum creatinine levels exceed 3 mg/100 mL
- Use lipid-based formulation of amphotericin B

Renal tubular acidosis occurs when the tubule cells are damaged and unable to fulfil their function of reabsorbing bicarbonate from the filtrate. Consequently the bicarbonate ions are lost in the urine and are not available to buffer body fluids, leading to metabolic acidosis, and the clinical features shown in Table 8.4. The drugs that commonly cause nephrotoxic renal tubular acidosis are acetazolamide, amphotericin, antibiotics, cisplatin, lithium, paracetamol (in overdose) and radiographic contrast media. Effects can be reduced by aggressive hydration with concomitant mannitol infusion to maintain a urine flow rate of 100 mL per hour (Cooley et al., 1994). Drugs such as hydralazine, quinine and quinidine may also cause renal tubular acidosis indirectly by inducing intravascular haemolysis and

Table 8.4 Clinical features of complete renal tubular acidosis

- Hyperchloraemic metabolic acidosis (serum bicarbonate < 24 mmol/L and venous blood < 7.34)
- Persistently alkaline urine (pH > 6.0) in the absence of a urinary tract infection
- Hypokalaemia
- Increased urinary excretion of potassium and calcium

haemoglobinuria. Pigment nephropathy, as it is termed, should be suspected if a patient has severe oliguric renal failure, a hypercatabolic state and disproportionate anaemia, and the urine contains pigment casts.

Renal tubular acidosis, together with glycosuria, aminoaciduria and phosphaturia are all symptoms of Fanconi's syndrome. This is a disorder of proximal tubular transport that is usually inherited. However, the anticancer drug 6-mercaptopurine, and the degradation products of tetracycline (owing to prolonged storage) can cause proximal tubular defects resembling a reversible Fanconi's syndrome. A separate and important deleterious effect of tetracyclines on the kidney relates to their anti-anabolic action. A rise in blood urea occurs with their use, and in patients with stable established kidney disease there may be a rapid deterioration in renal function with severe uraemia. Furthermore, tetracyclines tend to produce nausea, vomiting and diarrhoea that may lead to dehydration and worsening of an already compromised renal function (Evans, 1980). Thus, tetracyclines are to be avoided in renal failure, except for doxycycline, which is exceptional in not producing this effect.

Crystal obstruction

Some drugs such as sulphonamides and methotrexate are relatively insoluble and may cause crystal formation in the distal convoluted tubules, pelvis and ureter. The risk of crystalluria is rare with the more modern sulphonamides, provided they are taken at the prescribed dose and with a good fluid intake. However, in high dose methotrexate regimes crystalluria is a serious problem, which can be minimized by ensuring good hydration prior to, during and after treatment, alkalization of the urine with bicarbonate, and administration of folinic acid until methotrexate levels reach non-toxic concentrations (Lydon, 1986).

Cytotoxic drugs and radiotherapy if used for the destruction of neoplastic tissue may lead to uric acid deposition in the renal tubules and the collecting system. Treatment of leukaemia in particular, can result in the development of fatal urate nephropathy if the breakdown of nucleic acids, released by the destruction of leukaemic cells, results in large amounts of insoluble urate entering the tubular fluid (Laurence et al., 1997). This can be avoided by starting the patient on allopurinol before treatment for the leukaemia is commenced. Allopurinol inhibits xanthine oxidase, which is the enzyme responsible for converting xanthines to uric acid. Because of the inhibition of the enzyme, the more soluble precursor hypoxanthine is excreted.

Nephrogenic diabetes insipidus

In nephrogenic diabetes insipidus, the renal tubules are partially or totally resistant to anti-diuretic hormone (ADH), resulting in polyuria and polydipsia. The main causative drug of this condition is lithium, with toxicity being more common at higher plasma lithium concentrations and with prolonged treatment. During treatment with lithium, there is a progressive decline in the patient's ability to concentrate urine. About 5–20% of patients are eventually unable to concentrate above the osmolarity of plasma. Treatment with desmopressin is useless, as the tubules are non-responsive, so the only option is to discontinue the drug. Symptoms generally resolve within three months of stopping the lithium, but there is usually some residual impairment of urine concentrating ability.

Demeclocycline also produces a reversible, dose-dependent nephrogenic diabetes insipidus, an effect which has been used therapeutically in the management of hyponatraemia secondary to inappropriate antidiuretic hormone secretion (Hems and Lee, 1997).

Interstitial nephritis

Acute interstitial nephritis, is a non-dose-related hypersensitivity reaction. It is characterized by tubular atrophy and renal scarring, in association with an inflammatory infiltrate, which results in an inability to concentrate urine, obligatory sodium wasting and reduced acid secretion. Rashes, arthropathies, altered liver function and circulating antibodies are also found. Acute renal failure normally occurs within two weeks of drug exposure. Most patients present with oliguria and up to 35% require haemodialysis (Hems and Lee, 1997). Spontaneous recovery usually occurs following the withdrawal of the nephrotoxin but this can take several months and there may be residual damage. Steroids may be used in an attempt to shorten recovery time. NSAIDs are the main cause of this type of renal damage, in particular, fenoprofen (Rang et al., 1995). Other drugs that also have this effect are the ß-lactams, in particular methicillin and ampicillin, as well as rifampicin, sulphonamides, captopril and allopurinol (deShazo and Kemp, 1997).

Analgesic nephropathy

Analgesic nephropathy is a chronic disease that is characterized by renal papillary and medullary necrosis accompanied by renal tubule atrophy. The degenerative and fibrotic changes may extend to the cortex of the kidney and produce glomerular damage and chronic interstitial nephritis, leading to severe irreversible chronic renal failure, with the signs and symptoms shown in Table 8.5. Analgesic nephropathy is associated with prolonged and massive abuse of analgesics, i.e. six or more tablets a day for several years. The syndrome is most commonly associated with proprietary combinations containing aspirin, paracetamol, and phenacetin, with caffeine or codeine (Nanra, 1986). The role of caffeine in these combinations is not clear as the pathogenesis of analgesic nephropathy is not fully understood. Phenacetin was the main culprit in the past and for this reason has been taken off the market and replaced by its active metabolite paracetamol. Stopping analgesic use generally results in stabilization or improvement of renal function, while continued use leads to progressive renal damage.

The prevalence of analgesic nephropathy varies widely throughout the world. Surveys have shown that the percentage of patients with end stage renal failure associated with analgesic abuse is as high as 36% in Belgium and as low as 0.07–0.4% in Britain (Hems and Lee, 1997). The withdrawal of over-the-counter sales of compound analgesics led to a significant reduction in the incidence of analgesic nephropathy in Australia, Sweden and Canada. Consequently, it has been suggested that compound analgesics should only be available

Table 8.5 Signs and symptoms of chronic renal failure

- Anaemia
- Breathlessness
- Drowsiness and tiredness
- Electrolyte imbalance, in particular elevated plasma creatinine, hyperkalaemia, hypocalcaemia
- Hypertension
- Malaise
- Muscle cramps
- Nausea and vomiting
- Oedema
- Paraesthesia
- Polyuria
- Pruritus
- Renal bone disease
- Restless legs syndrome

on prescription and that all NSAIDs and compound analgesics should be clearly labelled with a warning about the risk of nephrotoxicity.

Retroperitoneal fibrosis

Retroperitoneal fibrosis has been described in patients taking bromocriptine, ergotamine, hydralazine, methyldopa and methysergide. It is characterized by fibrosis over the posterior abdominal wall and retroperitoneum. The ureters may become embedded in the fibrous tissue resulting in an obstructive uropathy. Other structures may also be involved, including the inferior vena cava, aorta, the mediastinal structures and the liver. Symptoms of retroperitoneal fibrosis may include back, abdominal or flank pain, malaise, fatigue, weight loss and dysuria. Early recognition of the problem is important because substantial, if not complete, resolution will occur on stopping therapy, although corticosteroids or surgery may be required. Because of the hazards, continuous therapy with methysergide should not exceed six months without a drug-free period of at least a month.

Rhabdomyolysis

Rhabdomyolysis (see Chapter 12) is a condition in which acute muscle damage leads to the release of cell contents, including myoglobin, enzymes and electrolytes, into the circulation. This muscle damage can in turn cause renal failure. The exact mechanism by which the damage is caused is not clear, although, at a pH below 5.6, as is found in the tubules of the nephron, myoglobin is converted to ferrihaeme. This may act as a direct tubular cell toxin or it may precipitate and obstruct the tubules. Alternatively, myoglobin may produce intrarenal vasoconstriction and acute renal failure by scavenging vasodilatory nitric oxide.

Assessment and general management of nephrotoxicity

As the damage caused to the kidney by drugs is reversible, it is important that nurses recognize the changes associated with nephrotoxicity, so that action can be taken to limit damage. In order to identify the changes induced by nephrotoxins a full assessment needs to be carried out before commencing the drug, so that the induced changes will be recognized from the patient's normal baseline state. Table 8.6 identifies laboratory and clinical test results that could be indicative of nephrotoxicity.

Table 8.6 Test results that may be a sign of nephrotoxicity (Casperson et al., 1995; Skinner 1996)

Parameter	*Normal value*	*Changes associated with nephrotoxicity*
Blood		
BUN (blood urea nitrogen)	2.5–6.7 mmol/L	Increases
Calcium	2.2–2.67 mmol/L	Decreases
Creatinine	60–120 (mol/L	Increases
Magnesium	0.7–1.1 mmol/L	Decreases
Phosphate	0.8–1.5 mmol/L	Increases
Potassium	3.4–5.0 mmol/L	Increases
Sodium	135–145 mmol/L	Increases or varies
Urine		
Cytology	Absent	Casts, renal tubular cells, red blood cells
Creatinine clearance	75–125 mg/min	Decreases
Osmolarity	500–800 mosmol/kg	Decreases
pH	4.3–8	Increases or decreases
Protein	10–140 mg/L	Increases
Specific gravity	1.001–1.025	Decreases
Fluid balance		
Intake and output	Intake & output equal	Intake and output unequal
Weight	Stable	Increasing or decreasing
Skin turgor	Normal	Signs of dehydration or oedema

When renal dysfunction occurs, the patient's medication should be carefully reviewed. If the patient is receiving any nephrotoxic drugs that may be responsible for the damage, they should, where possible, be discontinued, and if drug therapy is still required, an alternative medication prescribed. This however is not always possible, if the drug is the only available therapy for a life threatening condition, e.g. amphotericin for aspergillus infection. Fortunately, most drug-induced renal damage is reversible. Efforts should be made to minimize further renal damage by keeping the patient well hydrated and avoiding other nephrotoxic drugs. If the patient is receiving any other drugs that are primarily eliminated through the kidneys, dose adjustments may be necessary.

Drug therapy in renal failure

Since most drugs, or their metabolites, are eliminated from the body by the kidneys, it is to be expected that when renal function declines drug excretion is impaired. In fact, the pharmokinetics of two-thirds of all drugs depends on renal function (Keller et al., 1995). If an alteration is not made to the dose of drug administered, the drug will accumulate leading to toxicity. This includes generally innocuous drugs such as penicillin, as well as many essential drugs such as digoxin. Thus, the glomerular filtration rate needs to be measured before planning a dosing regimen, and dosage size and the interval between doses need to be adjusted according to the degree of renal failure. Alternatively, another drug is used that has similar activity but whose elimination is not dependent on kidney function, and whose metabolites do not exert serious side-effects (Vree et al., 1983). Wherever possible nephrotoxic drugs should be avoided, and if this is not possible the patient must be carefully monitored, and serum drug levels monitored.

In the case of patients receiving dialysis, it is important to know to what degree drugs dialyse out of the blood. This will depend on the drug's molecular weight and whether it is small enough to cross the semi-permeable membrane used. It will also depend on plasma-protein binding and water solubility. Generally, weak or non-protein bound, water-soluble drugs dialyse out easily. However, uraemia decreases the binding of drugs to albumin and so increases their dialysability (Choi and Johnson, 1987). Examples of drugs that will be removed by dialysis in significant amounts include aminoglycosides, isoniazid, lithium, methyldopa, and phenytoin (Grahame-Smith and Aronson, 1992). Dose size and timing in relation to dialysis thus needs to be adjusted accordingly. Table 8.7 suggests some guiding principles for management of drug therapy in patients with renal failure.

Table 8.7 Principles of drug therapy in renal failure

- Restrict drug administration in renal failure to absolute essentials
- Utilize pharmokinetic data to plan dosage regime
- Monitor plasma concentration of drug wherever possible. Drug response is individual despite recommended dosing schedules. The best time to measure plasma concentrations is just before the next dose
- Avoid nephrotoxic drugs
- Avoid catabolic agents (e.g. steroids, tetracyclines) which may aggravate uraemic state

As well as an alteration in drug pharmokinetics in renal failure, the actions of some drugs may be altered. Thus, the brain is more sensitive to the central nervous system depressant effects of tranquillizers, sedatives, and opiates. However, renal failure has to be quite advanced for this. Patients with renal failure have reduced cholinesterase activity and consequently are more sensitive to acetylcholinesterase inhibitors such as neostigmine, which is used in treatment of myasthenia gravis, paralytic ileus, post-operative urinary retention and to reverse muscle relaxants. The control of body fluids is disturbed in renal failure, and if patients become hypovolaemic, they become more sensitive to hypotensive agents, particularly α-adrenoceptor antagonists such as prazosin and ACE inhibitors such as captopril. Antibiotics used to treat urinary tract infections may fail because they are unable to achieve therapeutic urinary concentration. Nitrofurantoin and nalidixic acid should never be used in renal failure, as they are poorly excreted and prone to cause toxicity (Evans, 1980). Patients with uraemia have an increased tendency to bleed so the effect of anticoagulants is enhanced, and aspirin and NSAIDs are more liable to produce gastric bleeding. Drugs that cause sodium retention, e.g. NSAIDs, may produce fluid overload, oedema, and heart failure. It must be borne in mind that many drugs are presented as their sodium and potassium salts. Thus large doses of penicillin and carbenicillin contain substantial amounts of sodium, and even magnesium trisilicate mixture contains 10 mmol sodium bicarbonate in each 10 mL (Evans, 1980). Renal failure frequently results in hyperkalaemia, and this may be made worse by potassium sparing diuretics, potassium supplements and ACE inhibitors.

References and further reading

Bartucci MR (1994) Cyclosporin A nephrotoxicity. ANNA Journal 21: 162-3

Casperson DS, Zumsteg M, Mahon SM (1995) Focus on oncology: nephrotoxicity of chemotherapeutic agents for genitourinary cancers. Journal of Urological Nursing 14: 1110-19

Choi L, Johnson CA (1987) Dialyzability of drugs. Dialysis and Transplantation 16: 537-40

Cooley ME, Davis L, Abrahm J (1994) Cisplatin: a clinical review. Part II—Nursing assessment and management of side effects of cisplatin. Cancer Nursing 17: 283-93

Cove-Smith R (1995) Drugs and the kidney. Medicine 23: 165-71

de Shazo RD, Kemp SF (1997) Allergic reactions to drugs and biologic agents. Journal of the American Medical Association 278: 1895-906

Douglas S (1992) Acute tubular necrosis: diagnosis, treatment, and nursing implications. AACN Clinical Issues 3: 688-97

Evans DB (1980) Drugs and the kidney. British Journal of Hospital Medicine 24: 244-51

Finley RS (1992) Drug interactions in the oncology patient. Seminars in Oncology Nursing 8: 95-101

Hems S, Lee A (1997) Drug-induced renal disorders. The Pharmaceutical Journal 259: 214-19

Grahame-Smith DG, Aronson JK (1992). Oxford Textbook of Clinical Pharmacology and Drug Therapy 2nd edn. Oxford: Oxford University Press. Chapter 26.

Keller RF, Giehl M, Frankswitsch T, Zellner D (1995) Pharmokinetics and drug dosage adjustment to renal impairment. Nephrology, Dialysis and Transplantation 10: 1516-20

Knox DM, Martof MT (1995) Effects of drug therapy on renal function of healthy older adults. Journal of Gerontological Nursing 21: 35-40

Laurence DR, Bennett PN, Brown MJ (1997) Clinical Pharmacology. 8th edn. Edinburgh: Churchill Livingstone

Lydon J (1986) Nephrotoxicity of cancer treatment. Oncology Nursing Forum 13: 68-77

Mendyka BE (1992) fluid and electrolyte disorders caused by diuretic therapy. AACN Clinical Issues 3: 672-80

Miano-Mason T (1997) Mechanisms and management of amphotericin B-induced nephrotoxicity. Cancer Practice 5: 176-81

Nanra RS (1986) Drug-induced renal disease. Medicine International 2: 1366-76

Rang HP, Dale MM, Ritter JM (1995). Pharmacology 3rd edn. Edinburgh: Churchill Livingstone

Rust DM, Jameson G (1998) The novel lipid delivery system of amphotericin B: drug profile and relevance to clinical practice. Oncology Nurses Forum 25: 35-48

Skinner S (1996) Understanding Clinical Investigations: A Quick Reference Manual. London: Bailliere Tindall

Spilman P, Whelton A (1992) Nonsteroidal antiinflammatory drugs: effects on kidney function and implications for nursing care. ANNA Journal 19: 19-26

Stevens A, Lowe J (1995) Pathology. London: Mosby. p318-19

Vree TB, Hekster CA, Van Dalen R (1983) Some consequences of drug choice and dosage regimen for patients with impaired kidney function. Drug Intelligence and Clinical Pharmacy 17: 267-3

Chapter 9
Cardiovascular and respiratory effects

Cardiovascular disorders

Drugs, including extracardiac drugs, can have a variety of adverse effects on the cardiovascular system (Table 9.1). They can affect heart rhythm and function, cause heart failure and interfere with the regulation of blood pressure and blood flow (Ferner, 1994). Unfortunately, physicians often fail to consider that these adverse effects are drug-induced, but rather ascribe them to underlying disease (Kirch, 1995). Factors predisposing to cardiovascular toxicity include heart disease, electrolyte imbalance and poor renal function.

Table 9.1 Examples of drugs having adverse effects on the cardiovascular system

Disorder	*Associated drugs*
Disturbances of heart rhythm	Cisapride, digoxin, pentamidine, phenothiazines, terfenadine, tricyclic antidepressants
Heart failure	Antacids with a high sodium content, ß-blockers, calcium antagonists, doxorubicin, NSAIDs
Hypertension	Clonidine, corticosteroids, erythropoietin, ketoconazole, MAOIs, naloxone, oestrogens
Hypotension	α-blockers, ACE inhibitors, calcium antagonists
Myocardial infarction	Androgens, cocaine, ergotamine, thyroxine
Peripheral vasoconstriction	ß-blockers, ergotamine, methysergide
Valve lesions	Methysergide

Disturbances of heart rhythm

Digoxin is the obvious example of a drug that causes disturbances of heart rhythm, mainly due to its narrow therapeutic index. Digoxin can cause virtually any cardiac arrhythmia, but the commonest are those that include extra ventricular and supraventricular beats. Atrial-ventricular nodal conduction may be impaired leading to heart block. The combination of ectopic arrhythmias and heart block is indicative of glycoside toxicity. Digoxin can slow the conduction of atrial impulses so effectively as to render the patient dangerously bradycardic. This is the rationale for taking the patient's pulse before giving cardiac glycosides, and for omitting the dose if the pulse is less than 60 beats per minute. Digoxin should be used cautiously in patients with impaired renal function because it will accumulate, and as it has a narrow therapeutic window, it can rapidly lead to toxicity. The adverse effects of cardiac glycosides are enhanced by electrolyte disturbances, especially hypokalaemia, hypercalcaemia, and hypomagnesaemia. Care must be exercised when using cardiac glycosides with acetazolamide, amphotericin, β_2-agonists, corticosteroids, diuretics, and itraconazole as they lower plasma potassium levels, which sensitizes the myocardium to the action of digoxin (Lucas, 1999). Hypoxia, acidosis, hypothyroidism, and old age also increase adverse effects. Studies suggest that when hospitalized patients are treated with digoxin, between 6 and 23% develop toxicity, and of them up to 41% die (Li-Saw-Hee and Lip, 1998). Management of digoxin toxicity depends on its recognition, followed by drug withdrawal, correction of electrolyte imbalance, and treatment of life-threatening dysrhythmias with lidocaine (lignocaine) or phenytoin. In life-threatening cases, antibody fragments to digoxin (Digiband) have been shown to be effective in clearing the drug (Smith, 1991).

As well as digoxin, many other drugs can cause cardiac arrhythmias (Table 9.1). All antiarrhythmic drugs, e.g. sotalol, quinidine, disopyramide, may exacerbate pre-existing arrhythmias. They may also cause new ones, and these drugs have been estimated to cause between 5 and 10% of arrhythmias in patients (MacLean and Lee, 1999). Patients prescribed anti-arrhythmics should be carefully selected and monitored, and their doses increased slowly. Amiodarone appears to have a low arrhythmia profile, i.e. less than 3%.

Serious ventricular arrhythmias are occasionally found with other drugs including halofantrine, phenothiazines, pimozide, and tricyclic antidepressants. Overdose with tricyclics is an important cause of atrial fibrillation and cardiac arrest in young people. The non-sedating antihistamines, terfenadine and astemizole can prolong the QT-interval, as can the antiemetic cisapride, and so predispose the patient to potentially fatal ventricular arrhythmias. Both terfenadine and cisapride cause arrhythmias in overdose or when other drugs, such as imidazole antifungals, protease inhibitors, and macrolide antibiotics, inhibit their metabolism. These drugs should thus not be taken with preparations that prolong the QT interval or which inhibit metabolism, and for this reason terfenadine was returned to prescription-only status in 1997.

Heart failure

Cardiac failure occurs when the heart is unable to pump enough blood around the body to meet metabolic needs, leading to dyspnoea, oedema, tachycardia, and confusion. Several drugs can lead to heart failure, directly or indirectly. The cytotoxic drug doxorubicin can damage heart muscle directly and irreversibly. The effect is dependent on life-time dose so that 3% of patients who have a lifetime dose of 400 mg per square metre or less will develop overt heart failure, compared with 20% of those who have a total dose of 700 mg per square metre (Ferner, 1994). Similarly thyroid hormones, as well as causing arrhythmias, can provoke heart muscle wasting and increase the demand on the heart, thus precipitating failure.

More commonly heart failure occurs as a result of increasing cardiac pre-load, i.e. volume overload, as is illustrated by the precipitation of heart failure in the elderly on commencement of NSAIDs and corticosteroids. Both groups of drugs cause salt and water retention, and an increase in blood volume. This can result simply in swollen ankles, but may also cause life-threatening congestive cardiac failure in patients with unstable cardiac homeostasis (Feenstra et al., 1997). Liquorice and its now obsolete derivative carbenoxolone (used to treat stomach ulcers) will sometimes lead to water retention because of their mineralocorticoid effect.

ß-blockers or calcium antagonists are also common causes of heart failure. ß-blockers antagonize the effects of sympathetic agents on myocardial contractility and rate. This can be beneficial because it decreases myocardial oxygen requirements, but it can also lead to heart failure. Calcium entry into cells is necessary for the heart muscle to contract; it is also necessary for electrical conduction between cells. Calcium antagonists, particularly verapamil, can affect this process and cause heart failure and conduction deficits.

Table 9.2 Complications of hypertension

Organ	*Disease*
Blood vessels	Atherosclerosis and aneurysm formation
Brain	Microaneurysms, intracerebral haemorrhage
Eyes	Retinopathy, blindness
Heart	Left ventricular hypertrophy and failure, angina pectoris, cardiac arrhythmias, myocardial infarction
Kidneys	Ischaemic cortical damage, renal failure
Lungs	Pulmonary oedema due to left ventricular failure
Lung, colon, kidney, etc.	? cancer (see Hamet, 1996)

The other two categories of calcium antagonists, represented by nifedipine and diltiazem, have a much more marked effect on calcium entry into vascular smooth muscle than cardiac muscle, and so may be preferable for patients who are at risk of heart failure or heart block.

If cardiac failure is believed to be drug-induced the drug should be discontinued and the condition managed with a change in lifestyle, together with ACE inhibitors and diuretics. Over-the-counter medicines should be discouraged, particularly those antacids and effervescent preparations with a high sodium content and NSAIDs.

Hypertension

Primary or essential hypertension accounts for 90% of cases of raised blood pressure. However, drug-induced hypertension must be borne in mind as a possible cause of secondary disease. Sympathomimetic drugs such as adrenaline (epinephrine), noradrenaline (norepinephrine), dobutamine and dopamine can all cause systemic hypertension. Perhaps less obvious causes are the immunosuppressive drug cyclosporin, due to increased vascular resistance and impaired sodium excretion, and erythropoietin, due to increased red blood cell production and viscosity (MacLean and Lee, 1999). Any drug that causes water retention, e.g. corticosteroids, carbenoxolone, and NSAIDs, may also lead to an increase in blood pressure.

The antihypertensive clonidine is now rarely used because of the severe rebound hypertension that followed its abrupt withdrawal. This occurs because the number of inhibitory α_2-adrenoceptors decreases during treatment with clonidine. The hypertensive crisis that can follow clonidine withdrawal is severe enough to cause stroke, intracranial haemorrhage and death.

Another group of drugs that can precipitate a hypertensive crisis are the monoamine oxidase inhibitor (MAOI) antidepressants. This can occur when the patient takes the drug with foods rich in tyramine, e.g. mature cheese, pickled herrings, red wine, game, and yeast extracts. The MAOIs directly inhibit first-pass metabolism of the tyramine in the food and therefore increased concentrations of tyramine reach the systemic circulation and the sympathetic nervous system. The tyramine stimulates the release of intraneural noradrenaline (norepinephrine) causing sympathetic over-activity with severe hypertension, hyperpyrexia, excitement, delirium, and possible death. Not only do MAOIs interact with foodstuffs they also interact with other drugs, namely sympathomimetics such as dopamine agonists, amphetamines, ephedrine, and phenylpropanolamine. Several of these drugs are available in over-the-counter remedies, so patients must receive extensive education about the food and drugs that they must avoid, and they should carry a drug-warning card. It is interesting to note that the adverse effect between moclobemide (an MAO-A selective inhibitor) plus controlled amounts of Bovril (a tyramine-rich yeast extract) has been used successfully to treat a patient with central autonomic failure (Karet et al., 1994).

Hypotension

The screening and treatment of hypertension is important as it can decrease the incidence of a variety of serious complications, including those identified in Table 9.2. However, the treatment of hypertension can produce its own problems as antihypertensives, especially if given inappropriately, can cause postural hypotension. This is a serious side-effect, especially in the case of the elderly who are more at risk of falls and their consequences. It is thus imperative that screening for hypertension should involve accurate blood pressure measurement. Furthermore, the British Hypertension Society recommends that in older patients with isolated systolic hypertension, but no target organ damage, measurements should be made over 3–6 months (Sever et al., 1993). In addition, blood pressure should be measured in both the sitting and standing position. This is because there is frequently a drop of 20 mmHg in standing blood pressure in patients with a sitting pressure of 160 mmHg. Standing blood pressure measurements should be used to guide treatment decisions. If standing blood pressure is not used, there is a danger that the postural hypotension will be made worse. The British Hypertension Society recommends treatment thresholds of 160 mmHg systolic, or 90 mmHg diastolic, or both, for elderly patients of 60–80 years (Sever et al., 1993). However, not all elderly hypertensives should be treated. Account must be taken of the patient's overall medical condition. It may be better not to prescribe anti-hypertensive medication for the very sick or medically complicated (Medicines Resource Centre, 1993).

The hypotension resulting from the first dose of an antihypertensive can be severe enough to cause a stroke or a myocardial infarction (Ferner, 1994). This is particularly true for prazosin and the ACE inhibitors. In the latter case, severe first-dose hypotension occurs more commonly in patients who have high renin level. As diuretics raise renin levels, they should be stopped 24–48 hours before starting ACE inhibitors.

Myocardial infarction

Drugs can result in myocardial infarction through several processes. Firstly, sudden cessation of treatment with a ß-blocker can expose the heart to increased sympathetic stimulation, partly because chronic receptor antagonism leads to a compensatory increase in the number of ß-receptors. It can therefore precipitate angina or an infarction. A sudden increase in heart rate and metabolic needs can also precipitate angina or infarction if patients with hypothyroidism are commenced on too high a dose of thyroxine.

Recent research, which is still being hotly debated, suggests that calcium channel-blockers may increase the risk of myocardial infarction in a dose-dependent fashion (Psaty et al., 1995). This is supported by the finding that there is a greater risk of myocardial infarction and death following the use of short-acting nifedipine in patients with a history of angina, myocardial infarction and hypertension (Pahor et al., 1995). Dougall and McLay (1996) in their review of calcium channel blockers suggest that until further research has confirmed or refuted the results of these two studies, it would be prudent to limit the use of all short-acting calcium antagonists as first-line treatment in 'at risk' individuals.

Calcium channel blockers may also precipitate coronary artery spasm, if they are withdrawn suddenly. Some drugs can cause coronary vasospasm more directly. This is true of the anti-migraine drug ergotamine, which is potentially dangerous in patients with angina or ischaemic heart disease. Ergotamine can also cause generalized vasospasm, which leads to a corresponding increase in total peripheral resistance and strain on the heart. Abuse of cocaine, including 'crack', is known to induce myocardial infarction, and coronary artery spasm is one of the mechanisms proposed to explain the problem (Amin et al., 1991). The other two are increased myocardial oxygen demand in the presence of a fixed coronary stenosis and increased thrombogenesis.

Atherogenic drugs may also precipitate myocardial infarction. The aromatic retinoids, such as isotretinoin, used in the treatment of severe skin disease, are powerful inducers of hyperlipidaemia. They elevate plasma triglycerides in 25% of patients, possibly by a factor of ten in rare cases, as well as decreasing high-density lipoproteins in 16% and elevating cholesterol in 7% (Laudano et al., 1990; Swan and Ford 1997). Body builders who abuse anabolic steroids are also at risk of premature myocardial infarction (Council on Scientific Affairs, 1990). Although the mechanism by which androgenic anabolic steroids cause this effect is open to debate, one explanation is that these drugs alter lipoprotein concentrations in favour of atherogenesis (Melchert and Welder, 1995).

Another drug for which there is considerable debate regarding its ability to cause myocardial infarction is oestrogen. Grahame-Smith and Aronson (1992) suggest that oestrogens cause a sixfold increase in risk from myocardial infarction because of their effect on coagulation and development of thromboembolism. Conversely, Ferner (1994) suggests that the increased risk from oestrogens and related compounds like diethylstilbestrol (stilboestrol) is due to their atherogenic potential. Rang et al. (1995) however, suggest that the consensus is that low doses of oestrogen do not increase the risk of cardiovascular disease in women who have no pre-existing disease. Furthermore, they suggest that oestrogens reduce the risk of cardiovascular disease by protecting the arterial walls against atheromatous change, whilst pills containing the newer progestogens increase the levels of high-density lipoproteins which also have a protective effect. However, a study by Lidegaard (1993) concluded that oral contraceptives are associated with an increased risk of cerebral thromboembolic attack, although the risk decreases with lower oestrogen and progestogen doses and is not demonstrable with progestogen only pills.

Rang et al. (1995) also suggest that unopposed oestrogen (i.e. with no accompanying progestogen) reverses the postmenopausal 'atherogenic' lipid profile and is epidemiologically associated with a 45% reduction in the risk of ischaemic heart disease. This reduction may be partially reversed by the addition of progestogens to the HRT regime, which is necessary for women with an intact uterus (Lichtman, 1991).

Peripheral vasoconstriction

ß-blockers such as propranolol can antagonize the β_2-receptors which mediate dilation of peripheral vessels, leading to vasoconstriction. The anti-migraine drugs methysergide and ergotamine, and possibly bromocriptine may also produce vasoconstriction in susceptible individuals and in overdose. This should be borne in mind when assessing patients with leg ulcers, as the vasoconstriction can contribute to failure of these wounds to heal. Alternative drug therapy should therefore be considered.

Valve lesions

Methysergide, an antagonist at 5-HT_2 serotonin receptors, is occasionally used for migraine prophylaxis but more commonly for treating the symptoms of carcinoid tumours. A serious adverse effect of prolonged methysergide usage is abnormal fibrosis, which includes fibrosis of the tricuspid valves.

Haematological adverse effects

Adverse effects on the cells of the haemopoietic system represent some of the most serious and common adverse drug effects (Firkin, 1995). All components of the blood can be affected adversely by drugs, as Table 9.3 indicates. The main effects are either to inhibit haemopoiesis of one or more cell lines, which is referred to as blood dyscrasia, or to interfere with coagulation, either stimulating or inhibiting it. Hypersensitivity reactions (see Chapter 5) are responsible for many of these adverse effects, as are direct toxic effects.

Table 9.3 Examples of drugs having adverse effects on the blood

Disorder	*Associated drugs*
Agranulocytosis	Carbamazepine, carbimazole, chlorpromazine, clozapine, co-trimoxazole, dapsone, metronidazole, mianserin, NSAIDs, sulphonamides, sulphonylureas
Aplastic anaemia	Carbamazepine, carbimazole, chloramphenicol, chlorpromazine, diclofenac, gold, sulindac, tolbutamide
Deficiency anaemia	Antiepileptics, metformin, NSAIDs
Haemolytic anaemia	Dapsone, methyldopa, penicillins, quinine and quinidine, rifampicin, sulphonamides
Haemorrhage	Antifibrinolytics, heparin, warfarin
Megaloblastic anaemia	Methotrexate, nitrous oxide
Methaemoglobinaemia	Chloroquine, phenacetin, prilocaine-lidocaine (lignocaine) cream (EMLA), sulphonamides
Thrombocytopenia	Digoxin, gold, heparin, oestrogens, quinidine, rifampicin, sulphonamides, thiazide diuretics
Thrombosis	Oestrogen-containing oral contraceptives, diethylstilbestrol (stilboestrol)

Neutropenia and agranulocytosis

Drugs can cause a reduction in total white cell count (leucopenia) but selective reduction in granulocytes, which include neutrophils, eosinophils, and basophils, is more common. Neutropenia refers to a decrease in circulating neutrophils, whilst agranulocytosis refers to a severe decrease in the number of granulocytes, resulting in a neutrophil count of less than $0.5 \times 10^9/L$. Most cytotoxic agents and antimetabolites used to treat cancer and immunologically mediated disorders are capable of interfering with neutrophil formation in the bone marrow, leading to neutropenia, and this adverse effect is frequently the dose limiting factor for these drugs. Recovery of neutrophil counts usually begins within a few days or a week after withdrawal of the drug, but it can be delayed significantly with oral alkylating agents such as chlorambucil.

Agranulocytosis usually occurs as an idiosyncratic reaction. It can be quite common, affecting 1 in 400 patients taking antithyroid drugs such as carbimazole, for example (Firkin, 1995). Other high-risk drugs are sulfasalazine (sulphasalazine), high dose co-trimoxazole, clozapine, dapsone, and ticlopidine. The onset of idiosyncratic agranulocytosis is usually delayed, appearing 2–12 weeks after starting treatment. However, it can be quite sudden and usually presents with severe sore throat or mouth ulcers. Patients should be advised to report such events immediately and to stop taking the drug. However, they must not be frightened into non-compliance with important drug therapy. The use of regular blood counts to monitor for dyscrasia, is open to debate. In the case of cytotoxic drugs where there is a dose-dependent inhibition of marrow function, serial blood counts clearly have a role to play. They are of less value in idiosyncratic reactions since the blood dyscrasia can occur suddenly. In addition, the cost of blood tests can be prohibitive (Pokalo, 1991).

Management of idiosyncratic agranulocytosis is prompt drug withdrawal, which normally results in restoration of normal neutrophil count within a few weeks. Corticosteroid and haemopoietic growth factor therapy have been used, but their value is uncertain (Firkin, 1995). The essential factor for enhancing survival is rapid treatment of any infection with appropriate antibiotics. In some cases, recovery of neutrophil count is absent or incomplete, leaving the patient vulnerable to infection.

Anaemia

Drug-induced anaemia can result from a deficiency of metabolites required for the manufacture of red blood cells, injury to the erythrocyte precursor in the bone marrow, or damage to the red cell itself.

Deficiency anaemias are a common secondary consequence of drug administration. The most common is iron-deficiency anaemia caused by bleeding from the upper gastro-intestinal tract and precipitated by aspirin and other NSAIDs. Phenytoin and other antiepileptics can impair folate absorption, while metformin can impair vitamin B_{12} absorption.

Injury to the red cell precursor may occur with methotrexate. This cytotoxic drug is utilized for its ability to interfere with the intracellular folate metabolism within malignant cells. However, it can also affect red blood precursor cells, leading to megaloblastic anaemia. Megaloblastic anaemia, together with leucopenia, may also occur in patients exposed to nitrous oxide. This anaesthetic was believed for a long time to be free of any serious toxic effects, but it has now been shown to cause significant metabolic abnormalities due to its ability to oxidize and degrade enzyme-bound vitamin B_{12}. With a single dose of the anaesthetic adverse effects are not detected due to the bone marrow's reserve of erythrocytes. However, patients receiving the drug repeatedly or those receiving prolonged administration, as in the case of patients having cardiac surgery, may develop adverse effects (Schumann, 1990).

Erythrocyte injury presents as haemolytic anaemia, which is characterized by reduced red cell survival in the blood. This can be due to intrinsic defects in the red cells resulting in abnormal erythrocyte fragility, for example a deficiency of the enzyme glucose-6-phosphate dehydrogenase (see Chapter 5), or to an extrinsic defect such as autoimmune or mechanical trauma to cells. Autoimmune haemolytic anaemia is an example of a type II hypersensitivity reaction. It can occur with many drugs, but it is most commonly reported with sulphonamides and related drugs, and with the antihypertensive methyldopa. In the case of methyldopa significant haemolysis occurs in less than 1% of patients, but the appearance of antibodies directed against the surface of red blood cell is detected, by the Coombes test, in 15–20% of treated individuals (Rang et al., 1995).

Chloramphenicol, given systemically, is an example of a drug that leads to anaemia through both a direct and indirect effect. Firstly, there is a dose-related reversible depression in the proliferation of bone marrow cells when the antibiotic is administered in the maximum recommended dose of 4 g/day in the treatment of meningitis, or in lower doses in patients with impaired hepatic function. This occurs through the same mechanism by which chloramphenicol inhibits bacterial protein synthesis. There is also inhibition of incorporation of iron into haem. Secondly, a hypersensitivity reaction may result in aplastic anaemia, neutropenia, agranulocytosis, or thrombocytopenia. This adverse effect is uncommon, occurring in between 1 in 20000 and 1 in 400000, but carries a high mortality (Grahame-Smith and Aronson, 1992). Blood tests should therefore be carried out regularly on patients taking chloramphenicol and courses of treatment should not last more than 1 or 2 weeks.

Aplastic anaemia is a condition in which there is suppression of red and white cells together with platelets, and is due to hypoplasia of the bone marrow. It is characterized by symptoms of anaemia, infection and bleeding. The onset of drug-induced aplastic anaemia can be acute or more commonly chronic. It can be difficult to prove a causal association, particularly as there may be a significant delay between exposure to the drug and development of the reaction. The reaction can occur months after the drug has been stopped. Since the use of systemic chloramphenicol has declined, NSAIDs as a therapeutic group are the most frequent cause of drug-induced aplastic anaemia (McMurray and Lee, 1998). Due to its association with aplastic anaemia, phenylbutazone is restricted to hospital use in the treatment of ankylosing spondylitis unresponsive to other treatment.

Methaemoglobinaemia

Methaemoglobinaemia is a rare cause of cyanosis, which may be congenital or induced by certain chemicals, including drugs. Methaemoglobin is an abnormal haemoglobin in which the iron molecule is oxidized to the ferric state (Fe^{3+}) rather than the normal ferrous state (Fe^{2+}). Because of this extra positive charge, the molecule is unable to bind oxygen, leading to cyanosis. Under normal conditions, the enzyme systems in the red blood cell maintain equilibrium between haemoglobin and methaemoglobin. However, this delicate balance can be upset by a variety of drugs, as indicated in Table 9.3, as well as by silver nitrate used in the treatment of burns (Strauch et al., 1969) and prilocaine-lidocaine (lignocaine) cream (EMLA) which is used to reduce the pain of venepuncture in children. Frayling et al. (1990) studied the effects of EMLA on 48 children and found that although peak methaemoglobin concentrations were well within safe limits, there were still increased blood concentrations after 24 hours. This suggests that cumulative effects may occur in children receiving the cream daily and illustrates the need to give drugs at their minimum effective dose.

Methaemoglobinaemia should be suspected when cyanosis fails to respond to oxygen, the partial pressure of oxygen is normal or elevated in the presence of decreased oxygen saturation, and blood is dark brown in colour and remains so despite aeration (Pow, 1997). In mild cases of chemically induced methaemoglobinaemia no treatment may be necessary, but if methaemoglobinaemia is greater than 30% intravenous methylthioninium chloride (methylene blue) is given at 1–2 mg per kg over 5 minutes. Other treatments include blood transfusion or exchange transfusions, and hyperbaric oxygen, which can maintain life during preparation for exchange transfusions.

Thrombocytopenia

Reduction in platelet numbers, with subsequent increased risk of haemorrhage, occurs commonly with most cytotoxic agents and antimetabolites as they interfere with the formation of platelets by megakaryocytes in the bone marrow. Intravenous heparin, in doses used to treat thromboembolism, is also associated with a high incidence of thrombocytopenia. In 30% of patients there is a transitory decrease in platelet numbers within 24–36 hours of commencing treatment (Rang et al., 1995). This effect is due to a direct aggregatory effect of heparin on platelets, and is normally of little clinical significance. A more serious thrombocytopenia occurs 2–14 days after starting heparin and is rarer. This second reaction is mediated by an immune mechanism that causes platelet activation and aggregation. The activated platelets have themselves got potent aggregating activity and may initiate thrombus formation and disseminated intravascular coagulation, as well as thrombocytopenia. The risk depends on the duration of heparin therapy; it appears to be more common with bovine than porcine heparin and less common with lower-molecular weight heparin molecules (Kessler, 1991). Thrombosis is a serious sequel in some of these patients and can occur after re-exposure to relatively small amounts of heparin in patients with heparin antibodies, including low-dose heparin and low molecular weight heparin.

Type II hypersensitivity reactions and pseudo-allergic reactions may lead to thrombocytopenia after exposure to any of a large number of drugs, as indicated in Table 9.3. Management strategies for thrombocytopenia include discontinuation of the culprit drug, adrenal steroids in the case of hypersensitivity reactions, blood or platelet transfusions if haemorrhage occurs, and discontinuation of any drugs which precipitate gastro-intestinal bleeding.

Clotting changes

Inhibition of the clotting cascade increases the risk of haemorrhage and is the main side-effect of anticoagulants. Many drugs interact with the oral anticoagulants and increase their effects, as indicated in Table 9.4. There is a need to avoid interacting drugs in patients on warfarin and regularly to measure the patient's degree of anticoagulation, assessed as the international normalized ratio (INR). If haemorrhage occurs as a side-effect of oral anticoagulant therapy, treatment involves withholding the anticoagulant, and the administration of vitamin K, or fresh plasma, or coagulation factor concentrates. (It must also be remembered that some drugs, e.g. aminoglutethimide, barbiturates, carbamazepine, colestyramine (cholestyramine), oral contraceptives, phenytoin, rifampicin, vitamin K, can interact with warfarin to decrease the INR, and this could result in thrombus formation (Adams, 1998)).

Table 9.4 Examples of drugs that interact with oral anticoagulants to increase their effect

Mechanism	*Examples of drugs*
Inhibition of microsomal liver enzymes, leading to decreased metabolism of anticoagulant	Antifungals, cimetidine, co-trimoxazole, imipramine, metronidazole, sulfinpyrazone, tamoxifen
Impairment of platelet aggregation and function	Aspirin, carbenicillin, fibrates, NSAIDs, ticlopidine
Displacement of anticoagulant from its binding site on plasma albumin	Chloral hydrate, NSAIDs
Inhibition of reduction of vitamin K and hence formation of clotting proteins	Cephalosporins, disulfiram, quinidine

The main side-effect of injectable anticoagulants is also haemorrhage, which is treated by stopping therapy and giving a heparin antagonist, e.g. protamine sulphate. The other group of drugs which inhibits clotting and so can potentiate haemorrhage are the fibrinolytic agents which include streptokinase, anistreplase, urokinase and alteplase. Treatment consists of withdrawal of the drug, tranexamic acid and if necessary fresh plasma or coagulation factors.

The converse of haemorrhage is thrombus formation, which occurs as a result of damage to the blood vessel wall, changes in blood flow, and increased blood coagulability. Oestrogen-containing oral contraceptive therapy may lead to thrombosis by increasing blood coagulability, as it leads to an increase in the concentration of prothrombin and fibrinogen in the blood (Stevens and Lowe, 1995). Franklin (1990) suggests that the risk of deep vein thrombosis is four times greater for those on oral contraceptives, whilst a study by Petitti et al. (1996) could not find a correlation between the occurrence of strokes and use of low-oestrogen oral contraceptives. In the case of hormone replacement therapy with oestrogen, it is usually argued that thrombus formation is not a problem as the association with thromboembolic disorders is based on studies of synthetic oestrogens used in oral contraceptives (Scharbo-Dehaan, 1996). However, a study by Jick et al. (1996) found that the risk of venous thromboembolism was three times higher amongst users of post-menopausal oestrogen replacement than among non-users.

Respiratory disorders

A study of adverse drug effects leading to hospitalization found that 3% involved the respiratory system, and of those conditions considered life threatening, 12% were respiratory (Belton and Lee, 1997). Table 9.5 identifies examples of drugs that may have adverse effects on the respiratory system. It is not only drugs however, that can have adverse effects, but also other chemicals used by health care professionals. For example, chlorhexidine and alcohol aerosols have been associated with asthma (Waclawski et al., 1989) as has the vapour given off by rubber gloves (Seaton et al., 1988).

Upper respiratory tree

Drugs having adverse effects on the upper respiratory tree usually produce a cough, nasal congestion or rhinitis. The ACE-inhibitors, which are widely used to treat hypertension and heart failure, are associated with a cough. This adverse effect occurs in between 5% and 20% of patients taking the drug (Belton and Lee, 1997). The cough is typically dry, persistent and non-productive, and it can be quite debilitating leading to loss of sleep, sore throat and vomiting. ACE-inhibitors should generally be discontinued in patients to whom the cough becomes troublesome, and an angiotensin-II receptor antagonist such as losartan considered instead.

Table 9.5 Examples of drugs having adverse effects on the respiratory system

Disorder	*Associated drugs*
Alveolitis (interstitial pneumonitis)	Amiodarone, gold, methotrexate, nitrofurantoin, penicillamine, sulfasalazine (sulphasalazine)
Asthma	ß-blockers, ß-lactam antibiotics, cholinergic agonists, cholinesterase inhibitors, iodinated contrast media, muscle relaxants, NSAIDs, propafenone,
Cough	ACE inhibitors
Nasal congestion	Antihypertensives, e.g. methyldopa, propranolol, antidepressants, e.g. amitriptyline, oral contraceptives
Organizing pneumonia	Amiodarone, bleomycin, mitomycin, cyclophosphamide, penicillamine, sulindac
Pulmonary fibrosis	Bleomycin, busulfan (busulphan), cyclophosphamide, gold, nitrofurantoin
Pulmonary oedema	Amphotericin, aspirin (in overdose), cytosine arabinoside, opiates (in overdose), haloperidol, IV ß-agonists, streptokinase
Pulmonary thromboembolism	Oral contraceptive
Respiratory depression	Narcotic analgesics, barbiturates, H_1-histamine receptor antagonists
Rhinitis	Anticholinesterases, levodopa, reserpine

Nasal congestion and rhinitis are caused by a variety of drugs, as Table 9.5 indicates. The commonest cause of nasal congestion is the topical use of nasal decongestants that contain ephedrine and xylometazoline, and which are available in over-the-counter cold remedies. When the patient stops taking the decongestant, even after only a few days of use, rebound congestion occurs. The patient consequently takes more decongestant and a cycle of decongestant use and rebound congestion is set up. It is speculated that rebound congestion occurs due to down-regulation of the α-adrenoceptors or is due to damage to the nasal mucosa. Prevention is by avoiding decongestants, or taking them for no more than seven days at a time.

Asthma

Occasionally drugs will unmask occult asthma, or more commonly will cause exacerbation of established disease. Some drugs produce bronchoconstriction by virtue of their pharmacological effects. β_2-adrenoceptors are found on bronchial smooth muscle and if stimulated cause bronchodilation. Consequently, drugs that have antagonistic effects on β_2-adrenoceptors will cause bronchoconstriction, e.g. ß-blockers such as propranolol, and the anti-arrhythmic agent propafenone. Blaiss (1991) suggests that agents such as atenolol, that are cardioselective, i.e. have mainly β_1 activity, should be used to treat patients with obstructive lung disease when required. However, Higgins (1994) maintains that patients with significant respiratory disease should not be given ß-blockers, even in the form of eye drops, as deaths have occurred when this advice has been ignored.

Opposing the sympathetic system is the parasympathetic, which works via muscarinic receptors. Thus cholinergic or muscarinic agonists such as pilocarpine will cause the contraction of bronchial smooth muscle and lead to bronchoconstriction, as will cholinesterase inhibitors such as ecothiopate, which prevent the breakdown of acetylcholine.

Drug-induced airway obstruction may also occur as an idiosyncratic effect. Antibiotics, in particular penicillins and cephalosporins, can act as antigens and trigger allergic bronchospasm, together with pruritus, urticaria and angio-oedema. It has been estimated that antibiotics account for bronchospasm and severe dyspnoea once in every 1000–10000 treatment courses (Belton and Lee, 1997). As well as causing anaphylactic reactions, some drugs such as the muscle relaxants and iodinated contrast media, can directly stimulate the release of histamine from mast cells, resulting in an anaphylactoid reaction (see Chapter 5).

Aspirin and the NSAIDs are another common cause of bronchoconstriction, and it is estimated that aspirin sensitivity affects between 10% and 30% of asthmatics (Lee, 1993). In sensitive individuals, acute bronchospasm is accompanied by conjunctival irritation, rhinorrhoea, urticaria, and flushing of the face, usually within minutes or hours of ingesting the medication. The suggested mechanism is that the NSAID inhibits cyclooxygenase leading to an imbalance between prostaglandin and leukotriene synthesis. It is important that patients who exhibit signs of a hypersensitivity reaction to aspirin and NSAIDs are advised to avoid them, including in the form of cold remedies. They should use paracetamol and opioid analgesics instead. The majority of patients with aspirin sensitivity may be desensitized to aspirin by oral administration of increasing doses of aspirin (Lee, 1993).

Paradoxical bronchoconstriction can occur with a number of inhaled drugs, including ß-agonists, corticosteroids, ipratropium and sodium cromoglycate. The response probably results from a non-specific irritation of the bronchial smooth muscle. In recent years, this has become less of a problem as nebulizer solutions have been changed to make them isotonic, rather than hypotonic, and to free them of preservatives such as benzalkonium. However, the hydrofluorocarbon propellants used in metered dose inhalers have been implicated in bronchospasm, especially in the slower acting bronchodilators such as salmeterol. Faster acting bronchodilators may attenuate any bronchoconstriction that occurs.

Alveolitis and pulmonary fibrosis

Alveolitis (also termed interstitial pneumonitis) and pulmonary fibrosis are two ends of the spectrum of related, but poorly understood, disease states. They are the result of hypersensitivity reactions, and direct toxicity, with the latter being more commonly associated with fibrosis. The symptoms of alveolitis usually occur within hours or weeks of starting the therapy, and include breathlessness, coughing and wheezing. Chest X-ray will often reveal pulmonary infiltrates and a blood test will show eosinophilia. Withdrawal of the drug and corticosteroid therapy usually results in symptom resolution.

Fibrotic disease is usually the result of direct toxicity leading to inflammatory response and destruction of the alveoli. Symptoms are malaise, a dry cough and breathlessness, which becomes progressively worse with continued use of the drug. Unfortunately, withdrawal of the drug does not always result in resolution of the disease.

Organizing pneumonia

Despite the name, cryptogenic organizing pneumonia has been associated with the drugs listed in Table 9.5. This uncommon condition is a non-infective pneumonia characterized by breathlessness, sometimes fever, and consolidation on the chest X-ray. Patients usually recover with steroid therapy.

Pulmonary oedema

Non-cardiogenic pulmonary oedema is the result of increased vascular permeability, leading to extravasation of fluid and proteinaceous material in the alveoli. The symptoms include breathlessness, cough and frothy sputum. The reaction can occur at therapeutic doses with drugs like amphotericin, hydrochlorothiazide, and intravenous salbutamol or in overdose with drugs like aspirin, dihydrocodeine, and tricyclic antidepressants.

Pulmonary oedema is particularly a problem when intravenous ß-agonists are used to suppress uterine contractions in premature labour, with an incidence of 4% (Belton and Lee, 1997). Most cases occur during drug administration, or in the following 24 hours, and respond well to intravenous furosemide (frusemide) and oxygen therapy.

Pulmonary thromboembolism

A pulmonary thromboembolism occurs when a thrombus in the deep veins breaks free and moves through the circulatory system until it becomes caught in the narrowing pulmonary blood vessels. It is a serious condition characterized by sudden collapse, chest pain, breathlessness, cyanosis and haemoptysis. The drug usually associated with this problem is the combined oral contraceptive pill (COC). Until recently the causative agent was thought to be the oestrogen in the pill, but it is now suggested that the type of progestogen given also has an effect on risk, with the third generation progestogens, gestodene and desogestrel being the main culprits. The risk of non-fatal venous thromboembolism is estimated to be 5–11 per 100000 women per year in non-COC users compared with 30 for preparations containing gestodene and desogestrel (MacLean and Lee, 1999). These progestogens should therefore not be used on patients with a risk of developing deep vein thrombosis, e.g. those with obesity or varicose veins. Gestodene and desogestrel should be reserved for patients who cannot tolerate the older progestogens.

Respiratory depression

Many drugs, which have a depressant action on the central nervous system, cause some degree of respiratory depression, but usually only in overdose. They include barbiturates, H_1-histamine receptor antagonists, some antidepressants and alcohol. However, the narcotic analgesics such as morphine, cause some degree of depression even in therapeutic doses. As respiratory depression can be fatal, it is important to monitor the respiratory rates of patients receiving high doses of narcotics, for example post-operatively through a patient-controlled analgesic system, and to have the antidote naloxone available.

References and further reading

Adams P (1998) Drug interactions that matter (2) Warfarin. The Pharmaceutical Journal 261: 704-8

Amin M, Gabelman G, Buttrick P (1991) Cocaine-induced myocardial infarction. Postgraduate Medicine 90: 50-5

Belton KJ, Lee A (1997) Adverse drug reactions. (5) Drug-induced respiratory disorders. The Pharmaceutical Journal 259: 413-17

Blaiss MS (1991) Drug-induced pulmonary reactions in children. Respiratory Management 27: 10-14

Council on Scientific Affairs (1990) Medical and nonmedical uses of anabolic steroids. Journal of the American Medical Association 264: 2923-7

Dougall HT, McLay J (1996) A comparative review of the adverse effects of calcium antagonists. Drug Safety 15: 91-106

Feenstra J, Grobbee DE, Mosterd A, Stricker B (1997) Adverse cardiovascular effects of NSAIDs in patients with congestive heart failure. Drug Safety 17: 166-80.

Ferner R (1994) Which drugs can cause cardiovascular problems? Prescriber 5: 51-4

Firkin FC (1995) Haematological side-effects of drugs. Medicine 23: 534-6

Franklin M (1990) Reassessment of the metabolic effects of oral contraceptives. Journal of Nurse-Midwifery 35: 358-64

Frayling IM, Addison GM, Chattergee K, Meakin G (1990) Methaemoglobinaemia in children treated with prilocaine-lidocaine (lignocaine) cream. British Medical Journal 301: 153-4

Grahame-Smith DG, Aronson JK (1992). Oxford Textbook of Clinical Pharmacology and Drug Therapy 2nd edn. Oxford: Oxford University Press

Hamet P (1996) Cancer and hypertension. Hypertension 28: 321-324

Higgins B (1994) Which drugs can cause respiratory side effects? Prescriber 5: 80-6

Jick H, Derby L, Myers MW, Vasilakis C, Newton K (1996) Risk of hospital admission for idiopathic venous thromboembolism among users of postmenopausal oestrogens. Lancet 348: 981-3

Karet FE, Dickerson C, Brown J, Brown MJ (1994) Bovril and moclobemide: a novel therapeutic strategy for central autonomic failure. Lancet 344: 1263-5

Kessler CM (1991) The pharmacology of aspirin, heparin, coumarin, and thrombolytic agents. Implications for therapeutic use in cardiopulmonary disease. Chest Supplement 99: 97-112S

Kirch W (1995) Hemodynamic effects of extracardiac drugs. International Journal of Clinical Pharmacology and Therapeutics 33: 190-3

Laudano JB, Leach EE, Armstrong RB (1990) Acne: therapeutic perspective with an emphasis on the role of isotretinoin, Dermatology Nursing 2: 328-37

Lee T (1993) Mechanism of bronchospasm in aspirin-sensitive asthma. American Review of Respiratory Disease 148: 1442-3

Lichtman R (1991) Perimenopausal hormone replacement therapy. Review of the literature. Journal of Nurse-Midwifery 36: 30-48

Lidegaard O (1993) Oral contraception and risk of cerebral thromboembolic attack: results of a case-control study. British Medical Journal 306: 956-63

Li-Saw-Hee FL, Lip GYH (1998) How safe is digoxin? Adverse Drug Reaction Bulletin 188: 715-8

Lucas H (1999) Drug interactions that matter (6) Antiarrhythmics. The Pharmaceutical Journal 262: 28-31

MacLean F, Lee A (1999) Adverse drug reactions. (11) Drug-induced cardiovascular disorders. The Pharmaceutical Journal 262: 113-18

McMurray M, Lee A (1998)) Adverse drug reactions. (9) Drug-induced blood disorders. The Pharmaceutical Journal 261: 414-18

Medicines Resource Centre (1993) The treatment of hypertension in the elderly. Medicines Resource Centre Bulletin 4: 33-4

Melchert RB, Welder AA (1995) Cardiovascular effects of androgenic-anabolic steroids. Medicine and Science in Sports and Exercise 27: 1252-62

Pahor M, Guralnick JM, Corti M, Foley DJ, Carbonin P, Havlik RJ (1995) Long-term survival and use of antihypertensive medications in older persons. Journal American Geriatric Society 43: 1191-7

Petitti D, Sidney S, Bernstein A, Wolf S, Queensberry C, Zeil H (1996) Stroke in users of low-dose oral contraceptives. The New England Journal of Medicine 335: 8-15

Psaty BM, Heckbert SR, Koepsell TD, Siscovick DS, Raghunathan TE, Weiss NS, Rosendaal FR, Lemaitre RN, Smith NL, Wahl PW, Wagner EH, Furberg CD (1995) The risk of myocardial infarction associated with antihypertensive therapies. Journal of the American Medical Association 274: 620-5

Pokalo CL (1991) Clozapine. Benefits and controversies. Journal of Psychosocial Nursing 29: 33-6

Pow J (1997) Methaemoglobinaemia: an unusual blue boy. Paediatric Nursing 9: 24-5

Rang HP, Dale MM, Ritter JM (1995) Pharmacology 3rd edn. Edinburgh: Churchill Livingstone

Scharbo-Dehaan M (1996) Hormone replacement therapy. The Nurse Practitioner 21: 1-15

Schumann D (1990) Nitrous oxide anaesthesia: risks to health personnel. International Nurse Review 37: 214-17

Seaton A, Cherrie B, Turnbull J (1988) Rubber glove asthma. British Medical Journal 296: 531-2

Sever P, Beevers G, Bulpitt C, Lever A, Ramsay L, Reid J, Swales J (1993) Management guidelines in essential hypertension: report of the second working party of the British Hypertension Society. British Medical Journal 306: 983-7

Smith TW (1991) Review of clinical experience with digoxin immune Fab(ovine). American Journal of Emergency Medicine 9: 1-6

Stevens A, Lowe J (1995) Pathology. London: Mosby. p318-9

Strauch B, Buch W, Grey W, Laub D (1969) Successful treatment of methemoglobinemia secondary to silver nitrate therapy. The New England Journal of Medicine 281: 257-8

Swan DK, Ford B (1997) Chemoprevention of cancer: review of the literature. Oncology Nursing Forum 24: 719-27

Waclawski ER, McAlpine LG, Thomson NC (1989) Occupational asthma in nurses caused by chlorhexidine and alcohol aerosols. British Medical Journal 298: 929-30

Chapter 10
Neurological, sensory and endocrine effects

Neurological

Many drugs have the potential to cause adverse neurological effects (Table 10.1), and in 1997, 18% of reactions reported to the Committee on Safety of Medicines were of this type (Thomson and Lee, 1998).

Table 10.1 Examples of drugs having adverse effects on the central nervous system

Disorder	*Associated drugs*
Akathisia	Antipsychotics
Aseptic meningitis	Azathioprine, immunoglobulins, isoniazid, NSAIDs, penicillins
Benign intracranial hypertension	Corticosteroids, danazol, nalidixic acid, nitrous oxide, oral tetracyclines, vitamin A
Choreoathetosis	Amphetamines, anabolic steroids, antiepileptics, antipsychotic drugs, combination oral contraceptive, L-dopa
Coma	Alcohol, antidepressants, antipsychotics, benzodiazepines, cyclosporin, insulin, opioids, tacrolimus
Convulsions	Baclofen, cyclosporin, isoniazid, lithium, propofol, vaccines, vincristine
Guillain-Barré syndrome	Captopril, corticosteroids, gold, oxytocin, penicillamine, streptokinase, vaccines
Headache	Calcium channel antagonists, compound analgesics, nitrates, hydralazine, indometacin (indomethacin)
Neuromuscular junction disorders	Aminoglycosides, ß-blockers, lithium, penicillamine, phenytoin
Peripheral neuropathy	Alcohol, isoniazid, vinca alkaloids, zidovudine
Parkinsonism	Metoclopramide, phenothiazines
Sleep disorders	Alcohol, analgesics, antiepileptics, antidepressants, antihistamines, antihypertensives, antiemetics
Tardive dyskinesia	Withdrawal from long-term use of antipsychotics, withdrawal from prochlorperazine, metoclopramide; anticholinergics, antihistamines
Tremor	Antiepileptics, benzodiazepines, caffeine, lithium

Headache

Although only about 3% of headaches are drug-induced, this diagnosis should always be considered when investigating this common symptom. Analgesic rebound headaches in particular need to be considered. They occur when patients suffering with headaches overuse analgesics, i.e. take them for more than four days a week. As a result, and through an unknown mechanism, the patient suffers with a chronic headache, leading to dependency on analgesics. If the patient can be persuaded to stop the analgesic, the headache initially gets worse and then resolves. The problem appears more common with compound analgesics and so patients should always be recommended to take simple analgesics, i.e. aspirin and paracetamol, and to avoid mixtures and opioids.

The drugs that are usually associated with causing headaches are the vasodilators such as calcium channel antagonists, nitrates and hydralazine. Stretching of the pain-sensitive cerebral blood vessel walls precipitates these vascular headaches. Anti-inflammatory drugs such as indometacin (indomethacin) may also precipitate a vascular headache.

Ibuprofen and other NSAIDs have occasionally been reported as causing aseptic meningitis. The problem occurs most frequently in patients with systemic lupus erythematosus and other connective tissue diseases. Patients develop the classic signs of meningitis, but an infective cause cannot be found, and the symptoms resolve when the drug is withdrawn. Patients who have previously suffered this disorder should be advised to avoid over-the-counter medications containing ibuprofen. Aseptic meningitis has also been described following therapy with azathioprine, immunoglobulins, isoniazid and penicillins.

A variety of drugs (Table 10.1) can cause benign intracranial hypertension, with its associated symptoms of headache, papilloedema, visual disturbances, nausea, vomiting, and tinnitus. The symptoms result from increased intracranial pressure possibly due to salt and water retention, and usually develop within days or months of commencing treatment. Although not life threatening, optic nerve damage and loss of vision can occur. The diagnosis is confirmed by measuring cerebrospinal fluid pressures, and treatment requires discontinuation of the drug. Symptoms usually resolve, although in some cases there may be permanent visual loss.

Sleep

Sleep is a vital biological process that is made up of 90-minute cycles of REM (rapid eye movement) sleep when dreaming occurs, and non-REM sleep. Non-REM sleep consists of four progressively deeper stages of sleep with stages 3 and 4 being known as deep or slow wave sleep (SWS). The first sleep cycle of the night may contain only two or three minutes of REM sleep and it is followed by the deepest sleep of the night. Later in the night, the REM periods are longer, lasting up to 45 minutes, and the non-REM periods are mostly stage 2 sleep. It is suggested that REM sleep is essential for restoration of the brain whilst non-REM sleep is important for growth and repair of the body, including wound healing (Adam and Oswald, 1983). More recently it has been suggested that the alternating bouts of REM and non-REM sleep are involved with learning and memory (Phillips, 1999).

A number of drugs can affect sleep architecture and are a common cause of daytime drowsiness and other sleep-related problems (Table 10.2), although in some cases, e.g. schizophrenia and Parkinson's disease, it can be difficult to know whether the drug treatment or disease is causing the problems. Highly lipophilic drugs, e.g. benzodiazepines and first generation antihistamines, which easily cross the blood-brain barrier and those that act on cholinergic, dopaminergic and histaminergic receptors in the central, rather than the peripheral, nervous system are most likely to cause daytime drowsiness. This can be a serious problem for someone who works with machinery or drives a vehicle. People are not allowed to drive under the effects of alcohol, but the law does not prevent them from driving under the effects of drugs, which can affect their coordination, judgement and response times more than alcohol. Hindmarsh (Anon, 1999) asked volunteers on driving simulators to hit the brakes whenever a brake light flashed, and found that antidepressants delayed reaction times by 120 milliseconds – twice that expected from drinking the legal limit of alcohol. Furthermore, the patients did not realize that they were impaired. Thus, patients should be very clearly warned if prescribed any drug that might cause daytime drowsiness. They should also be prescribed the minimal dose necessary to control their symptoms, in order to keep the sedative effect to a minimum.

Table 10.2 Drugs that have an adverse effect on sleep (Dietrich, 1997; Novak and Shapiro 1997; Cender et al., 1998)

Disorder	*Associated drugs*
Insomnia	Amphetamines, ß-agonists, clonidine, corticosteroids, hypnotics, SSRIs, thyroxine
Nightmares (occur particularly when REM sleep is increased)	ACE-inhibitors, ß-blockers, clonidine, corticosteroids, levodopa, tricyclics, MAOIs
Sedation	α-agonist, α-antagonists, ß-blockers, amitriptyline, opioid analgesics, phenothiazines, vitamin A overdose
Sleepwalking (occurs particularly when slow wave sleep is increased)	Amitriptyline, lithium, thioridazine
Decreased slow wave sleep	Aspirin, corticosteroids, fluoxetine
Sleep apnoea	Alcohol, anabolic steroids, benzodiazepines, opioids

When considering which drugs are causing a patient to be drowsy during the day it is important to ask about over-the-counter remedies that the patient may be taking, as well as herbal remedies. Many herbs, e.g. almonds, camomile, fennel, ginseng, marjoram, melissa, orange blossom and valerian are traditionally thought to be sedatives (Idzikowski and Shapiro, 1993). Because they are freely available and 'natural', they are often thought to be safe and healthy, and may be taken in substantial quantities.

It is not only drugs which cause sedation that can result in fatigue and daytime drowsiness. This problem can also occur with drugs that affect sleep quantity and quality, e.g. levodopa and high dose dexamethasone, which can cause vivid nightmares, and theophylline which may cause insomnia. Also sudden withdrawal of drugs, e.g. opioids, phenobarbital (phenobarbitone), antihypertensives, can lead to restless sleep, insomnia and nightmares for weeks afterwards, so they should be withdrawn slowly using tapering doses. The longer the patient has been on the drug the longer the withdrawal period. In the case of the benzodiazepines, rebound insomnia may be more evident with shorter-acting agents, e.g. oxazepam, temazepam, triazolam, while daytime sedation is more common with longer-acting agents, e.g. diazepam. In some cases, the insomnia caused by the drug or its withdrawal may need to be treated in turn by night sedation (Turner and Elson, 1993).

Medications that cause a decrease in slow wave sleep such as the antiepileptic ethosuximide should be used with care in young children. Decreased slow wave sleep can affect the amount of growth hormone produced and possibly stunt somatic growth (Lee and Stotts, 1990).

Convulsions

Drugs can precipitate convulsions, especially in patients with epilepsy. Firstly, this may be because of rapid, or inappropriate, withdrawal of antiepileptics and consequently withdrawal should be gradual. Withdrawal syndromes associated with other drugs, such as alcohol, barbiturates and benzodiazepines, have also been implicated in causing fits in non-epileptic patients. Secondly, fits may occur as a result of lowering blood levels of antiepileptics through drug interactions. Thus, the concomitant use of drugs such as alcohol, barbiturates, and carbamazepine, in an epileptic controlled with phenytoin, may increase the metabolism of the antiepileptic, resulting in convulsions.

Thirdly, fits can be a side-effect of drug use. Antihistamines, cimetidine, lidocaine (lignocaine), phenothiazines, theophylline and tricyclic antidepressants can all cause fits, usually through drug overdose (Burns and Schultz, 1993). Convulsions have occurred in both epileptic and non-epileptic patients taking quinolones at therapeutic doses. Rarely, isolated cases of neurological toxicity or convulsions have been described with ciprofloxacin taken together with theophylline or an NSAID, and consequently the combination of theophylline and quinolone should be avoided (Thomson and Lee, 1998). It has been shown that quinolones competitively inhibit the binding of the inhibitory neurotransmitter GABA to its receptor. As GABA binding is involved in preventing fits, this may account for their epileptogenic effect.

Coma and encephalopathy

Most cases of drug-induced coma are caused by overdoses of drugs used therapeutically for their effects on the central nervous system. These include benzodiazepines, antipsychotics, antidepressants and opioids. Alcohol may have an additive or synergistic effect with these drugs, and will increase central nervous system depression (Ferner,

1998). Altered metabolism or elimination of the active drug may cause drug accumulation and so contribute to the neurotoxicity.

Cyclosporin has been reported to cause coma as well as other neurological adverse effects including convulsions, encephalopathy and movement disorders. The mechanism is unknown. Coma and convulsions have also been reported with the immunosuppressant tacrolimus. A number of cytotoxic drugs including cisplatin and high dose methotrexate may cause direct toxicity resulting in convulsions and encephalopathy. Also, severe and prolonged hypoglycaemia may cause coma, so drugs which can precipitate hypoglycaemia, such as alcohol, insulin, sulphonylureas, high dose salicylates, pentamidine and quinine, may cause convulsions, coma and permanent brain damage.

Neuropathies

Drugs can have toxic effects on the cranial nerves or the peripheral nerves. The symptoms of cranial nerve toxicity depend on which of the twelve are affected, and the effects of drugs on the eye (cranial nerves II and III) and the ear (cranial nerve VIII) are addressed later in the Chapter.

Peripheral neuropathy can result in a number of features depending on the type of nerve damaged, i.e. sensory, motor or autonomic. Risk factors for drug-induced neuropathy include alcoholism, diabetes mellitus, vitamin deficiency, and impaired renal and hepatic function leading to accumulation of the active drug. Table 10.1 indicates some of the drugs commonly associated with peripheral neuropathy. Where possible drugs suspected of causing neuropathy should be withdrawn, although the effect is not always reversible. However, early withdrawal improves the prognosis.

Occasionally Guillain-Barré syndrome (GBS) may be drug-induced. This is a rare immune-mediated disorder in which the myelin of peripheral nerves is damaged, leading to severe peripheral nerve dysfunction. The syndrome usually starts with paraesthesia of the fingers and toes followed by upper and lower limb, and finally body weakness. These symptoms may develop within days of starting the drug or up to a year later. Drugs associated with this syndrome include captopril, hepatitis B, influenza and MMR vaccine, penicillamine and streptokinase. Zimeldine, a serotonin reuptake inhibitor was withdrawn in 1983 after 200000 prescriptions had been dispensed and 10 cases of GBS reported (Thomson and Lee, 1998).

Neuromuscular junction disorders

Some drugs (Table 10.1) can affect the nervous transmission from a motor neurone to its skeletal muscle cell, and so can produce what is termed drug-induced myasthenic syndrome. This particularly occurs post-operatively, when drugs such as aminoglycosides, clindamycin and tetracyclines, which are used during the operation, prevent the re-establishment of spontaneous respiration, and cause a myasthenic crisis. Symptoms include generalized weakness and paralysis of respiratory muscles, and treatment consists of assisted ventilation and the use of anticholinesterase drugs such as neostigmine.

Myasthenia gravis is an autoimmune disease in which antibodies to acetylcholine receptors prevent transmission of impulses at neuromuscular junctions, leading to muscle weakness, ptosis, dysphagia, dysphonia, dyspnoea and respiratory failure. Some drugs, such as high dose corticosteroids, aminoglycosides, anticholinergics, neuromuscular blocking agents, phenytoin and quinine can worsen existing disease. Consequently, myasthenic patients should avoid these drugs, and the small amount of quinine in tonic water. A variant of the disease occurs in patients with rheumatoid arthritis and Wilson's disease when given penicillamine (Wittbrodt, 1997). Nearly all these patients have receptor antibodies, but the disease remits within a year of discontinuing the penicillamine.

Drug-induced myasthenic syndrome is uncommon, and is associated with aminoglycosides, ß-blockers and phenytoin. It is distinguished from true myasthenia gravis by the absence of antibodies and remits promptly on drug withdrawal.

Movement disorders

A variety of movement disorders (Table 10.3) can be the result of drug usage. The drugs most commonly implicated in movement disorders are the antipsychotics and metoclopramide, as well as antidepressants, including tricyclics and selective serotonin re-uptake inhibitors, antiepileptics, anti-parkinsonism drugs and lithium. High potency depot antipsychotics have been particularly implicated (Committee on Safety of Medicines and Medicines Control Agency, 1994). It is not unusual for two or more drug-induced movement disorders to coexist in one patient, and a particular drug may cause more than one type of movement disorder.

Table 10.3 Definition of movement disorders

Movement disorder	*Definition*
Akathisia	Motor restlessness
Choreoathetosis	A combination of jerky (choreiform) and writhing (athetoid) movements
Dystonia	Abnormal postures or muscle spasm caused by altered muscle tone
Myoclonus	Spasmodic contraction of the muscles
Parkinsonism	Tremor, rigidity and akinesia
Tardive dyskinesia	Consists of choreiform, athetoid, or rhythmic stereotyped movements involving the tongue, jaw, trunk or extremities
Tics	Spasmodic twitching of muscles, usually those of the face and neck
Tremor	An involuntary muscular quivering

What most of these drugs have in common is that they interact directly or indirectly with the neurotransmitter dopamine. This neurotransmitter is released from the substantia nigra in the midbrain to allow messages to pass to the basal nuclei along the nigro-striatal pathway. This pathway and the basal nuclei are concerned with regulating voluntary movement. Drugs which antagonize dopamine, particularly at the D_2-receptor subtype, such as the phenothiazines, will thus lead to movement disorders, as will overuse of dopamine agonists in the treatment of Parkinson's disease (Robertson and George, 1990). Reduction of the dosage of the drug concerned, and if necessary the substitution of a drug with less effects on D_2-dopamine receptors, (e.g. risperiodone or clozapine) will reduce symptoms (Launer, 1996). In addition to dopamine, the basal nuclei also contain the chemical transmitter acetylcholine. The function of dopamine is to inhibit the action of acetylcholine, and an increase in acetylcholine can lead to movement alterations because of over-excitation of the muscles. Thus, the phenothiazines, such as thioridazine, which have considerable anticholinergic effects produce fewer movement disorders than phenothiazines, such as fluphenazine, which have fewer anticholinergic effects. Another neurotransmitter involved in this balancing act is GABA (gamma amino butyric acid), the production of which is stimulated by acetylcholine and which in turns inhibits dopamine release (Sims, 1995). As many antiepileptics work by enhancing the action of GABA, it is not surprising that they also can cause movement disorders.

Sensory

The two main sense organs affected by adverse drug reactions are the eye and the ear. Taste is dealt with in Chapter 7.

The eye

Adverse drug reactions can affect all the tissues of the eye, including the conjunctiva, cornea, lens, retina and optic nerve (Table 10.4). They are of particular concern because they can result in impaired eyesight and even blindness.

Table 10.4 Examples of drugs having adverse effects on the eye

Disorder	*Associated drugs*
Cataracts	Busulfan (busulphan), corticosteroids, ergot
Conjunctivitis	Aspirin, atropine, barbiturates, ß-blockers, neomycin, sulphonamides
Diplopia and nystagmus	Aspirin, barbiturates, carbamazepine, corticosteroids, indometacin (indomethacin), lithium, phenytoin, propranolol, sodium valproate, tricyclic antidepressants
Eye drop allergy	Atropine, neomycin
Glaucoma	Anticholinergics, adrenal agonists, monoamine oxidase inhibitors, tricyclic antidepressants
Myopia	Acetazolamide, anticholinesterases, pilocarpine, prochlorperazine, sulphonamides, thiazide diuretics, tetracycline
Opaque corneal deposits	Amiodarone, chlorpromazine, chloroquine, indometacin (indomethacin)
Optic neuritis	Chloramphenicol, ethambutol, ibuprofen, isoniazid, sulphonamides
Stevens-Johnson syndrome	See Chapter 5

Supporting structures

Starting with the supporting structures of the eye, antihistamines and anticholinergic drugs can affect the quality and quantity of the tears. This may cause feelings of dry eye and pain. Patients using contact lenses should be advised not to wear their lenses until after they have discontinued these drugs. Many drugs are also excreted in the tears. The antituberculous drug rifampicin is an important example as it can discolour contact lenses and patients should be warned of this. Wearers of soft contact lenses should also be warned not to put eye drops containing benzalkonium chloride into their eyes while wearing their lenses as the benzalkonium chloride causes irreversible opacity of these lenses (Burton, 1989).

Conjunctivitis

The next structure to consider is the conjunctiva, the mucous membrane that lines the inner surface of the eyelid and the exposed surface of the eyeball. Allergic reactions can occur to a multitude of ophthalmic drops and ointments. The main culprits are neomycin and atropine, although allergy to the preservatives, such as benzalkonium, found in many eye drops can also occur. The patient typically presents with irritation, redness and conjunctival oedema (chemosis) of the eye(s) being treated. This can progress to gross periorbital swelling and sometimes a characteristic skin rash can develop under the eye due to the antigen running down the face in the tears. It is usual to discontinue the medication and allow the allergic reaction to settle on its own, although in severe cases preservative-free steroids may be used. The use of systemic medications such as aspirin, barbiturates, ß-blockers, and sulphonamides can also very occasionally result in conjunctivitis.

Corneal deposits

Beneath the conjunctiva is found the cornea, a transparent fibrous coat, which refracts light into the lens of the eye. It can be affected adversely by opaque corneal deposits that can result from the administration of a number of systemic drugs, including amiodarone, chlorpromazine, chloroquine, and indometacin (indomethacin).

Accommodation

Behind the cornea is the muscular iris, with its central hole, the pupil. The iris consists of two smooth muscles, the constrictor activated by parasympathetic nerves and which makes the pupil smaller, and the dilator activated by the sympathetic nerves, which makes it larger. Altering the curvature of the lens brings about focusing for near and far vision (accommodation), and the ciliary muscles, which are activated by parasympathetic nerves, perform this function. Drugs which mimic or antagonize the sympathetic and parasympathetic nervous system will change pupil size and may alter accommodation, thus producing either miosis (small pupil) or mydriasis (large pupil), accommodative spasm or accommodative paralysis (cyloplegia). Thus, the clinical use of atropine-like drugs either topically as mydriatics, or systemically, can result in loss of accommodation for near vision, and hence inability to read. Tricyclic antidepressants like amitriptyline which have anticholinergic properties may also do this, particularly in elderly patients who have already lost much of their accommodative ability. Conversely, drugs with cholinergic activity or parasympathomimetic properties can cause myopia (shortsightedness). A transient idiosyncratic myopia occurs in patients taking acetazolamide, prochlorperazine, sulphonamides and tetracycline and disappears within a few days of stopping medication.

Glaucoma

Glaucoma is a disease in which eyesight is lost due to retinal damage, secondary to raised intraocular pressure. Pressure within the eye is exerted by aqueous humour that is secreted by cells within the ciliary processes. This fluid normally drains into the venous system and the canal of Schlemm at the angle between the iris and the cornea. Intraocular pressure becomes raised when drainage is impaired. Clinically glaucoma presents either as the simple glaucoma in which pressure rise and visual loss are insidious, or as the rarer acute glaucoma where the pressure rise is sudden and painful, and in which blindness can result within a few hours. Both topical and systemic drugs can precipitate acute-angle closure glaucoma in susceptible individuals with shallow anterior chambers and narrow angles. Possible culprits include anticholinergic drugs such as atropine, adrenergic agonists such as adrenaline (epinephrine), and less commonly the monoamine oxidase inhibitors and tricyclic antidepressants. Patients at risk of this adverse effect are usually elderly and long-sighted (hypermetropic). They are unlikely to have any previous history of glaucoma, as chronic open-angle glaucoma is not a risk factor.

Corticosteroids are another drug group that can cause raised intraocular pressure. When applied directly to the eye, corticosteroids will cause some degree of raised intraocular pressure in more than a third of the population (Menage, 1994), and even when taken by other routes, including the skin and inhalation, they can have the same effect. Consequently, patients on long-term corticosteroid treatment should have their intraocular pressure monitored periodically.

Cataracts

The lens of the eye may be affected by several drugs, including ergot and busulfan (busulphan), which can result in cataract formation. The most common culprit is corticosteroids. The effect is dose-dependent and can result from both topical and systemic treatment. Friedlaender et al. (1990) argue that the use of corticosteroids should be avoided in the treatment of mild allergy, due to their long-term side-effects, in particular cataract formation. The authors suggest that cataract formation may begin after 600 drops or six months treatment. However, it is unusual for cataracts to form with less than one or two years of oral treatment with 15 mg of prednisolone or equivalent per day (Menage, 1994).

The retina

The retina can be damaged by the use of chloroquine and hydroxychloroquine. The effect does not occur with the low doses used in the treatment of malaria, but is reported in the long-term treatment of collagen diseases. The toxicity is dose-related and rarely occurs in patients receiving less than 25 mg daily, or a total cumulative dose of less than 300 g (Menage, 1994). The damage takes the form of a bull's eye maculopathy, so called because there is a ring of depigmentation around the fovea, surrounded by a ring of more pigmented retina. As considerable irreversible loss of vision can occur before it becomes noticeable to the patient, it is important that patients treated with chloroquine have a baseline eye examination and then regular monitoring of colour vision, visual fields and fundal examination. They should be advised to stop taking the drug if any visual disturbances occur.

Phenothiazines can cause a granular pigmentary retinopathy with prolonged use. The main symptoms are brownish colouring of vision, night-blindness, and decreased visual acuity. Improvement in vision is usual when the drug is stopped.

Visual disturbances are common with cardiac glycosides like digoxin, and are usually a sign of overdosing. They include the perception of halos around objects, dancing figures, coloured tinges to objects, flashes of light and photophobia (Goldstein, 1986).

Optic and oculomotor nerves

Inflammation of cranial nerve II (optic neuritis) can be caused by many drugs, including chloramphenicol, ethambutol, ibuprofen, isoniazid, and the sulphonamides. Chloramphenicol in a daily dose greater than 100 mg can cause a severe bilateral optic neuritis leading to optic atrophy and irreversible loss of vision. Some patients, experience warning signs of paraesthesia, numbness and cramps before the onset of the optic nerve damage. Ethambutol can cause retrobulbar neuritis. The adverse effect is avoided if doses less than 15 mg per kg per day are used. Patients should be warned to discontinue treatment and seek medical advice if they develop visual disturbances. These are usually reversible in the early stages. Patients requiring higher doses should have periodic checks of visual acuity, colour vision and visual field.

Optic neuritis leading to optic atrophy has also been reported with isoniazid. Because of the potential effect of vitamin deficiency on the neurotoxicity, vitamin B6 is often prescribed simultaneously.

Diplopia (double vision) and nystagmus (involuntary rapid eye movement) have been attributed to a number of drugs (Table 10.3). The drugs appear to interfere with the centres in the brain which coordinate eye movement. Toxic effects on cranial nerve III, the oculomotor nerve, occurs in 1–10% of patients receiving vinca alkaloids, and results in drooping eyelids (ptosis) and paralysis of the eye muscles (Thomson and Lee, 1998).

The ear

Drugs that have adverse effects on the ear do so by producing reversible or irreversible damage to the auditory nerve (cranial nerve VIII). As Table 10.5 indicates there are two types of ototoxicity: cochlear (hearing) and vestibular (balance) toxicity. The former is characterized by tinnitus and sensorineural hearing loss (deafness), and the latter by loss of equilibrium. As extensive damage to the inner ear cannot be reversed, it is important to be aware and on the

Table 10.5 Examples of drugs that have the potential to cause ototoxicity (Haybach, 1993)

Drug	*Type of damage*	*Site of damage*	
		Cochlear	Vestibular
Chloroquine	Reversible	✓	–
Cisplatin	Reversible or irreversible	✓	✓
Furosemide (frusemide)	Reversible or irreversible	✓	✓
Gentamicin	Reversible or irreversible	✓	✓
Minocycline	Reversible or irreversible	–	✓
Neomycin	Irreversible	✓	–
Quinine	Reversible	✓	–
Salicylates	Reversible	✓	✓
Streptomycin	Reversible or irreversible	✓	✓
Vancomycin	Reversible or irreversible	✓	–

look out for ototoxic symptoms. Cochlear toxicity is associated with ringing, roaring or blowing noises, ear pain, and a feeling of aural fullness. Dizziness, blurred or bouncing vision, unsteadiness, or motion intolerance is indicative of vestibular toxicity.

Symptom manifestation and severity vary markedly with the individual. Those most at risk are the very young and very old and those with a history of hearing loss. Other risk factors include renal or hepatic disease, concurrent use of two or more potentially ototoxic drugs or an ototoxic drug with a nephrotoxic drug, previous use of ototoxic drugs, dehydration, bacteraemia, and previous cranial radiation.

Ototoxicity is most commonly associated with salicylates, such as aspirin, and cinchona alkaloids such as the antiarrhythmic agent quinidine and the antimalarials chloroquine and quinine. When associated with these drugs, ototoxicity can become part of two larger syndromes, namely salicylism and cinchonism. Salicylism is characterized by tinnitus, hearing loss, vertigo, headache, perspiration, nausea, vomiting and diarrhoea. It can lead to disturbances of vision, lassitude, confusion, thirst and hyperventilation. Cinchonism can include symptoms of both cochlear and vestibular toxicity as well as abdominal pain, flushed sweaty skin, rash, headache, blurred vision and diarrhoea. If ototoxicity is suspected it may be necessary either to stop the medication or to modify the regimen by reducing the dosage or substituting an alternative drug.

Endocrine

A wide range of drugs can affect the functioning of the endocrine system (Table 10.6), usually by modifying hormone synthesis or release. However, drugs may also interfere with the tests used to identify endocrine disease, and it is important to recognize this if incorrect diagnoses are not to be made. Fortunately, in the case of the endocrine system most adverse drug effects are dose-related rather than idiosyncratic, and so should be easier to predict.

Table 10.6 Examples of drugs having adverse effects on the endocrine system

Disorder	*Associated drugs*
Adrenal suppression	Ketoconazole, corticosteroids
Diabetes insipidus	Lithium
Gynaecomastia	Cimetidine, digoxin, ketoconazole, marijuana, metoclopramide, phenytoin, verapamil
Hyperthyroidism	Amiodarone, interferon-α, lithium, radiographic contrast media
Hyperprolactinaemia	Cimetidine, cocaine, methyldopa, metoclopramide, phenothiazines, tricyclic antidepressants, verapamil
Hypothyroidism	Amiodarone, interferon-α, lithium
Ovarian and testicular dysfunction	Glucocorticoids
Syndrome of inappropriate ADH secretion	Carbamazepine, chlorpropamide, cisplatin, cyclophosphamide, tricyclic antidepressants, vincristine
Virilization	Danazol

Drugs affecting the pituitary and its hormones

The pituitary gland produces at least nine different hormones, but only four of them are significantly affected by drug therapy.

Prolactin

Prolactin is a protein hormone secreted by the anterior pituitary gland. Its principal role in humans is in breast development and to stimulate milk production. Its release is increased by serotonin and decreased by dopamine, thus drugs that interfere with these two systems can lead to hormone imbalance, in particular hyperprolactinaemia. This condition appears clinically in women as amenorrhoea, infertility, galactorrhoea and occasionally hirsutism, whilst impotence is the major feature in men. Many drugs can cause hyperprolactinaemia either through increased serotonergic stimulation, most commonly the selective serotonin reuptake inhibitors (SSRIs), such as paroxetine and fluoxetine, and more rarely the tricyclic antidepressants, or through decreased dopamine inhibition, for example the phenothiazine antipsychotics, reserpine, methyldopa and metoclopramide. Oestrogen-containing preparations, cimetidine and verapamil can also cause hyperprolactinaemia, but the mechanism by which they do so is not entirely clear. Cohen and Davies (1998) suggest that serum prolactin levels should be measured before commencing treatment with drugs liable to cause hyperprolactinaemia to avoid extensive pituitary evaluation if hyperprolactinaemia occurs later. Drug-induced hyperprolactinaemia and galactorrhoea usually resolve within weeks of stopping the offending drug.

Drugs that suppress prolactin release include levodopa, bromocriptine, pergolide, and the serotonin antagonist metergoline. (Yeung and Cockram, 1993). They are effective in reversing galactorrhoea and restoring ovulation and fertility in patients with hyperprolactinaemia.

Antidiuretic hormone

The posterior pituitary stores antidiuretic hormone (ADH). This is made in the hypothalamus and released by the pituitary in response to an increase in plasma osmolarity and dehydration. Some drugs can result in inappropriate ADH secretion, i.e. secretion when the plasma osmolarity is low or normal. This is termed the syndrome of inappropriate secretion of ADH (SIADH) and is characterized by hyponatraemia, with the patient complaining of lethargy, weakness and weight gain. These symptoms can progress to headaches, nausea, vomiting, and, if untreated, to confusion, convulsions and death. This syndrome has been linked to carbamazepine where it has an incidence of up to 22% (Millar and Lee, 1998), as well as to chlorpropamide, the phenothiazines, tricyclic antidepressants and cytotoxic drugs. The drugs appear to exert their effect by stimulating the release of ADH, although the dry mouth stimulated by some antipsychotic and antidepressants may trigger polydipsia. Smoking is another factor associated with the development of SIADH, and the risk may increase with age (Spigset and Hedenmalm, 1995). Management of SIADH includes discontinuation of the drug, in severe cases, the possibility of fluid restriction until the hyponatraemia has resolved. In patients with life threatening symptoms, it may be appropriate to administer hypertonic saline solution intravenously, but over-rapid correction of hyponatraemia can result in osmotic demyelination syndrome, which is characterized by bulbar palsy, paralysis of all limbs and death. In chronic SIADH, where other methods of treatment have failed, demeclocycline which inhibits the effects of ADH on the kidney can be effective. Patients being initiated on carbamazepine or antipsychotics would benefit from having serum sodium levels measured at the start of treatment and again a month later.

Decreased ADH levels result in diabetes insipidus, characterized by the production of copious dilute urine and severe thirst. Lithium has been related to this condition and is believed to result from direct inhibition of ADH production.

Drugs affecting the thyroid

Thyroxine and triiodothyronine are synthesised from dietary iodine and are released from the thyroid gland in response to thyroid stimulating hormone (TSH) produced by the pituitary gland. Many drugs can interfere with biochemical tests of thyroid function (Table 10.7) by interfering with the synthesis, transport and metabolism of thyroid hormones or by altering the synthesis and secretion of TSH. Only rarely, however, do these cause clinically apparent thyroid disease, although it is important to be aware of the influence of drugs so that test results can be interpreted correctly. The administration of iodine-containing preparations can lead to the development of hyperthyroidism, with common causes being radiographic contrast media, the anti-arrhythmic amiodarone, and over-the-counter vitamin preparations. Hyperthyroidism more commonly occurs in patients with an underlying goitre and in iodine deficient areas.

Amiodarone may also cause hypothyroidism, usually in iodine-replete areas. It is often associated with an increase in thyroid anti-

Table 10.7 Drugs that may interfere with thyroid function tests (Gittoes and Franklyn, 1995)

- Amiodarone
- Anabolic steroids
- Aspirin
- ß-blockers
- Carbamazepine
- Corticosteroids
- Fenclofenac
- Heparin
- Iodine contrast media
- Oestrogens
- Phenobarbital (phenobarbitone)
- Phenylbutazone
- Phenytoin

body titres, and Walker (1994) suggests that amiodarone unmasks autoimmune hypothyroidism, while Harjai and Licata (1997) identify other possible mechanisms in their review of amiodarone. Thyrotoxicosis usually resolves if the drug is stopped, but this can take up to eight months due to the drug's long half-life. In patients with serious cardiac arrhythmias, stopping the drug may not be an option, and antithyroid drug therapy in the form of carbimazole or propylthiouracil may be given. Prednisolone may also be useful, particularly in patients with no previous history of thyroid disease (Harjai and Licata, 1997).

Lithium also affects thyroid function, usually leading to hypothyroidism because of its ability to inhibit the release of thyroxine. Clinical hypothyroidism affects 5–15% of patients on long-term lithium treatment and as many as 30% have sub-clinical hypothyroidism (Millar and Lee, 1998). Rarely lithium causes thyrotoxicosis. The mechanism is unclear but in the majority of patients, there is evidence of autoimmune thyroid disease. Long-term treatment with interferon alfa may also cause both hyperthyroidism and hypothyroidism, with the highest incidence being in patients with hepatitis C.

Drugs affecting the adrenal glands

The two adrenal glands are divided up into an inner medulla and an outer cortex. The former is functionally part of the sympathetic nervous system and produces adrenaline (epinephrine) and noradrenaline (norepinephrine), while the latter produces three hormone groups, namely the mineralcorticoids, glucocorticoids, and adrenal sex hormones. Adverse drug effects occur most commonly in relation to the glucocorticoids, as they are commonly used therapeutically, particularly as anti-inflammatory drugs and immunosuppressants. Administration of pharmacological doses of glucocorticoids causes iatrogenic Cushing's syndrome. Symptoms usually occur at daily doses of more than 50 mg hydrocortisone and may begin to appear within two weeks of starting therapy. Symptoms can include 'moon face', 'buffalo hump', weight gain, a tendency to bruising, psychiatric symptoms, osteoporosis, skin thinning, posterior cataracts, pancreatitis and aseptic necrosis (Walker, 1994).

Administration of doses greater than 5 mg prednisolone or 20 mg hydrocortisone for more two weeks leads to suppression of the hypothalamic-pituitary-adrenal (HPA) axis. In the absence of ACTH the adrenals atrophy and do not synthesize and release glucocorticoids. If drug therapy is ceased abruptly, hypoadrenalism can occur. Signs and symptoms include lethargy, anorexia, weight loss, hyponatraemia and hyperkalaemia. Patients must be counselled not to stop treatment abruptly, and patients stopping therapy after long-term treatment should have their medication gradually tailed off. In addition, the adrenals respond inadequately to stress so increased doses of steroids must be given during serious illness or surgery, and the patient must be advised to carry a steroid card to inform people of their therapy. This card may need to be carried for up to two years as it can take this long for the HPA axis to recover in patients who have been on glucocorticoids for 18 months or more.

Metyrapone and aminoglutethimide are both used to treat Cushing's disease, as they work by blocking corticosteroid biosynthesis. They can therefore lead to hypoadrenalism when used in excess. Ketoconazole is a potent inhibitor of adrenal glucocorticoid synthesis, and adrenal insufficiency has been reported with oral doses as low as 20 mg twice daily after two days treatment (Millar and Lee, 1998). Patients may be treated by withdrawing the drug or by corticosteroid replacement therapy.

The anti-tuberculosis drug rifampicin has been reported as precipitating acute adrenal insufficiency in patients with pre-existing hypoadrenalism, probably as a result of induction of microsomal enzymes. It is recommended that such patients should have their doses of replacement corticosteroids increased on commencing rifampicin.

Drugs affecting gonadal hormones

The hypothalamus produces gonadotrophin-releasing hormones that stimulate the pituitary to produce follicle stimulating hormone (FSH) and luteinising hormone (LH). In women, they stimulate follicular maturation and oestrogen and progesterone production, while in men they stimulate spermatogenesis and testosterone production. High doses of corticosteroids inhibit pituitary gonadotrophin release, resulting in ovarian and testicular dysfunction. Ketoconazole inhibits testicular production of testosterone, whilst danazol decreases the ability of testosterone to bind to its transport protein, leading to an increase in the free active testosterone. This may explain the virilization and hirsutism observed in patients taking danazol.

Gynaecomastia

Gynaecomastia is the abnormal accumulation of tissue in the male breast. It can occur physiologically because of changing hormone levels in the neonatal period, at puberty and in old age. Gynaecomastia can also occur as an adverse effect of drug therapy, when the underlying mechanism is usually either increased oestrogen-like activity or reduced testosterone effects. Breast enlargement is common in men treated for prostatic cancer with the synthetic oestrogen diethylstilbestrol (stilboestrol) (DES). Other drugs producing gynaecomastia because of their oestrogenic activity are anabolic steroids, clomifene (clomiphene), digoxin, and conjugated or synthetic oestrogens. Drugs that produce gynaecomastia by reducing testosterone synthesis or effect include cimetidine, ketoconazole, penicillamine, and phenytoin. Some drugs, e.g. spironolactone both inhibit androgen production and block its action (Turner, 1997). In some cases the mechanism of action is not clear, e.g. calcium channel blockers, cannabis, isoniazid, methadone, antipsychotics and tricyclic antidepressants. Drug-induced gynaecomastia usually develops soon after drug therapy is started and resolves when the drug is stopped.

References and further reading

Adam K, Oswald I (1983) Protein synthesis, bodily renewal and the sleep-wake cycle. Clinical Science 65: 561-7

Anon (1999) Drugged driving. New Scientist 162: 5

Burns RJ, Schultz DW (1993) Drug-induced neurological disorders. The Medical Journal of Australia 159: 624-6

Burton S (1989) Drugs and the eye. Nursing 3: 24-6

Cender D, Gelhot A, Phillips B, Anstead M, Khawaja I, Pinto JS (1998) Daytime drowsiness: is a drug to blame? Journal of Respiratory Diseases 19: 617-29

Cohen MA, Davies PH (1998) Drug therapy and hyperprolactinaemia. Adverse Drug Reaction Bulletin 190: 723-6

Committee on Safety of Medicines and Medicines Control Agency (1994) Drug induced extrapyramidal reactions. Current Problems in Pharmacovigilance 20: 15-16

Dietrich B (1997) Polysomnography in drug development. Journal of Clinical Pharmacology 37(Supp): 70-78S

Ferner RE (1998) Interactions between alcohol and drugs. Adverse Drug Reaction Bulletin 189: 719-22

Friedlaender MH, Udell IJ, Wagoner MD (1990) Ocular allergy: nuisance or hazard? Patient Care 24: 60-74

Gittoes NJL, Franklyn JA (1995) Drug-induced thyroid disorders. Drug Safety 13: 46-55

Goldstein J (1986) Ocular side effects of systemic drugs: A physical assessment guide for ophthalmic medical assistants. Journal of Ophthalmic Nursing and Technology 5: 103-6

Harjai KJ, Licata AA (1997) Effects of amiodarone on thyroid function. Annals of Internal Medicine 126: 63-73

Haybach PJ (1993) Tuning into ototoxicity. Nursing 93 23: 34-40

Idzikowski C, Shapiro CM (1993) Non-psychotic drugs and sleep. British Medical Journal 306(6885): 1118-21.

Launer M (1996) Selected side effects of dopamine receptor antagonists. Prescriber Journal 36: 37-41

Lee KA, Stotts NA (1990) Support of the growth hormone-somatomedin system to facilitate healing. Heart and Lung 19: 157-64

Menage M (1994) Adverse drug reactions that affect the eye. Prescriber 5: 25-30

Millar J, Lee A (1998) Adverse drug reactions. (6) Drug-induced endocrine disorders. The Pharmaceutical Journal 260: 17-21

Novak M, Shapiro CM (1997) Drug-induced sleep disturbances. Focus on nonpsychotropic medications. Drug Safety 16: 133-49

Phillips H (1999) Perchance to learn. New Scientist. 163: 27-30

Robertson DRC, George CF (1990) Adverse effects and long-term problems of antiparkinsonian therapy. Adverse Drug Reaction Bulletin 145: 544-7

Sims J (1995) The extrapyramidal effects of phenothiazines on patients. Nursing Times 91: 30-1

Spigset O, Hedenmalm K (1995) Hyponatraemia and the syndrome of inappropriate antidiuretic hormone secretion (SIADH) induced by psychotropic drugs. Drug Safety 12: 209-25

Thomson F, Lee A (1998) Adverse drug reactions (7) Drug-induced neurological disorders. The Pharmaceutical Journal 260: 269-74

Turner H (1997) Gynaecomastia. Medicine 25: 41-3

Turner R, Elson E (1993) Steroids may cause sleep disturbances. British Medical Journal 306: 1477-8

Walker M (1994) What effect do drugs have on the endocrine system? Prescriber 5: 29-32

Wittbrodt ET (1997) Drugs and myasthenia gravis. An update. Archives of Internal Medicine 157: 399-407

Yeung VTF, Cockram CS (1993) Drug-induced gynaecomastia and galactorrhoea. Adverse Drug Reaction Bulletin 162: 611-14

Chapter 11
Psychological effects

In 1997, 8.6% of yellow card reports submitted to the Commission on the Safety of Medicines featured suspected psychiatric reactions to drugs (Bishop and Lee, 1998). However, as drug-induced mental health disorders are by their nature difficult to recognize and diagnose, and because these disorders are stigmatized and so not freely admitted, the true incidence is difficult to envision. A number of factors can increase the likelihood of a person developing a psychiatric reaction to a drug, as indicated in Table 11.1. This chapter examines the possible adverse psychological effects of drugs, as well as briefly touching on drug abuse and dependence.

Table 11.1 Factors that increase the risk of a person developing a psychiatric reaction to a drug

1. They already suffer from mental illness
2. They have impaired cerebral function, as in the elderly or patients with brain damage
3. They abuse alcohol or other drugs
4. They are in a stressful environment such as an intensive care unit

Confusion and delirium

Acute confusion and delirium have a rapid onset, often within a 24-hour period. Attention, memory and concentration become poor, conversation is disjointed and patients are easily distracted. They are unable to carry out everyday tasks, may appear generally unwell, and may develop a tendency to fall. Consciousness is clouded, patients are less aware of their surroundings, may be disoriented, misinterpret reality, and be restless and agitated. The patient's mental state may vary throughout the day, and may deteriorate in the evening. The causes of confusion and delirium are myriad, but drug therapy must always be considered as a possible cause when assessing the patient. Many drugs can cause confusion either alone (Table 11.2) or through interaction with other drugs (Table 11.3), particularly in the elderly (McMinn, 1995). Effective management of confusion and delirium is early recognition of the condition and treatment of the cause, which in the case of an adverse drug effect, requires identification and withdrawal of the causative drug. While waiting for the confusion and delirium to abate, it is necessary also to manage any disruptive behaviour and agitation. Sedatives and physical restraint should be avoided if possible, as they can make matters worse as well as complicate diagnosis. If sedatives must be used diazepam or lorazepam and a short-acting anti-psychotic are the preferred choice.

Table 11.2 Drugs commonly causing confusion

Drug type	*Examples*
Antibiotics	Penicillin, streptomycin, sulphonamides
Anticholinergic drugs	Atropine, hyoscine, tricyclic antidepressants
Antiepileptics	Carbamazepine, phenytoin, sodium valproate
Cardiovascular drugs	Digoxin, diuretics, ß-blockers
Dopamine antagonists	Amantadine, bromocriptine, levodopa
Tranquillizers and hypnotics	Benzodiazepines, barbiturates, phenothiazines
Others	Corticosteroids, opioid analgesics, cimetidine, oral hypoglycaemics, lithium

Depression

Depression is a common symptom with 10% of the population being depressed enough to warrant professional care (Neese, 1991). Symptoms of depression include a general feeling of misery, apathy and pessimism, sleep disturbances, loss of appetite, low self-esteem, loss of motivation, retardation of thought and action, and suicide. Medical disorders, e.g. endocrinopathies, malignancies, strokes, Parkinson's disease, electrolyte imbalance (reduced serum sodium and potassium levels) and viral disease can all precipitate depressive disorders, as can the drugs used to treat them. A study by Hall et al. (1980) found that 8% of cases of depression were due to drug toxicity or withdrawal. Some drugs that have consistently been associated with depression are shown in Table 11.4.

Table 11.3 Examples of drug interactions which may produce confusion (Newbern, 1991)

Interaction between		*Effect*
Drug	*Drug*	
Alcohol	Sedative	Additive suppressant effect on central nervous system
	Oral hypoglycaemic	Potentiates effect of both drugs
Antacids	Cimetidine	Reduced cimetidine clearance
	Morphine	Reduced morphine clearance
Diuretics	Digoxin	Digoxin toxicity due to hypokalaemia
Phenylbutazone	Oral hypoglycaemic	Potentiates hypoglycaemia
Quinidine	Digoxin	Enhanced risk of digoxin toxicity

Table 11.4 Drugs that may cause mental health disorders

Disorder	*Associated drugs*
Dementia	Alcohol, amphetamines, centrally acting anticholinergics, antiepileptics, benzodiazepine
Depression	Amphetamines (withdrawal), benzodiazepines, ß-blockers, calcium-channel blockers, ciprofloxacin, corticosteroids, digoxin, fluphenazine, indometacin (indomethacin), isotretinoin, levodopa, pravastatin, ranitidine
Mania	Baclofen, bromocriptine, chloroquine, corticosteroids, dopaminergics, isoniazid, MAOIs, tricyclic antidepressants
Psychosis	Amantadine, amphetamines, anticholinergics, antiepileptics, bromocriptine, cimetidine, cocaine, digoxin, isoniazid, levodopa, mefloquine
Serotonin syndrome	Dextromethorphan, MAOIs, pethidine, SSRIs, tricyclic anti-depressants

The main biochemical theory to explain depression is the monoamine hypothesis. This suggests that depression is caused by a reduction/deficiency in noradrenaline (norepinephrine) and/or serotonin transmission in the central nervous system. This theory underpins the use of tricyclic antidepressants, monoamine oxidase inhibitors, and clomipramine in the treatment of depression, as they all increase the amount of noradrenaline (norepinephrine) and serotonin in the synaptic cleft. It also explains why drugs like methyldopa, which cause depletion of noradrenaline (norepinephrine), may cause depressive symptoms in up to 10% of patients (Bishop and Lee, 1998), and consequently should not be used in the treatment of hypertension in people suffering from depression. However, there are 'some glaring inconsistencies' with the monoamine theory (Rang et al., 1995, p 579) resulting in other theories being proposed (Brasfield, 1991).

The data to support the idea that depression is a regular or frequent concomitant of therapeutic treatment with a particular drug is often lacking (Smith and Salzman, 1991). This combined with the absence of an explanatory underlying mechanism means that it is difficult to anticipate and diagnose depression as an adverse drug effect. Thus, the diagnosis of drug-induced depression is based on identifying the quality and quantity of the depressive effect and by ruling out other causes. One of the best hints that mood disorder is organic in aetiology is the age of onset. If depression becomes manifest for the first time after the age of 45, it should be assumed to be organic until proven otherwise (Lane and Gelenberg, 1993). Similarly, if a child develops depression, organic causes should be sought, including drug therapy, as these can cause depression in children, as illustrated by epileptic children prescribed barbiturates (Anon, 1983). If the mood alteration is so severe that it interferes with social or occupational functioning and if there is a close temporal association between the initiation of a drug or a dosage change and the onset of depression, then drug-induced depression is the likely diagnosis (Lane and Gelenberg, 1993). Typically, the mood change occurs within a period of a few days to two months following drug initiation or change, and resolution of symptoms after withdrawal of the drug confirms the diagnosis.

It must always be borne in mind, however, that more than one of the patient's drugs may precipitate depression. Thus for example, it is generally accepted that many of the antihypertensive drugs used to control blood pressure have the capacity to cause depression, i.e. reserpine, clonidine, propranolol, guanethidine and methyldopa, although not all authors agree (Bright and Everitt, 1992). Consequently, there is a tendency to attribute any symptoms of depression to these drugs. However, Okada (1985) relates eight case histories of patients treated with thiazide diuretics in which there was a clear link between depression and use of the diuretic. Thus, as it is common to treat patients with hypertension with both an antihypertensive and a diuretic, it is important if patients present with depression as an adverse effect, to consider both groups of drugs.

It must also be recognized that in rare cases tricyclic antidepressants can induce depression (Anon, 1987). This is important, because increasing the dose will just exacerbate the symptoms. Most cases of tricyclic-induced depression have occurred in the elderly, but it may also occur in younger age groups. In order to recognize this problem plasma drug levels should be measured routinely for any patient taking tricyclics. A high drug level in combination with worsening depression suggests tricyclic-induced central anticholinergic toxicity. Treatment is dosage reduction or withdrawal of the tricyclic drug. To minimize the problem of tricyclic-induced depression, dosage increases should always be made gradually and concurrent use of two or more medications with anticholinergic properties should be avoided whenever possible.

Psychosis

Acute psychosis can be caused by various factors including neurological (head injuries), psychiatric, endocrine (thyrotoxicosis) and post-operative states. It can also be caused by numerous drugs (Table 11.4), as well as by withdrawal from alcohol and central nervous depressants. The symptoms of psychosis include distorted personality, delusions, and hallucinations, which in the case of drug-induced psychosis are more commonly visual than auditory.

Corticosteroids have been known for a long time to cause changes in mental status, including euphoria, depression, mood swings and psychosis. Thus any of the causes of Cushing's syndrome, including drug therapy, can precipitate psychosis. Travlos and Hirsch (1993) describe two case studies where high-dose methylprednisolone was used in the treatment of acute spinal cord injury and resulted in acute psychosis. They suggest that conservative reports put the incidence of high-dose steroid-induced psychosis at 5.7%, and express concern as these reactions put their patients at increased risk of spinal cord injury and worsening neurological damage.

Chloroquine has been known, for many years, to cause psychosis and behavioural toxicity, especially in the high doses used to treat malaria. It also has the problem that in many areas of the world the malarial parasite has become resistant to it. It was thus with great anticipation that mefloquine (Lariam) was introduced in 1985. Mefloquine is now considered the most effective antimalarial drug on the market, and it has been widely prescribed as prophylaxis for people travelling to areas where malaria is resistant to chloroquine. Unfortunately, mefloquine has been shown to produce a variety of neuropsychiatric symptoms including depression, anxiety, panic attacks, confusion, hallucinations, paranoid delusions and convulsions. The manufacturers of Lariam maintain that based on large observational studies these serious side-effects only affect 1 in 10000 people who take prophylactic mefloquine (Bishop and Lee, 1998). However, many doctors believe that the true number of Lariam takers who develop serious side-effects is much higher (Thompson, 1996), and much media attention has been given to the debate over this issue. Side-effects such as those associated with mefloquine may be acceptable in the treatment of malaria, but they are unacceptable with preventative medicine.

Recreational drugs can also cause psychosis. This includes Ecstasy, one of the top recreational drugs taken by young people in this country. The current emphasis on the symptoms of the drug and the advice (Table 11.5) might suggest that the dangers are purely physical. However, Lehane and Rees (1996) identify that out of 390 admissions to their hospital's psychiatric intensive care unit, 50 (13%) were drug-related. Of these 35 (70%) were because of taking Ecstasy and eight (23%) of these patients admitted were still receiving psychiatric treatment eight months after their admission.

Mania

Drug-induced mania is rare. Symptoms include elevated mood, overactivity, insomnia, rapid speech, grandiose ideas and disinhibition. Mania is believed to result from overactivity of noradrenergic transmission and so drugs, such as MAOIs, tricyclics and levodopa, that enhance transmission can cause mania. Mania may be precipitated by the introduction of an antidepressant, especially tricyclic antidepressants, or, more commonly, by increasing the dose. On rare occasions, withdrawal of an antidepressant can cause mania (Bishop and Lee, 1998). Treatment involves withdrawal of the offending drug and the treatment of any residual symptoms with antipsychotic drugs.

Table 11.5 Advice to minimize the adverse effects of Ecstasy (Cook, 1995)

Adverse effect	*How to minimize*
Pyrexia	Chill out – take breaks from the dance floor during the night and go outside and cool down, or go to a quiet room and relax for a while
Dehydration	Rehydration – drink plenty of non-alcoholic drinks throughout the night. Fruit juices and cola are particularly useful as they also replace lost electrolytes
'Bad trips', psychosis	Rest – sleeping before taking Ecstasy can reduce the risk of unwanted psychological problems Spacing – leave at least six hours between doses to allow the first dose to be freed from the serotonin receptors. This will allow the psychological effects to subside, so avoiding dangerous compounding effects
Collapse – cardiac arrest, grand mal convulsions	Inform – tell friends exactly what you have been taking, so that if you do collapse they can provide helpful information to A & E staff in order that they can treat you rapidly

The use of anabolic steroids such as testosterone by sports competitors and body builders is estimated to be relatively common in the Western World. Case studies, interviews and clinical studies indicate that that these drugs may lead to mood swings, increased irritability, aggression, mania and dependence, especially when high doses have been used. The antisocial behaviour which can result from the effects of anabolic steroids can be seen in road rage, wife battering and animal cruelty, and this behaviour can cause much long-term suffering for the person's family. However, the research results are often conflicting as to whether anabolic steroids are the main cause of the antisocial behaviour in the people who use them. The alternative view is that other confounding variables such as individual variation in response to the drug or its dose, expectations, personality, diet, other drug use and family history are more important (Korkia, 1998).

Dementia

Dementia presents as deterioration of the intellect, memory and personality, and it can be caused by a number of drugs (Table 11.4). Dementia can occur due to levodopa. However, dementia is also known to affect some people with Parkinson's disease, so it is difficult to know whether the dementia is a result of the disease or the treatment.

Symptoms of depression in the elderly can sometimes be mistaken for dementia. This is known as pseudo-dementia and this diagnosis should be excluded before considering drugs as the cause of the dementia (Bishop and Lee, 1999).

Alcohol abuse can lead to Wernicke-Korsakoff syndrome, which can be mistaken for dementia (Geller, 1996). This condition is due to thiamine deficiency and can manifest as Wernicke encephalopathy, which is an acute or subacute disorder characterized by severe mental confusion, apathy or drowsiness with some oculomotor impairment. About half these patients will also have Korsakoff psychosis, which is a chronic amnesic state with profound loss of the ability to store new information. Many more alcoholics are neurologically asymptomatic but have impairments in problem-solving ability and visual-spatial disorganizations, as well as learning and memory problems. Functional deficits improve with abstinence but they do not necessarily resolve.

Serotonin syndrome

This is a rare condition, which occurs in patients receiving combinations of serotonergic drugs. It is characterized by a variety of symptoms, including confusion, disorientation, abnormal movement, muscle rigidity, fever, sweating, diarrhoea and hypotension. Symptoms commonly start within hours of starting the second drug, and are usually minor, although deaths have occurred. The diagnosis is made if three or more symptoms are present together and no other cause can be found. Symptoms usually resolve when the offending drugs are discontinued, although in severe cases treatment with intravenous fluids, activated charcoal, intravenous ß-blockers and neuromuscular blockade may be necessary (Anon, 1995). Most severe reactions have occurred with the combination of a selective serotonin reuptake inhibitor (SSRI) and a monoamine oxidase inhibitor (MAOI). Serotonin syndrome can easily be prevented by not using two serotonergic drugs simultaneously, and by allowing a washout period of two weeks or more between stopping one serotonergic drug and the next. This is especially important with drugs such as fluoxetine, which have long-half lives. Patients should also be advised regarding over-the-counter cough and cold remedies containing dextromethorphan, as serotonin syndrome has been reported when this is given in combination with MAOIs and SSRIs.

Drug abuse and dependence

Drugs are not used solely to treat medical disorders. They are also used for a variety of other purposes, including relaxation, to provide mystical/religious experiences, for excitement and to enhance performance on the sports field, and even in the bedroom (Aldridge and Measham, 1999). The drugs that are generally used for recreational purposes can be divided into three groups, as shown in Table 11.6. As can be seen they are frequently non-medicinal substances, e.g. LSD, Ecstasy, tobacco and solvents, but also include prescription drugs, most commonly stimulants, analgesics, tranquillizers and sedatives (Geller, 1996). The abuse of drugs is usually seen as a problem of adolescence, but it must be recognized that it is also an increasing problem of the elderly (Seibert, 1990).

Table 11.6 Drugs of abuse

Sedatives	*Stimulants*	*Hallucinogens*
Alcohol Barbiturates Benzodiazepines Opioids (codeine, methadone, morphine, heroin)	Amphetamines Caffeine Cocaine Nicotine	Cannabis Inhalants (glue, anaesthetic gases, amyl nitrite) LSD Mescaline Phencyclidine (PCP)

As with any drug, recreational drugs have adverse effects that range from the minor to the severe. One of the problems of illicit drugs is that they are not manufactured to any quality standard, and consequently adverse effects can occur from any contaminants that may be present. These constituents may be added on purpose, for example talcum powder and bathroom cleaner added to heroin to increase its bulk, or be accidental. For example in 1976, a 23-year-old attempted to manufacture some pethidine. The chemistry went wrong and he ended up injecting himself with MPTP (methylphenyltetrahydropyridine), which selectively destroys the dopamine-producing cells in the substantia nigra. Consequently, he developed severe parkinsonism three days after injecting himself, which fortunately responded to dopamine treatment.

Throughout this book in the appropriate chapters, the adverse effects of drugs of abuse have been included. However, it must be appreciated that the adverse effects of drug abuse are not just physical and psychological, but also social. For example, alcohol abuse contributes to 50% of all traffic deaths, suicides and homicides (Bartholomew, 1990). Furthermore, drug abuse can lead to dependence and the problems that that entails.

Drug dependence arises from repeated use of a drug, either continuous or intermittent use, and it can arise in both drug abusers and in those on prescribed long-term therapy, especially benzodiazepines (Seivewright, 1998). It is characterized by psychological dependence, i.e. emotional distress and craving if the drug is withdrawn, physical dependence, i.e. physical symptoms such as sweats and tremors if the drug is withdrawn, and tolerance, i.e. the need for increasing amounts of the drug in order to have the same effect. The degree to which these three characteristics are present depends on the drug type involved (Table 11.7). As well being defined in terms of withdrawal, addiction can also be defined by the three Cs: Compulsion, loss of Control, and Continued use despite adverse consequences (Anon, 1998a).

A major issue for addicts, health care professionals and the government is the treatment of addiction. The management of this problem is not just a medical one as there are many social and ethical issues involved. One possibility is to treat addiction just like any

Table 11.7 Types of drug dependence

Type	*Psychological dependence*	*Physiological dependence*	*Tolerance*
Alcohol	Severe	With prolonged heavy use	Occurs
Amfetamine (amphetamine)	Severe	Slight	Occurs
Barbiturates	Severe	Very severe	Occurs
Cannabis	Occurs	Dubious	Slight
Cocaine	Severe	Slight	Slight
Morphine	Severe	Severe	Marked
Tobacco	Strong	Slight	None

other chronic disease with long-term medication. This serves to limit the harm of addiction by helping addicts to switch from street drugs to less dangerous substitutes. The familiar example of this is the use of methadone, but it is as addictive as heroin and it requires daily clinic visits as it is metabolized within 24 hours. Other alternatives are being developed that last longer, e.g. levomethadyl acetate hydrochloride (LAAM), and are less addictive, e.g. buprenorphine (Mestel and Concar, 1994). Other therapeutic options are nicotine replacement patches and gum for smokers, disulfiram (Antabuse) which makes drinking alcohol a nauseating experience by disabling an enzyme essential for breaking down alcohol in the liver, and naloxone an antagonist of heroin which prevents the addict from experiencing any effect when using the drug. As well as pharmacological treatments there are also various behavioural therapies utilizing rewards in the form of vouchers to stay off drugs, and relaxation therapy.

A major problem of discontinuing drug usage is the withdrawal reaction that can ensue. For example delirium tremens, characterized by disorientation, hallucinations, convulsions and increased psychomotor and autonomic activity, is experienced within 48–72 hours of stopping chronic excessive alcohol intake. These very unpleasant symptoms not surprisingly serve to encourage the addict to resume their drinking. Withdrawal reactions are not confined to long-term drug use or to recreational drugs but can occur, for example, after short-term use of benzodiazepines when withdrawal leads to insomnia and anxiety. Furthermore, withdrawal reactions are not confined to drugs of addiction. For example, the antidepressants are particularly well known for causing psychological effects on withdrawal. Thus, sudden stoppage of tricyclic antidepressants can lead to symptoms of anxiety, nightmares, nausea, dizziness, headache and muscular aches, while abrupt withdrawal of monoamine oxidase inhibitors (MAOIs) can lead to delirium, auditory and visual hallucinations, and schizophreniform psychosis (Bishop and Lee, 1999). These symptoms usually arise within two weeks of stopping the drug. In the case of selective serotonin re-uptake inhibitors, sudden cessation of the drug can lead to sleep disturbances, dizziness, behavioural disturbances, tremor and dyskinesia.

It has been argued that the decriminalization of drug usage would make it appear less alluring to young people and would therefore decrease the problems of addiction. It is certainly true that pumping money into law enforcement has not made the problem of addiction go away (Concar and Spinney, 1994). The experience in Holland where cannabis use has been decriminalized for over 20 years has demonstrated that the fears that the population will become either stoned on cannabis or progress on to harder drugs is unfounded. In fact, the converse is true. Holland has fewer drug addicts per capita than Italy, Spain, Switzerland, France and Britain, and far less than the United States (Anon, 1998b). Furthermore cannabis is now believed to have a medicinal role, as it can help patients with multiple sclerosis, spinal injuries, glaucoma, cancer, epilepsy, anorexia, and the pain and nausea of chemotherapy (Shamash, 1998). Consequently, there is increasing pressure for cannabis to be legalized so that it can be used therapeutically.

One major problem for people using illicit drugs is that there is no requirement for drug companies to warn patients about the dangers of mixing prescribed drugs with illicit ones. Concar (1997) describes the case of Philip Kay a 32-year-old tax inspector who died after taking Ecstasy. His blood levels suggested that he had swallowed 22 tablets, yet his friends insisted that he had only taken two pills. They suggest that the reason for Kay's high levels of Ecstasy was that the two tablets interacted with a newly approved prescription drug called Ritonavir that Kay was taking to control his HIV. Unfortunately, although most prescribed drugs and over-the-counter medicines come with safety notices warning about potentially hazardous interactions with other prescribed medicines, pharmaceutical companies hardly ever issue warnings about mixing their products with illicit substances. Drug companies argue that if they clarify the dangers of illicit drug interactions they would be seen to be condoning drug abuse. This defence is not helpful and puts people at risk of considerable danger. This is especially true in the case of drugs used to treat HIV, as many sufferers use illegal drugs. Table 11.8 gives examples of interactions between illicit and medicinal drugs.

As well as warning people about the interactions of illicit drugs with medicinal compounds, it is also important to warn them of the adverse effects of the drugs they choose to take, and how they can minimize their effects. Table 11.5 gives an example of the advice that can be given to someone using Ecstasy.

Table 11.8 Examples of medicines that interact with illegal drugs

Medicine	*Recreational drug*	*Mechanism*
Monoamine oxidase inhibitors (MAOIs)	Ecstasy (MDMA)	MAOIs block the clearance of neurotransmitters released by MDMA
Tricyclic antidepressants	LSD	Increase brain's response, resulting in unpleasant trips
Rifampicin	Heroin and other opiates	The antibiotic increases the synthesis of an enzyme which metabolizes opiates, so causing addicts to increase their dose in order to get the same effect
Prozac, Ritonavir	Ecstasy (MDMA)	The medicinal drug inhibits the liver enzyme that metabolizes Ecstasy

References and further reading

Aldridge J, Measham F (1999) Sildenafil (Viagra) is used as a recreational drug in England. British Medical Journal 318: 669

Anon (1983) Barbiturate-induced depression in epileptic children. Nurses' Alert 7: 42

Anon (1987) Depressive reaction from an antidepressant. Nurses' Alert 11: 51

Anon (1998a) Marijuana. A safe high? New Scientist 157: 24-9

Anon (1998b) The Dutch experiment. Vraag een politieagent... New Scientist 157: 30-1

Anon (1995) Prozac-associated serotonin syndrome. Nurses' Drug Alert 19: 18

Bartholomew S (1990) Chemical dependence. Recognition and intervention. Physician Assistant 14: 15-28

Bishop S, Lee A (1998) Adverse drug reactions (10) Drug-induced mental health disorders. The Pharmaceutical Journal 261: 935-9

Brasfield KH (1991) Practical psychopharmacologic considerations in depression. Nursing Clinics of North America 26: 651-63

Bright R, Everitt D (1992) ß-blockers and depression: evidence against an association. Journal of the American Medical Association 267: 1783-7

Concar D (1997) Deadly combination. New Scientist 155:20-1

Concar D, Spinney L (1994) The highs and lows of prohibition. New Scientist 144: 38-41

Cook A (1995) Ecstasy (MDMA): alerting users to the dangers. Nursing Times 91: 32-3

Geller A (1996) Common addictions. Clinical Symposia 48: 1-32

Hall RC, Gardner ER, Sticknet SK (1980) Physical illness manifestations as psychiatric disease. Archives General Psychiatry 37: 989

Korkia P (1998) Anabolic-androgenic steroid series: part II. Psychological effects of anabolic steroid use: a review. Part 2. Journal of Substance Misuse 3: 106-13

Lane RD, Gelenberg AJ (1993) Recognizing and managing drug-induced depression. Physician Assistant 17: 62-5

Lehane M, Rees C (1996) When Ecstasy means agony. Nursing Standard 10: 24-5
McMinn B (1995) Drug-related confusion in the elderly: the role of the mental health nurse. Australian and New Zealand Journal of Mental Health Nursing 4: 22-30
Mestel R, Concar D (1994) How to heal the body's craving? New Scientist 144: 32-7
Neese JB (1991) Depression in general hospital. Nursing Clinics of North America 26: 613-22
Newbern VB (1991) Is it really Alzheimer's? American Journal of Nursing 91: 51-4
Okada F (1985) Depression after treatment with thiazide diuretics for hypertension. American Journal of Psychiatry 142: 1101-2
Rang HP, Dale MM, Ritter JM (1995) Pharmacology 3rd edn. Edinburgh: Churchill Livingstone
Seibert J (1990) Understanding chemical abuse and dependence in the elderly. Journal of Home Health Care Practice 2: 27-31
Seivewright N (1998) Theory and practice in managing benzodiazepine dependence and misuse. Journal of Substance Misuse 3: 170-7
Shamash J (1998) Purely medicinal. Nursing Standard 12: 12
Smith B, Salzman C (1991) Do benzodiazepines cause depression? Hospital and Community Psychiatry 42: 1101-2
Thompson C (1996) Malaria pill stands accused. New Scientist 150: 14-15
Travlos A, Hirsch G (1993) Steroid psychosis: a cause of confusion on the acute spinal cord injury unit. Archives of Physical Medicine and Rehabilitation 74: 312-5

Chapter 12
Effects on the skin and musculoskeletal system

Almost without exception, any drug that is taken systemically is capable of causing a skin eruption, making cutaneous eruptions the most common indication of an adverse drug reaction (Sauer and Hall, 1996). However, as the cutaneous reactions mimic many skin diseases, diagnosis can be difficult. In contrast musculoskeletal disorders only account for 3.4% of all adverse drug reactions reported to the Committee on the Safety of Medicines (Young and Lee, 1998), however they too can be difficult to diagnose.

Skin disorders

As Table 12.1 indicates, dermatological drug reactions are diverse, and they can range the entire gamut of skin disorders from acne to a fatal exfoliative dermatitis. The commonest form of adverse skin reaction is a rash and can be produced by some of the most commonly prescribed drugs. It is difficult to predict who will develop a rash, as these reactions are usually idiosyncratic, but certain factors increase the risk (Table 12.2).

Rashes

When considering whether a dermatological condition is the result of an adverse reaction it is imperative to take a full drug history including non-prescribed medicines and injections, e.g. contrast media. It is also necessary to consider the morphology and distribution of the presenting rash, although it must be appreciated that the same drug can produce different rashes in different people. The most common reaction is an exanthematous rash, which can occur any time up to three weeks after drug administration. The lesions

Table 12.1 Examples of drugs that can cause dermatological adverse effects

Disorder	*Associated drugs*
Acne	Androgens, corticosteroids, iodine, lithium, antiepileptics, antituberculous agents
Alopecia	Allopurinol, amfetamine (amphetamine), androgenic steroids, anticoagulants, cytotoxics, gold, oral contraceptives, retinoids, tricyclics
Bullae (large blisters)	ACE-inhibitors, barbiturates, chlorpropamide, sulphonamides
Contact dermatitis	Antihistamines, bacitracin, chloramphenicol, local anaesthetics, penicillins, phenothiazines, preservatives such as parabens found in some creams and paste bandages, sulphonamides
Exanthematous rash	ACE inhibitors, allopurinol, antiepileptics, cephalosporins, diuretics, hypnotics
Fixed drug eruptions	Analgesics, cephalosporins, NSAIDs, laxatives, penicillins, tetracyclines
Hirsutism	Androgens, antiepileptics, oral contraceptives
Hypertrichosis	Acetazolamide, corticosteroids, cyclosporin, interferon, penicillamine, phenytoin, psoralens, streptomycin
Lichenoid (rash that resembles lichen)	Antimalarials, ß-blockers, gold, NSAIDs
Photosensitive rashes	Amiodarone, antiepileptics, nalidixic acid, NSAIDs, phenothiazines, sulphonamides, sulphonylureas, tetracyclines, thiazide diuretics, tricyclic antidepressants
Pigmentation	Antiepileptics, oral contraceptives, tetracyclines, vitamin A
Purpura	Barbiturates, corticosteroids, salicylates, quinine, sulphonamides, sulphonylureas, thiazides
Pruritus – not associated with a rash	Alkaloids, oral contraceptives, phenothiazines, morphine, rifampicin (cholestatic reaction)
Urticarial rash	ACE-inhibitors, analgesics, antiepileptics, diuretics, H_2-histamine antagonists, NSAIDs, penicillins

Table 12.2 Factors that increase the risk of developing a rash

Patient	Female, elderly, genetics, e.g. slow acetylators
Disease	Hepatic and renal disease, systemic lupus, AIDS
Drug	Cross-sensitivity, polypharmacy (four drugs or more)

may be morbilliform (measles-like), rubelliform (German measles-like), or scarlatiniform (scarlet fever-like) or may be macular (flat spots) or papular (raised spots). The eruption is usually symmetrical and found on the trunk and extremities, including the palms, soles and interdigital areas (Roberts and Bunker, 1993a). The rash may be accompanied by an erosive stomatitis, and if the drug is continued, an exfoliative dermatitis may develop.

Urticarial rashes, or hives, present as smooth, elevated patches (weals) that are redder or whiter than the surrounding skin and sometimes they are surrounded by a halo. They usually cause severe itching. Angio-oedema is a similar eruption, but the oedematous areas are larger and deeper, involving the subcutaneous as well as dermal layers. Drugs are the most frequently identified cause of urticaria, and so a drug reaction should always be sought (Durgin, 1983). They may be the result of a pseudo-allergic reaction to codeine and aspirin that results in mast cell degranulation, or a type I or type II hypersensitivity reaction, as described in Chapter 5.

Fixed drug eruptions are round, well-demarcated, erythematous plaques that are associated with local pigmentation. They develop between 30 minutes and eight hours after drug administration. The reddish lesions turn brown and blistering may follow. The lesions heal with crusting and scaling and are followed by persistent pigmentation. The hands, feet, genitalia and perianal areas are common sites, while the limbs are more common than the trunk. The reaction recurs at the same body site with re-administration of the drug.

Lichen planus is an uncommon, chronic, pruritic disease characterized by violaceous flat-topped papules that have a shiny hyperkeratotic lichenified surface. The lesions are typically seen on the flexor aspects of the limbs, particularly of the wrists and the legs. Mucous membrane lesions on the cheeks or lips are whitish. Rashes with many of the features of lichen planus can occur in patients taking the three 'Cs' – chloroquine, chlorpropamide, chlorothiazide – as well as the drugs in Table 12.1.

Photosensitivity rashes may be phototoxic or photoallergic. The former are common and can be produced by sufficient exposure to the drug, particularly tetracyclines, chlorpromazine, and psoralens, combined with ultraviolet light, in most people (Roberts and Bunker, 1993a). The rash appears within 5–20 hours of exposure and resembles exaggerated sunburn, which is confined to areas that were exposed to light. Photoallergic reactions, in contrast, occur with 24 hours of re-exposure to the sensitizing drug, in particular phenothiazines, sulphonamides, and griseofulvin, and to ultraviolet light. Sensitization may be topical, and photocontact dermatitis may ensue, as can occur with sunscreens containing para-aminobenzoic acid. Systemic drugs can also act as sensitizers, and cross-reactivity with chemically related substances is common. Unfortunately, persistent light reactivity may occur in the absence of the precipitating drug.

Acne

Drug-induced acneiform eruptions (blackheads and whiteheads) usually begin within a week of exposure to the offending drug. Androgens act as a stimulus to sebaceous gland development and secretion, and so women who take oral contraceptives, which contain androgenic stimuli from progesterone may develop an acneiform condition (Durgin, 1983). Post-pill acne has also been noted in women on discontinuation of oral contraceptives. Iodine, bromine, and related compounds may cause acneiform eruptions, and as these are found in many multivitamin and mineral preparations, long-term use of these supplements can precipitate an inflammatory acne. Iodides are also present in some sedatives, in asthma and cold preparations and in thyroid medication. Management is by drug withdrawal, but where this is not possible, the drug-induced eruption can be counterbalanced by 250 mg of tetracycline twice daily, together with a simple topical application such as a preparation containing 2.5% or 5% benzoyl peroxide.

Purpura

Purpura is a deposit of blood or blood pigment in the skin. It can occur as a result of inhibition of the clotting process, in particular inhibition of platelet activity or thrombocytopenia, or of inflammation of skin blood vessels (vasculitis), or be due to shearing of the capillaries due to defective supporting connective tissue. The last commonly occurs in the elderly as a part of altered collagen synthesis, as well as being an adverse drug effect, particularly seen with long-term corticosteroid treatment.

Blisters

Blisters or bullae are raised fluid-filled lesions that may occur as an adverse drug effect. They may be localized and develop rapidly, as in the case of allergic reactions to topical medications, or they may be widespread. Fixed drug eruptions can develop bullae, as indicated above, and some drugs can cause a generalized bullous eruption, especially barbiturates (particularly in overdose), captopril, furosemide (frusemide) (may be phototoxic), penicillamine, penicillins (which produce pemphigus-like bullae), and sulphonamides. The blisters usually clear on discontinuing the drug.

Pigmentation

Drugs can cause pigmentation of the skin by either inducing hypermelanosis or through deposition of the drug or its metabolites in the skin. Melanin hyperpigmentation, which may be an adverse reaction to phenytoin or some cytotoxic drugs for example, appears slowly over many months and fades equally slowly, if at all. Drugs, or their metabolites, deposited in the skin may resolve with removal of the drug if it is rapidly metabolized but may also persist if the deposits bind to tissues. The pigmentations that can result from drug reactions are diverse. For example, the skin may appear yellow with mepacrine, orange with vitamin A, green with senna abuse, blue-grey with silver and gold salts, and blue-black in the case of lead poisoning.

Pruritus

Pruritus is a generalized term for itching of the skin, whatever the cause. It is associated with a variety of dermatological conditions including eczema, allergic reactions, lichen planus, and blistering disorders. If no dermatological lesions are present, systemic disorders must be sought, which can include endocrine disorders such as diabetes, liver and renal failure, malignancy, and parasitophobia, as well as adverse drug effects.

Contact dermatitis

The skin normally acts as an effective barrier, but if the barrier is overcome and substances penetrate the epidermis, an inflammatory response may occur, leading to epidermal damage and possibly contact dermatitis. This may simply be due to an irritant effect, or may be due to an allergic response to a specific substance acting as a sensitizer.

Allergic dermatitis occurs only after previous exposure to the drug concerned; symptoms take 48–96 hours to develop after contact. Symptoms are unrelated to the quantity of the allergen, and they may develop both at the site of contact with the allergen as well as in areas that were previously sensitized by drug contact. In contrast, in irritant dermatitis there is no predictable time interval between contact and the appearance of symptoms. Dermatitis occurs soon after exposure, and the severity varies with the quantity, concentration, and length of exposure to the drug concerned.

Although the clinical appearance of both allergic and irritant dermatitis may be similar, there are differences that help to distinguish them. Allergic dermatitis or eczema tends to produce erythema, oedema and vesicles, with the more chronic lesions being lichenified. Irritant dermatitis may present as slight scaling and itching or extensive epidermal damage resembling a superficial burn.

Allergic dermatitis is a particular problem in patients with venous leg ulcers. Many of the preparations used to treat these ulcers contain chemicals that may act as sensitizers, e.g. neomycin, lanolin, formaldehyde, parabens, tars, clioquinol or chlorquinaldol (the 'C' of many proprietary steroids). Chloramphenicol and sulphonamides from ophthalmic preparations can also cause dermatitis around the eyes. Nurses and pharmacists who prepare and administer penicillin injections and dentists who prepare and administer local anaesthetics are often susceptible to contact dermatitis caused by these agents.

Porphyrias

The synthesis of haemoglobin in the haemopoietic organs of the liver and bone marrow is a complex process involving a series of enzyme-controlled chemical reactions. Genetic abnormality of a single enzyme in the synthetic pathway means that haem is not produced and that the chemical the enzyme should have acted upon accumulates, leading to various toxic effects, depending on the particular enzyme abnormality involved. As the chemicals involved in haem synthesis are porphyrins, the group of genetic diseases are referred to as porphyrias, with specific names depending on the enzyme affected, e.g. acute intermittent porphyria, variegate porphyria, porphyria cutanea tarda. The symptoms of the disease depend upon the particular genetic abnormality, and consist of both cutaneous and extra-cutaneous manifestations. If porphyrins collect in the skin, they can cause skin fragility leading to blisters from exposure to the sun or minor trauma. They can also cause severe photosensitivity, even to long wavelength ultraviolet light that penetrates window glass, as they absorb light energy, which damages the tissues, leading to oedema, scarring and thickening. Another symptom of the disease is excessive hair growth on the forehead, cheeks and arms, and this together with being nocturnal and disfigured may be the origin of the werewolf legend (Billett, 1988).

The nervous system is also sensitive to excessive porphyrins and ALA synthase (the first enzyme in the biosynthetic pathway), and these may cause variable psychiatric and neurological symptoms, including acute abdominal pain, neuropathy and psychosis. King George III suffered from porphyria, which accounts for his bouts of insanity. Some porphyrins are hepatotoxic causing decreased liver function, siderosis, fatal liver disease and gallstones. Other extra-cutaneous symptoms include red teeth and haemolytic anaemia.

Drugs may cause an acute attack of porphyria in one of four ways. Firstly, some drugs may cause a decrease in the enzymes involved in haem biosynthesis, leading to a decrease in the haem, and a compensatory increase in ALA synthase. Griseofulvin may act in this way. Secondly, direct increases in ALA synthase can occur with steroids and oestrogens, which may explain why acute intermittent porphyria usually presents after puberty when these hormones are present in greater abundance. The 'oestrogen effect' may also account for premenstrual attacks of acute intermittent porphyria (Billett, 1988). A third method of increasing ALA synthase is increased breakdown of haem, which may be stimulated by iron supplements. However, the main effect is through the drug metabolizing cytochrome P450 group of enzymes, which contain haem. Consequently, drugs that induce these enzymes produce an increased demand for haem and an attempt by the body to stimulate its synthesis. Due to the absence of one of the synthetic enzymes in this pathway, porphyrins collect and cause acute attacks of porphyria. The best treatment is to avoid drugs known to precipitate acute attacks in people who suffer from porphyria (Table 12.3). Haematin infusion, which replenishes haem and so removes the stimulus for the synthetic pathway can be useful. Intravenous infusion with fructose during acute attacks of porphyria inhibits the formation of ALA-synthase, the main enzyme for regulat-

Table 12.3 Drugs associated with acute attacks of porphyria (Laurence et al., 1997)

- Alcohol
- Barbiturates
- Carbamazepine
- Chloramphenicol
- Chlordiazepoxide
- Enalapril
- Erythromycin
- Flucloxacillin
- Furosemide (frusemide)
- Griseofulvin
- Halothane
- Imipramine
- Lisinopril
- Methyldopa
- Metoclopramide
- Pentazocine
- Phenytoin
- Prilocaine
- Progesterone
- Sulfasalazine (sulphasalazine)
- Tamoxifen
- Terfenadine
- Verapamil
- Vibramycin

ing, and hence stimulating haem synthesis. Chloroquine has also been used as this drug is believed to bind hepatic porphyrins in a water-soluble complex that is excreted in urine (Demian, 1988). The use of sunscreens with UVA and UVB protection can be useful (Bielan, 1996).

Hair growth

Drugs can influence hair growth by promoting both alopecia and hirsutism. Both can be of great concern to the sufferer as alteration of hair growth can have a major impact on a person's body image, regardless of the fact that the change may be temporary.

Hair loss (alopecia) has many causes, and it is necessary to observe the scalp to see whether the hair loss is diffuse or patchy, and whether or not the scalp appears scarred. Drug-induced alopecia is usually of the diffuse, non-scarring type. It occurs when the normal development of hair and follicle is interfered with resulting in inadequate growth and the hairs being shed earlier than usual. Alopecia is clearly and dramatically associated with cytotoxic drugs, but many other drugs may induce alopecia, and a few are listed in Table 12.1. Treatment consists of stopping the drug if that is possible, after which hair normally grows back, although it may occasionally be a different colour or texture. In the meantime, a wig may help to maintain the person's body image.

Excessive hair growth can take the form of hirsutism or hypertrichosis. Hirsutism is characterized by the excessive growth of androgen-dependent terminal hairs, which are dark, thick and coarse, on the face, chest, back, abdomen, axilla and pubic regions (Azziz et al., 1998). Hypertrichosis is the excessive growth of fine, soft, light-coloured vellus hair. Drugs than can induce both forms of excessive hair growth are shown in Table 12.1. When assessing drug history, it is important to remember that surreptitious androgen use is not unknown in women athletes, especially those at a high level of competition (Griffing and Melby, 1991). Treatment is by withdrawal of the offending drug, if that is appropriate, together with some method of hair removal such as shaving, depilatories, bleaching, plucking, waxing or electrolysis.

Muscle disorders

Muscular aches and pains are common and usually the result of exercise and minor injury. However, it must be recognized that some drugs can have adverse effects on the muscular system (Table 12.4). Muscle cramps, particularly in the legs and mainly at night, can occur as a result of minor metabolic disturbances such as hyponatraemia, hypokalaemia and hypomagnesaemia. Drugs that commonly cause this problem include the loop and thiazide diuretics, calcium antagonists and oral β_2-adrenoceptor agonists such as salbutamol.

Table 12.4 Examples of drugs having adverse effects on the muscular system

Disorder	*Associated drugs*
Eosinophilia-myalgia syndrome	Tryptophan
Muscle cramps	ACE inhibitors, β_2-agonists, calcium antagonists, diuretics
Myalgia	Carbimazole, cimetidine, danazol, fibrates, statins (HMG-CoA reductase inhibitors), quinolone antibiotics, suxamethonium, zidovudine
Myopathy	Barbiturates, cimetidine, cyclosporin, danazol, diuretics, enalapril, laxatives, nalidixic acid, vincristine, zidovudine
Myositis	Penicillamine
Rhabdomyolysis	Amphotericin B, barbiturates, benzodiazepines, fibrates, statins (HMG-CoA reductase inhibitors), opioids, phenothiazines, retinoids

Myalgia (muscle pain) can occur with a number of drugs (Table 12.4). One of the main culprits is suxamethonium, which can cause myalgia in up to 50% of patients following surgery (Young and Lee, 1998). The problem seems to occur more commonly in women and it affects mainly the neck, shoulders, back and chest. Giving a small dose of a non-depolarizing muscle relaxant, e.g. vecuronium just before suxamethonium is administered can reduce the incidence and severity of the myalgia. In the case of patients who have been on the equivalent of 10 mg or more of prednisolone for more than 30 days, withdrawal of the corticosteroids can lead to severe and widespread myalgia.

Rhabdomyolysis

Minor muscular damage can occur as the result of drug usage. Local damage can occur following intramuscular injection with chlorpromazine, diclofenac, or repeated opioid injections. It is rarely severe but does lead to a spurious rise in serum creatine phosphokinase, which can confuse the interpretation of diagnostic tests.

Of more concern is rhabdomyolysis, a rare condition in which there is acute muscle damage, which results in the release of cell contents, including myoglobin, enzymes and electrolytes, into the circulation. The presenting symptom of rhabdomyolysis is muscle pain, with elevated creatine phosphokinase and myoglobinuria. Alcohol has been implicated in about 20% of cases, while drugs such as barbiturates, benzodiazepines, opioids, and phenothiazines account for most of the rest. Rhabdomyolysis may also be a complication of neuroleptic malignant syndrome (Staab, 1994) (see Chapter 5). The fibrates (e.g. bezafibrate) and statins (e.g. lovastatin), used to lower blood lipid levels, have been identified by the Committee on Safety of Medicines (1995) as a particular group of drugs for which rhabdomyolysis is a risk. The risk may be increased in renal impairment, hypothyroidism, where a fibrate and statin are used in combination, or with concurrent cyclosporin, erythromycin, or nicotinic acid treatment. Levels of creatine phosphokinase should be monitored in a patient taking a statin or fibrate with any of these interacting drugs (Pedersen and Tobert, 1996). Other drugs associated with the development of a myopathy are listed in Table 12.4, and adverse drug reactions that affect the neuromuscular junction are discussed in Chapter 10.

Eosinophilia-myalgia syndrome (EMS)

Eosinophilia-myalgia syndrome is a disabling illness associated with severe myalgia and a raised eosinophil count (more than 1.0 × 10 cells/L) (Swygert et al., 1990). Other symptoms include arthralgia, rash, cough, dyspnoea, oedema, abnormal liver function tests and fever. It has been associated with the dietary supplement L-tryptophan. The clinical course tends to be unpredictable with the majority of patients progressing to a severe and disabling illness despite stopping the L-tryptophan. In 1990, the Committee on Safety of Medicines recommended the withdrawal of products containing tryptophan. However, it has now been reintroduced for the adjunctive treatment of resistant depression. It should only be prescribed by a hospital specialist and treatment must be closely monitored.

Bone disorders

Drugs that have adverse effects upon bone do so by affecting calcium metabolism. Serum calcium homeostasis depends upon the interplay between intestinal calcium absorption and renal excretion, and bone formation and resorption. Parathyroid hormone, calcitonin, and vitamin D all regulate these processes.

Osteoporosis

Osteoporosis is a condition in which there is diminished bone mass, resulting in an increased susceptibility to fractures. It has received considerable media attention in recent years, as a complication of the menopause, but also as an adverse effect of corticosteroids. As little as 5 mg daily is enough to cause a state of net bone loss (Borg and Walker, 1994), and rates of loss are in the region of 4–10% per year (Young and Lee, 1998). Corticosteroids bring about their effect by both decreasing bone formation, because they decrease both osteoblast activity and sex hormone secretion, and by increasing bone resorption, because they reduce calcium absorption from the gut and calcium reabsorption by the kidney (Jones and Sambrook, 1994).

Patients, who require long-term corticosteroid therapy should be advised to stop smoking, limit their alcohol intake, to take regular exercise and have adequate calcium dietary intake in order to minimize the complication. Patients who have substantial bone loss due to corticosteroid treatment may be treated with bisphosphonates, nasal calcitonin or calcitriol.

Other drugs that can cause osteoporosis are shown in Table 12.5. Heparin-related osteoporosis appears to be related to both dose and duration of therapy. Symptomatic bone disease usually occurs with a daily dose of greater than 10000 U given for longer than three months (Jones and Sambrook, 1994). Bone density should be monitored in patients on long-term heparin, and it appears that bone loss may be reduced by use of low weight molecular weight heparin, and possibly vitamin D and calcium supplements. Bone loss appears reversible, with 70% of patients having radiological improvement 6–12 months after ceasing heparin (Dahlman et al., 1990).

Table 12.5 Examples of drugs having adverse effects on the bones

Disorder	*Associated drugs*
Avascular bone necrosis	Corticosteroids
Idiopathic skeletal hyperostosis	Retinoids
Osteomalacia	Aluminium salts, barbiturates, bisphosphonates, phenytoin, total parenteral nutrition
Osteoporosis	Corticosteroids, cyclosporin A, heparin, methotrexate
Osteosclerosis	Excessive intake of vitamins A and D and fluorine

In the case of the other drugs causing osteoporosis, adverse effects can be reduced by minimizing dose and duration of therapy, and it is suggested that cyclosporin G may be less toxic than its molecular analogue cyclosporin A.

Osteomalacia

Osteomalacia is a condition that results from lack of vitamin D, or a disturbance of its metabolism. Severe calcium deficiency or hypophosphataemia can also result in osteomalacia, and the characteristic symptoms of bone pain and tenderness and muscle weakness. It can result from the ingestion of large quantities of aluminium-containing antacids. Aluminium impairs bone mineralization and affects osteoblast function (due to phosphate depletion). In patients on haemodialysis, excessive aluminium in the dialysate has a toxic effect on bone mineralization with an increased risk of fracture. Use of aluminium salts to bind phosphates in chronic renal failure can also lead to osteomalacia. Osteomalacia is most common with long-term administration of barbiturates, phenytoin and carbamazepine. Bisphosphonates used to treat Paget's disease, hypercalcaemia of malignancy and osteoporosis can inhibit bone mineralization when given continuously for periods longer than 6–12 months. In addition, osteomalacia is a potential complication of long-term total parenteral nutrition (TPN) with an incidence ranging from 42–100% (Young and Lee, 1998). Possible causes include inadequate calcium and phosphate supplementation, aluminium overload and hypercalciuria.

Avascular necrosis of bone is an uncommon problem usually affecting the femoral heads. The most common iatrogenic cause is systemic steroids or ACTH, which, it has been suggested, cause vasculitis of the small blood vessels affecting the femoral head.

Osteosclerosis may result from the ingestion of excessive amounts of vitamins A and D and fluorine. Chronic vitamin D poisoning can also result in ectopic calcification of muscles, tendons and ligaments. Long-term treatment of psoriasis with retinoids has been associated with ossification disorder resembling diffuse idiopathic skeletal hyperostosis (DISH).

Joint disorders

Joint pain or arthralgia can be caused by a variety of drugs (Table 12.6), but fortunately it subsides soon after cessation of treatment. Arthralgias in the form of reactive arthropathy have also been reported in a number of patients receiving vaccination with influenza, hepatitis B and BCG. In the case of the later, cross-reaction between BCG and the HLA-B27 (an antigen found on white blood cells) has been postulated as a possible mechanism for this reaction (Borg and Walker, 1994).

Quinolone antibiotics have been linked with arthropathy, and although the mechanism has not been confirmed, this has led to restrictions in their use. They are contraindicated in children, growing adolescents and during pregnancy. The adverse effect usually affects people under 30 years of age, with an incidence around 1% (Young and Lee, 1998). Stiffness, pain and synovial swelling are the

Table 12.6 Examples of drugs having adverse effects on the joints

Disorder	*Associated drugs*
Arthralgia	ß-blockers, captopril, carbimazole, cimetidine, iron-dextran complex, phenytoin, prazosin, sulphonamides, vaccines
Arthropathy	Quinolones
Drug-induced systemic lupus erythematosus	Chlorpromazine, hydralazine, isoniazid, methyldopa, minocycline, penicillamine, procainamide, quinidine, sulfasalazine (sulphasalazine)
Gout	Alcohol, cytotoxics, cyclosporin, diuretics, ethambutol, laxative abuse, nicotinic acid, omeprazole, pyrazinamide, low-dose salicylates
Haemarthrosis	Warfarin

main symptoms which occur within a few days of starting treatment, and which usually resolve on stopping treatment.

Quinolones can also cause tendonopathy, which carries a risk of immediate, or secondary tendon rupture and prolonged disability (Hayem and Carbon, 1995). The risk is increased if the patient has renal damage or is on corticosteroids. The main site affected is the Achilles tendon although the shoulder, hand and knee have also been affected. Any patient with tendon pain who is taking quinolones should stop them immediately and rest the limb until symptoms resolve.

In patients on oral anticoagulants haemarthrosis may occur without a history of trauma, even in patients who have been well controlled for years. This is commonly due to the concurrent prescription of drugs that displace warfarin from its plasma protein binding site, e.g. the sulphonamides, or reduces its rate of metabolism, e.g. alcohol. As the number of drugs that increase the anticoagulant effect of warfarin is quite extensive it is important before prescribing a drug to a patient on warfarin to check whether an adverse interaction is known to exist.

Gout

Gout is probably the most common adverse reaction resulting in musculoskeletal manifestations. It occurs when blood levels of uric acid are raised (hyperuricaemia). This occurs because there is either an over-production of uric acid due to high cell turnover as occurs with cytotoxics, or under excretion of uric acid, which is associated with hyperlipidaemia, renal failure, alcohol consumption and some drugs (Table 12.6). Urate crystals are deposited in certain joints, especially those of the foot and elbow, stimulating an acute inflammatory reaction leading to a painful arthritis. Management involves either stopping the drug, or if that is not feasible, using a uricosuric agent such as allopurinol, together with a high fluid intake and an agent to make the urine alkaline (e.g. sodium bicarbonate), to promote urate excretion.

Drug-related systemic lupus erythematosus (D-RSLE)

This condition is becoming increasingly common and 5–10% of systemic lupus erythematosus (SLE) may be drug-induced (Young and Lee, 1998). Symptoms resemble those of SLE and include fever, arthralgia, polyarthritis, pleurisy and pericarditis, and, in 25% of sufferers, erythema of the hands and face. This may take a form ranging from a classical butterfly rash on the face to a red scaly plaque with follicular plugging and atrophy (Roberts and Bunker, 1993b). The more serious features of idiopathic lupus such as nephritis and cerebral disease are rare in drug-induced disease (Price and Venables, 1995). The syndrome develops between one month and five years after starting the drug and usually resolves when the drug is discontinued, although treatment with corticosteroids may be necessary for some patients. Hydralazine and procainamide are the most common causes of D-RSLE and patients taking these drugs long-term should have a three-monthly blood count, together with measurement of their erythrocyte sedimentation rate (ESR) and serum anti-nuclear antibodies.

References and further reading

Azziz R, Redmond G, Wheeland R, Glaser V (1998) Excessive hair growth: diagnosis and therapy. Patient Care 32: 157-68

Bielan B (1996) What's your assessment? Dermatology Nursing 8: 170-3

Billett H (1988) Porphyrias: inborn errors in heme production. Hospital Practice 23: 41-60

Borg A, Walker D (1994) Effects of drugs on the musculoskeletal system. Prescriber 5: 73-6

Committee on Safety of Medicines (1995) Rhabdomyolysis associated with lipid-lowering drugs. Current Problems in Pharmacovigilance 21: 3

Dahlman T, Lindval N, Heegren M (1990) Osteopenia in pregnancy during long-term heparin treatment. British Journal of Obstetrics and Gynaecology 97: 221-8
Demian PL (1988) Case report: porphyria cutanea tarda. Physician Assistant 12: 87-96
Durgin JM (1983) Dermatologic-drug reactions. The Journal of Practical Nursing 33: 21-5
Griffing GT, Melby JC (1991) Hirsutism. Causes and treatment. Hospital Practice 26: 43-58
Hayem G, Carbon C (1995) A reappraisal of quinolone tolerability. Drug Safety 13: 338-42
Jones G, Sambrook P (1994) Drug-induced disorders of bone metabolism. Incidence, management and avoidance. Drug Safety 1: 480-9
Laurence DR, Bennett PN, Brown MJ (1997) Clinical Pharmacology 8th edn. Edinburgh: Churchill Livingstone
Pedersen TR, Tobert JA (1996) Benefits and risks of HMG-CoA reductase inhibitors in the prevention of coronary heart disease. Drug Safety 14: 11-24
Price E, Venables P (1995) Drug-induced lupus. Drug Safety 12: 283-90
Roberts N, Bunker C (1993a) Identifying adverse drug reactions: skin (part one). Prescriber 4: 57-62
Roberts N, Bunker C (1993b) Identifying severe skin reactions to drugs. Prescriber 4: 47-50
Sauer GC, Hall JC (1996). Manual of skin diseases 7th edn. New York: Lippincott-Raven
Staab W (1994) Neuroleptic malignant syndrome: critical factors. Critical Care Nurse 14: 77-81
Swygert L, Maes E, Sewell L, Miller L, Falk H, Kilbourne E (1990) Eosinophilia-Myalgia Syndrome. Journal of the American Medical Association 264: 1698-703

Chapter 13
Effects on the reproductive system and sexuality

Loss of sexual appetite is rarely reported as a side-effect by the yellow card system, probably because general practitioners (GPs) do not enquire too closely about it and patients are even less likely to mention it. However, many drugs taken medicinally or for recreational purposes can adversely affect sexual function, as indicated in Table 13.1. This chapter will look at the effects of drugs on the reproductive system as well as the problem of drugs causing cancer. This latter problem may seem inappropriate for a chapter on sexual problems, but one of the three main mechanisms by which drugs are believed to be involved in carcinogenesis is through hormonal effects. As hormonal manipulation of the reproductive system is very common, i.e. contraception and hormone replacement therapy, it therefore seems appropriate to include carcinogenesis here.

Studying the effects of drugs on sexual appetite and performance is very difficult, as sex is as much psychological as physical. Consequently, there is considerable variation in whether sexual adverse effects are experienced (Siegel, 1982). It is also very difficult to identify whether claimed effects are the result of the drug, the disease it is being used to treat, some problem with the sexual organs themselves, or some other factor (Beaumont, 1977). For example recent studies have demonstrated that eating 7 g liquorice daily for four days can lead to an average decrease in testosterone levels of 44% (Armanini et al., 1999). Furthermore, knowledge or belief that certain drugs can interfere with sexual function can in itself lead to loss of libido and impotence (Fuentes et al., 1983).

Table 13.1 Examples of drugs having adverse effects on the male and female sexual function

Adverse effect	*Associated drugs in men*	*Associated drugs in women*
Ejaculation/orgasm	Antidepressants	Clonidine, fluoxetine
Erectile function/ vaginal lubrication	Anti-androgens, antipsychotics, cimetidine, digoxin, hypoglycaemic agents, ketoconazole, methyldopa, reserpine, thiazide diuretics, vasodilators	Labetalol, spironolactone, thiazide diuretics
Libido	CNS depressants, digoxin, oestrogenic drugs, spironolactone	CNS depressants, fluoxetine, guanethidine, methyldopa, oral contraceptive, reserpine
Spermatogenesis/ ovulation	Aminoglycosides, androgens, antimalarials, co-trimoxazole, cytotoxics, nitrofurantoin, oestrogens, progestogens, reserpine, sulfasalazine (sulphasalazine)	Drugs which increase prolactin levels, cytotoxics

It will be noted from Table 13.1 that many more drugs have been identified as affecting male sexuality in comparison with female. This is probably because the effects on men are more obvious and have also been studied more, and it seems likely that the extent of sexual dysfunction caused by drugs in women has been underestimated, rather than there being a true difference (Duncan and Bateman, 1993). Separating out the aspects of sexual function into four categories has been done for convenience, and it must be noted that this separation is somewhat artificial, as there is considerable overlap between the categories.

Libido

Libido or sexual desire is a complex psychological phenomenon. It is influenced by reproductive hormones, the emotional and physical health of the person, and the interest and sexual attractiveness of the partner. Reduction in libido is associated with many drugs that have a depressant effects on the central nervous system, including neuroleptics, lithium, benzodiazepines, and socially used agents such as alcohol. The effect is more marked if these drugs are used in combination. Libido also appears to be affected by drugs that alter hormonal function, in particular drugs that increase prolactin levels, e.g. methyldopa. However, as many of these drugs are actually centrally acting dopamine antagonists, e.g. chlorpromazine, metoclopramide, domperidone, it is not clear whether the effects on libido are primarily due to the rise in prolactin levels or the other effects of these drugs on the central nervous system.

Oestrogenic drugs are believed to reduce libido in men and this includes drugs such as digoxin and spironolactone which have a steroid structure with oestrogenic properties (Bateman, 1994). The use of anti-androgens is believed to affect the libido of both men and women. This is demonstrated by drugs such as cyproterone acetate, flutamide, and luteinizing hormone releasing hormone (LHRH) analogues, e.g. goserelin and leuprorelin, which are being increasingly used in the treatment of hormone-sensitive prostate cancer, with impotence as a common side-effect. The oral contraceptive, much blamed for releasing an epidemic of sexual licence, can in fact depress the libido in some women (Durie, 1987). In others, the freedom from worry of pregnancy has a liberating influence. A study by Shen and Hsu (1995) identified that the selective serotonin reuptake inhibitors (SSRIs) have a greater effect on female sexuality than had previously been thought. They found in a study of 33 women, that SSRIs caused loss of libido either alone in 27% of the women, or in combination with delayed orgasm in a further 27%. Fluoxetine was the worst culprit.

Erectile failure

Impotence is defined as the consistent inability to maintain an erect penis of sufficient rigidity for sexual intercourse. The process of erection involves a combination of hormonal, vascular and neurogenic factors, including the autonomic nervous system and the production of nitric oxide by the penis. Consequently, a variety of drugs can interact with the process and cause impotence or erectile failure. A study of 1180 men attending medical outpatients found that 34% were suffering with impotence, and of the 188 (47%) who agreed to be investigated for their problem, medication was thought to be the cause in 25% of cases (Slag et al., 1983).

The group of drugs most commonly associated with impotence is the antihypertensives, and this is the main reason for non-compliance with these drugs (Bansal, 1988; Slag et al., 1983). The Medical Research Council (MRC) trial of treatment for mild hypertension found impotence occurred in 13.8% of patients after 12 weeks of treatment with propranolol compared with 8.9% in the control group (Medical Research Council Working Party on Moderate Hypertension (MRCWPMH, 1981). The reason for the high incidence in the control group is probably the fact that hypertension itself causes impotence.

The mechanism by which ß-blockers cause impotence is unclear, but it has been shown that they can reduce testosterone levels. This effect is seen maximally with propranolol for which the incidence of impotence is quoted as up to 15% (Burns-Cox and Gingell, 1997). Furthermore, many hypertensive patients will have atherosclerosis and stenoses of their pelvic vessels and therefore reduced penile blood flow. ß-blockers will further reduce this flow by lowering systolic blood pressure. It has been shown that the newer ß-blockers, e.g. atenolol, metoprolol, and nadolol have a lower incidence of impotence, with obvious implications for prescribing.

Centrally acting antihypertensives, such as methyldopa and clonidine, inhibit sympathetic outflow and therefore reduce blood pressure. A study was carried out in which 381 men were treated for hypertension with 50 mg of hydrochlorothiazide and 500–2000 mg of methyldopa daily. Impotence was reported by 13% whilst the incidence of impotence was 15% for the 133 men treated with the same diuretic in combination with 0.2–1 mg of clonidine (Hogan et al., 1980).

Other drugs used to treat hypertension that are associated with impotence are the thiazide diuretics probably because they have a direct inhibitory effect on relaxation of the smooth muscle in the corpora cavernosum preventing erection (Burns-Cox and Gingell, 1997). Their effect may also be secondary to reduced intravascular volume or hypokalaemia, which they can cause. A placebo-controlled trial demonstrated a significant increase in impotence in the thiazide diuretic-treated group (Chang et al., 1991), while the Medical Research Council trial demonstrated a rate of 16.2% with bendroflumethiazide (bendrofluazide) (MRCWPMH, 1981). The less commonly used aldosterone antagonist and potassium-sparing diuretic spironolactone is associated in many reports with gynaecomastia, reduced libido and an incidence of impotence of between 4 and 30% (Brock and Lue, 1993). It is thought to act as an anti-androgen by inhibiting the binding of dihydrotestosterone to its receptor.

The use of vasodilators such as hydralazine and prazosin are also a major cause of impotence (Slag et al., 1988). In a double-blind study sexual difficulties were frequently reported after addition of prazosin or hydralazine therapy in hypertensive patients receiving thiazides and were relatively more common with prazosin (27.7%) than hydralazine (17.8%) (Veterans Administration Cooperative Study Group on Antihypertensive Agents, 1981). Conversely, 15 of the 19 hypertensive diabetic men who had been experiencing impotence on methyldopa or clonidine noted improvement of sexual function when blood pressure was controlled with prazosin (Lipson, 1984).

The antipsychotic drugs are the second main group to be associated with impotence, with rates of 25% rising as high as 60% with thioridazine (Brock and Lue, 1993). They have anticholinergic effects and consequently interfere with the parasympathetic nerve supply to the penis. This side-effect can occur within 24 hours of starting treatment and resolve when treatment ceases (MRCWPMH, 1981). Similarly, antidepressants of all classes may alter erectile function, particularly the tricyclics, e.g. imipramine and amitriptyline, and the monoamine oxidase inhibitors (MAOIs), e.g. phenelzine. The newer selective serotonin re-uptake inhibitors (SSRIs), e.g. fluvoxamine, paroxetine, sertraline have a reduced sedative and anticholinergic effect and therefore should have a lower incidence of impotence. However, some studies have suggested that sertraline causes sexual dysfunction in as many as 17% of patients who take it (Bateman, 1994).

Other drugs associated with impotence are cimetidine, which has an anti-androgenic action and is associated with gynaecomastia (Peden et al., 1979). The incidence of impotence is lower with ranitidine, which has implications for prescribing (Vian, 1983). The hypolipidaemic agent clofibrate also has an anti-androgenic action with reduced libido and impotence, while digoxin has been reported to have anti-androgenic and oestrogenic action with reduced libido and impotence in long-term use. Alkylating agents such as chlorambucil or cyclophosphamide have been associated with erectile dysfunction and reduced libido (Balducci et al., 1988). However, patients receiving these drugs are likely to be stressed by their disease and its symptoms, and it is difficult to define the role their medication plays in their impotence.

Recreational drugs can also lead to impotence. Despite the fact that advertisements for cigarettes try to imply they are 'sexy', this is not the case. Nicotine affects the smooth muscle of the vascular walls leading to vasospasm and increases the tone of erectile tissue in the corpora cavernosum thereby reducing patentcy. Long-term nicotine abuse is associated with atherosclerosis of the internal pudendal arteries involved in the blood supply to the penis, and it has been shown that smokers are twice as likely to be impotent as age-matched controls (Burns-Cox and Gingell, 1997). Furthermore, a study of 1290 men revealed that current cigarette smoking exacerbates drug effects. Current smoking increased the age-adjusted probability of complete impotence in those taking cardiac drugs (from 14 to 41%), antihypertensive medications (from 7.5 to 21%) and vasodilators (from 21 to 52%) (Feldman et al., 1994).

Alcohol also has its problems. Acute intoxication leads to sedation and transient impotence, whilst long-term use leads to liver cirrhosis and associated abnormalities of steroid metabolism. These abnormalities of metabolism result in increased levels of oestrogen and reduced testosterone levels, which in turn lead to reduced libido and associated impotence. An alcoholic polyneuropathy affecting the nerves of the penis may also occur leading to neurogenic impotence.

Not only can drugs diminish erection, they can do the reverse and cause persistent, painful erection. A number of drugs have been reported to be associated with priapism, including chlorpromazine, thioridazine, fluphenazine, pericyazine, haloperidol, and trazodone (Segraves, 1988). It is also worth noting that anticholinergic drugs such as diphenhydramine and benztropine may reverse drug-induced priapism.

Vaginal lubrication

The antihypertensive labetalol was shown to reduce vaginal lubrication significantly in a controlled study of six healthy volunteers compared with propranolol and a placebo (Riley and Riley, 1981).

However, there are no studies in patients receiving the drug therapeutically (Duncan and Bateman, 1993). Thiazide diuretics and spironolactone have also been reported to cause reduced vaginal lubrication. The effect may be due to inhibition of dihydrotestosterone binding to androgen receptors.

Alcohol is a vasodilator that can divert blood away from the genitals to the body core during arousal, and therefore it can interfere with vaginal lubrication. McEnany (1998) suggests that vaginal dryness may be associated with blockade of muscarinic cholinergic receptors and so will occur with any drugs that have antimuscarinic effects, including the tricyclic antidepressants and the monoamine oxidase inhibitors (MAOIs).

Ejaculation

Traditional antidepressants and probably SSRIs impair the process of ejaculation. This may result in retrograde ejaculation with semen passing into the bladder at orgasm and making the urine cloudy when voided. A study by Smith et al. (1984) found that among long-term users 65% believed cocaine to be an aphrodisiac while 35% felt it impaired ejaculatory ability.

Orgasm

Clonidine and methyldopa have both been reported to impair orgasm and it is certainly possible that other centrally acting agents could have a similar effect. Women taking selective serotonin reuptake inhibitors (SSRIs) such fluoxetine, and paroxetine report an inability to achieve orgasm (Vallone, 1997), whilst a controlled study by Riley and Riley (1986) demonstrated a dose relationship between diazepam and difficulty of orgasm attainment.

Spermatogenesis

Oestrogens, androgens and some progestogens can inhibit spermatogenesis. Cytotoxic drugs damage testicular function and produce oligospermia. The anti-inflammatory drug sulfasalazine (sulphasalazine) has also been shown to produce a fall in sperm count with associated infertility. Monoamine oxidase inhibitors also cause a fall in sperm count although the mechanism is not clear. Cannabis enhances sensory experiences, and so is described by some as an aphrodisiac, but it does so at the cost of disrupting sperm production and the menstrual cycle. Cimetidine, as well as leading to problems of loss of libido and impotence, has also been shown to be associated with oligospermia (Peden et al., 1979).

Ovulation

In women, drugs that increase prolactin levels may impair ovulation. Drugs known to induce hyperprolactinaemia include drugs that block dopamine receptors, e.g. phenothiazines, haloperidol, metoclopramide, or which affect dopaminergic function, e.g. methyldopa. A study of high dosage spironolactone (400 mg/day) indicated an incidence of menstrual irregularities in 100% of women (Spark and Melby, 1968). In another study six out of nine women developed amenorrhoea while on 100–200 mg/day. Normal menstruation returned within two months after spironolactone was stopped (Levity, 1970). Cytotoxic drugs also impair reproductive function.

Carcinogenesis

Carcinogenesis is the process by which healthy cells become malignant. Agents which act as carcinogens are radiation, viruses and chemicals. Carcinogenic chemicals include environmental pollutants e.g. soot, recreational drugs, e.g. tobacco smoke, and medicinal drugs e.g. cyclophosphamide. Currently, there are three main mechanisms by which drugs are believed to be involved in carcinogenesis. Firstly, chemicals act as carcinogens in a complicated multistep process, in which a chemical acts as an initiator and provokes an irreversible change in cellular DNA, whilst another, or the same, chemical acts as a promoter and modifies the expression of the altered genes. Some chemicals, called complete carcinogens, can act as both initiator and promoter whereas others – incomplete carcinogens - can only fulfil one action. Sometimes a carcinogen needs to be converted from an inactive procarcinogen to an active ultimate carcinogen. The P450 enzyme system unfortunately sometimes fulfils this function, and drugs which induce this enzyme system can therefore increase the risk of malignancy developing.

It has long been known that cytotoxic agents used in the treatment of cancer can lead to the development of a second malignancy many years after the treatment of the first. Secondary malignancies are seen especially after multi-agent chemotherapy regimens using alkylating agents in the treatment of Hodgkin's disease (Vora, 1996). Table 13.2 indicates some of the drugs known to act as carcinogens.

As well as causing mutations, some drugs can allow cancer development by suppressing the immune system. A major role of the immune system, particularly the T cells, is to destroy foreign cells, including cancer cells. It is therefore not surprising that suppression of this system with drugs such as azathioprine and corticosteroids can lead to malignancy. It has particularly been noted that there is a greatly increased risk of developing lymphomas after renal transplantation. In immunosuppressed patients there also seems to be an increased risk of cancers of the liver, biliary tree and bladder, of soft tissue sarcomas, bronchial adenocarcinoma, squamous carcinoma of the skin and malignant melanoma. There is probably an association between the occurrence of lymphoma and long-term use of phenytoin (Grahame-Smith and Aronson, 1992).

The third mechanism by which drugs may play a role in carcinogenesis is hormonal. Whether the use of hormones, in particular oestrogen, actually generate cancer formation or whether they promote the growth of tumours which are already present is not entirely clear.

Table 13.2 Drugs believed to act as carcinogens

- Busulfan (busulphan)
- Cannabis (Campbell, 1999)
- Chlorambucil
- Cyclophosphamide
- Diethylstilboesterol (Sundaram, 1995)
- Griseofulvin
- Melphalan
- Phenolphthalein–an ingredient of many laxatives
- Phenacetin

Oral contraceptives

One group of drugs that is repeatedly making the news headlines as a cause of cancer is the oral contraceptives. They have been associated with breast, endometrial, cervical and ovarian cancers as well as with the rarer liver, pituitary and skin cancers (Knowlden, 1990). The first indication that the combined oral contraceptives might have a role in breast cancer came with the study by Pike et al. (1983), which found that pills with a high progestogen potency carried a substantial risk of breast cancer. In 1992 the WHO reviewed the available research and concluded that 'there appears to be no overall association between oral contraception and the risk of breast cancer'. However, they did note that some recent studies have found a weak association between long-term use of oral contraceptives and breast cancer diagnosed before the age of 36 (Chilvers et al., 1989; Kay and Hannaford, 1988), and perhaps up to the age of 45 (Meirik et al., 1986; Schlesselman, 1989; Thomas, 1991). For example, the UK National Case-control Study Group (1989) found that of all women diagnosed with breast cancer before age 36 there was a highly significant trend in risk of breast cancer, for both parous and nulliparous women, with total duration of oral contraceptive use. Relative risks were 1.43 for 49–96 months use and 1.74 for 97 or more months. However, such cancers represent a very small proportion of all breast cancers and it is unclear whether this observed association is attributable to bias, the development of new cases of cancer, or accelerated growth of existing cancers.

The World Health Organization (1992) identifies that there is a relationship between use of combined oral contraceptives and risk of cervical squamous cell carcinoma, with a usage of more than 5 years being associated with a modest increase in relative risk ranging from 1.3–1.8 (p15). However, it is not clear whether this is a biological reaction to the pill itself, or whether it is the result of the increased sexual freedom which oral contraceptives permit. There is a strong association between cervical cancer and both the herpes simplex and the human papilloma viruses. The use of oral contraceptives means that a barrier to these viruses is not used, so increasing the risk of cancer when compared with barrier methods of contraception. Whilst considering the risk of malignancy from oral contraceptives it must be borne in mind that these drugs reduce the risk of ovarian cancer (Franklin, 1990).

Hormone replacement therapy

Case-control studies published since 1975 have demonstrated an increased risk of endometrial cancer associated with the use of exogenous oestrogen. Duration of use has been the single most important factor in determining the magnitude of the risk, with increasing risk occurring with increasing duration (Hulka, 1980). Unopposed oestrogens in the form of hormone replacement therapy and high dose sequential pills have a proliferative effect on endometrial tissue, but a course of at least 6 days per month progestogen treatment can reverse the effect of the oestrogen.

References and further reading

Armanini D, Bonanni G, Palermo M (1999) Reduction of serum testosterone in men by licorice. The New England Journal of Medicine 341: 1158

Balducci L, Phillips DM, Gearhart JG, Little DD, Bowie C (1988) Sexual complications of cancer treatment. American Family Physician 37: 159-72

Bansal S (1988) Sexual dysfunction in hypertensive men. A critical review of the literature. Hypertension 12: 1-10

Bateman N (1994) Which drugs can cause sexual dysfunction? Prescriber 5: 98-102

Beaumont G (1977) Sexual side-effects of clomipramine (Anafranil). Journal of International Medical Research 5 Supplement: 37-44

Brock GB, Lue TF (1993) Drug-induced male sexual dysfunction. Drug Safety 8: 414-26

Burns-Cox N, Gingell C (1997) Erectile dysfunction: is medication to blame? Prescriber 8: 77-80

Campbell J (1999) Cannabis: the evidence. Nursing Standard 13: 45-7

Chang SW, Fine R, Siegel D, Chesney M, Black D, Hulley SB (1991) The impact of diuretic therapy on reported sexual function. Archives of International Medicine 151: 2402-8

Chilvers C, McPherson K, Peto J, Pike MC, Vessey MP (1989) Oral contraceptive use and breast cancer risk in young women. Lancet i: 973-82

Duncan L, Bateman DN (1993) Sexual function in women. Do antihypertensives have an impact? Drug Safety 8: 225-34

Durie B (1987) Drugs and sexual function. Nursing Times 83: 34-5

Feldman HA, Goldstein I, Hatzichristou DG, Krane RJ, McKinlay JB (1994) Impotence and its medical and psychological correlates: results of the Massachusetts male ageing study. The Journal of Urology 151: 54-61

Franklin M (1990) Reassesment of the metabolic effects of oral contraceptives. Journal of Nurse-Midwifery 35: 358-64

Fuentes RJ, Rosenberg JM, Marks RG (1983) Sexual side effects. What to tell your patients, what not to say. RN 46: 35-41

Grahame-Smith DG, Aronson JK (1992). Oxford Textbook of Clinical Pharmacology and Drug Therapy 2nd edn. Oxford: Oxford University Press.

Hogan MJ, Wallin JD, Baer RM (1980) Antihypertensive therapy and male sexual dysfunction. Psychosomatics 21: 234-7

Hulka BS (1980) Effect of exogenous estrogen on postmenopausal women: the epidemiologic evidence. Obstetrical and Gynaecological Survey. Supplement 35: 389-99

Kay CR, Hannaford PC (1988) Breast cancer and the pill – a further report from the Royal College of General Practitioners' oral contraception study. British Journal of Cancer 58: 675-80

Knowlden HA (1990) The pill and cancer: a review of the literature. A case of swings and roundabouts. Journal of Advanced Nursing 15: 1016-20

Levity JL (1970) Spironolactone therapy and amenorrhoea. Journal of the American Medical Association 211: 2014-5

Lipson LG (1984) Treatment of hypertension in diabetic men: problems with sexual dysfunction. American Journal of Cardiology 53: 46-50A

McEnany G (1998) Sexual dysfunction in the pharmacological treatment of depression: when 'don't ask, don't tell' is an unsuitable approach to care. Journal of the American Psychiatric Nurses Association 4: 24-9

Medical Research Council Working Party on Mild to Moderate Hypertension (1981) Adverse reactions to bendroflumethiazide (bendrofluazide)and propranolol for the treatment of mild hypertension. Lancet 2: 540-3

Meirik O, Lund E, Adami Ho, Bergstom R, Christoffersen T, Bergs OP (1986) Oral contraceptive use and breast cancer in young women. Lancet 2: 650-4

Peden NR, Cargill JM, Browning MC, Saunders JHB, Wormsley KG (1979) Male sexual dysfunction during treatment with cimetidine. British Medical Journal 1: 659-60

Pike MC, Henderson BE, Krailo MD, Duke A, Roy S (1983) Breast cancer in young women and use of oral contraceptives: possible modifying effect of formulation and age of use. Lancet 2: 926-9

Riley AJ, Riley EJ (1981) The effect of labetalol and propranolol on the pressor response to sexual arousal in women. British Journal of Clinical Pharmacology 12: 341-4

Riley AJ, Riley EJ (1986) The effect of single dose diazepam on female sexual response induced by masturbation. Sexual and Marital Therapy 1: 49-53

Schlesselman JJ (1989) Cancer of the breast and reproductive trap in relation to use of oral contraceptives. Contraception 40: 1-38

Segraves RT 1988) Sexual side-effects of psychiatric drugs. International Journal Psychiatry in Medicine 18: 243-52

Siegel RK (1982) Cocaine and sexual dysfunction: the curse of Mama Coca. Journal of Psychoactive Drugs 14: 71-4

Shafer RB (1983) Impotence in medical clinic outpatients. Journal of the American Medical Association 249: 1736-40

Shen WH, Hsu JH (1995) Female sexual side effects associated with selective serotonin reuptake inhibitors: a descriptive clinical study of 33 patients. International Journal of Psychiatry in Medicine 25: 239-48

Slag MF, Morley JE, Elson MK, Trence DL, Nelson CJ, Nelson AE, Kinlaw WB, Beyer S, Nuttall FQ, Shafer RB (1983) Impotence in medical clinic outpatients. Journal of the American Medical Association 249: 1736-40

Smith DE, Wesson DR, Apter-Marsh M (1984) Cocaine and alcohol induced sexual dysfunction in patients with addictive disease. Journal of Psychoactive Drugs 16: 359-61

Spark RF, Melby JC (1968) Aldosteronism in hypertension. Annals of Internal Medicine 69: 685-91

Sundaram B (1995) Tackling the aftermath faced by the daughters of DES. Nursing Times 91: 34-5

Thomas DB (1991) Oral contraceptives and breast cancer: a review of the epidemiological literature. Contraception 43: 597-642

UK National Case-control Study Group (1989) Oral contraceptive use and breast cancer in young women. Lancet. i: 973-82

Veterans Administration Cooperative Study Group on Antihypertensive Agents (1981) Comparison of prazosin and hydralazine in patients receiving hydrochlorothiazide: a randomized double-blind clinical trial, Circulation 64: 772-9

Vallone DC (1997) When comforting words are not enough: SSRIs. Nursing 97 27: 50-2

Vian L (1983) Probable case of impotence owing to ranitidine. Lancet ii: 635-6

World Health Organization (1992) Oral contraceptives and neoplasia. WHO Technical Report Series 817. Geneva: WHO

Chapter 14
Drug resistance

Bacterial resistance

The discovery of penicillin in 1928 by Alexandra Fleming led on to the antimicrobial era and great optimism that infection had been conquered. However, antibiotics are losing their effectiveness, as illustrated by the fact that in 1992 13300 people died in American hospitals from bacterial infections that would not respond to antibiotics (Valigra, 1994). The main reason that antibiotics are losing their magic touch is that bacteria are developing resistance to them, and this is now a major public health threat (Department of Health, 1999). This is not a new problem, for in 1944 penicillin resistance was reported in *Staphylococcus aureus*, and by1952 75% of hospital isolates were found to be resistant to penicillin (Finland, 1955). It is however becoming an increasingly serious problem. Currently the chief drug-resistant nosocomial pathogens are methicillin resistant *S. aureus* and coagulase-negative staphylococci, vancomycin-resistant *Enterococcus faecalis* and *E. faecium*, and multidrug-resistant species *Pseudomonas aeruginosa, Stenotrophomonas maltophilia.* In May 1996 the first documented case of infection caused by a strain of *S. aureus* with intermediate levels of resistance to vancomycin was reported from Japan, and it is expected that strains of *S. aureus* with full resistance to vancomycin will emerge soon (Domin, 1998). It may thus not be long before we witness the development of nosocomial pathogens for which there are no antibiotic solutions.

The problem of resistance is not constrained to the hospital setting, for the community also has its problems of antimicrobial resistance, with the main bacterial problems being multidrug-resistant *Mycobacterium tuberculosis, Neisseria gonorrhoea*, salmonella, and penicillin-resistant *Streptococcus pneumoniae* (Swartz, 1997). Looking more globally, multidrug resistant cholera has arisen in Ecuador, while *Shigella dysenteriae* is a serious problem in Africa as one strain has become resistant to all the usual microbial treatments and is only susceptible to the fluoroquinolones which are potentially toxic (Godfrey, 1997). Resistant organisms do not stay in their country of origin, as demonstrated by multi-resistant *Salmonella typhi*, which has spread around the world (Rowe et al., 1997). Furthermore, resistance to antimicrobials is not confined to bacteria but is found in all groups of microbes. Examples of resistance in other organisms include: fungi (fluconazole-resistant *Candida* species), viruses (zidovudine-resistant HIV) and parasites (metronidazole-resistant *Trichomonas* species and chloroquine-resistant *Plasmodium falciparum*) (Cohen and Tartasky, 1997). The latter accounts for the resurgence of malaria in the past twenty years (Kain, 1993).

What is antibiotic resistance?

A microorganism can be defined as resistant if it is not inhibited or killed by a drug at concentrations of the drug achievable in the body after normal dosage (Mims et al., 1993). Some species of bacteria are naturally resistant to some families of antibiotics, because they lack the target that the drug is aimed at, or because they are impermeable to the drug. For example *Pseudomonas aeruginosa* has always been resistant to flucloxacillin (Neal, 1997). Natural resistance is not a problem, and it allows specific antibiotics to be chosen to treat specific bacterial infections without destroying all the bacteria in the body. Many bacteria found on the human body are not pathogenic and form a symbiotic relationship with us, protecting us from harmful bacteria. It is preferable when treating a patient with an infection not to kill the commensal or symbiotic bacteria. This can often be achieved by using an antibiotic which is selective for the bacteria causing the infection, rather than using a broad-spectrum antibiotic.

How does resistance develop?

In order to understand how bacterial resistance develops it is necessary to know something of bacterial anatomy. Bacterial cells are very different from human cells, which is fortunate because it is the differences that are targeted by antibiotics. If there were no differences between bacterial and human cells, it would be very difficult to kill the bacteria causing the infection without harming the person in which they are growing. One of the main differences between human and bacterial cells is the genetic material. In mammalian cells, the genetic material is found in the nuclei in the form of chromosomes. Bacteria do not have nuclei and their genetic material is contained in the cytoplasm as chromosomal deoxyribonucleic acid (DNA) and as plasmids. The latter are small circles of DNA containing genetic information not required for growth and replication.

A bacterium may develop resistance either by chromosomal mutation and selection, or by plasmid transfer. Mutation involves a chance change in the genetic code of the chromosome. Because of the alteration in the genetic code an abnormal protein is formed. Usually the abnormal protein is harmful and the bacterium dies. However, bacteria can double in number every twenty minutes, so from the millions of bacteria that can be produced from one parent in a few days, there is a good possibility that one of these mutations gives rise to a useful protein. If this new protein protects the bacterium from a particular antibiotic, the bacterium is resistant. For example, the production of an altered ribosomal protein accounts for the resistance of some bacteria to streptomycin (Friedland and McCraken, 1994).

Plasmid determined resistance is more common than chromosomal resistance, possibly because genes located on plasmids may evolve independently of the chromosome, and genes carried on plasmids are intrinsically more mobile than those on chromosomes. Some plasmids are indiscriminate and cross species barriers so that the same resistance gene is found widely in different species. For example, studies by Salyers (Wuethrich, 1994) showed that the gene for tetracycline resistance has been transferred from bacteria that live in the guts of pigs, sheep and cows to distantly related intestinal and periodontal bacteria living in the human gastro-intestinal tract.

Plasmid based resistance may be transferred to other bacteria by three mechanisms, namely conjugation, transformation, and transduction. Conjugation involves cell to cell contact whereby DNA is transferred from a donor bacterium to a recipient via a cytoplasmic bridge called a sex pilus. Many Gram-negative and some Gram-positive bacteria, notably streptococci, staphylococci and clostridia are able to conjugate. Conjugation is probably significant in the dissemination of resistance genes among bacteria that are normally found at high population density and hence are likely to come into frequent contact with each other, e.g. *Enterobacteriaceae*.

Transformation is a process whereby bacteria are able to take up naked DNA and incorporate it into their genome. In general, bacteria do not discriminate foreign DNA during the uptake process. Consequently, transformation is an ideal mechanism for transferring useful genes across generic boundaries in the laboratory and in genetic engineering. There is some evidence that gonococci, which are highly transformable, can become transformed simply by growing donor and recipient bacteria in mixed laboratory culture. Although transformation occurs naturally in some species, there is no convincing evidence that it is important clinically in the dissemination of resistance, but it is conceivable that transformation may occasionally allow resistance genes to enter new species (Saunders, 1984).

Transduction is the transfer of genes by bacteriophages, a type of virus that infects bacteria. As part of their replication cycle the virus may pick up pieces of DNA from one bacterium and transfer them to another bacteria, generally a related species. There is evidence that transduction plays a significant role in the natural transmission of resistance genes between strains of *Staphylococcus aureus* and between strains of *Streptococcus pyogenes* (Saunders, 1984).

The mechanism of resistance

Antibiotics are bacteriostatic or bactericidal and they generally exert their effect through one of five mechanisms (Table 14.1). Bacteria develop resistance to antibiotics either by altering the target site of the drug, inhibiting its access to the target site, or by production of enzymes that inactivate the drug (Kelly and Chivers, 1996). For example, in order to damage bacteria antibiotics usually need to enter the cell to have an effect. Consequently, if the access of the drug can be inhibited the bacteria will be resistant. This can be achieved by increasing the impermeability of the cell wall or by pumping the drug out of the cell. This mechanism is found in Gram-negative cells where betalactams, e.g. penicillins and cephalosporins, gain access to their target enzymes by diffusion through porins in the outer cell membrane. Mutations in porin genes result in a decrease in permeability of the outer membrane and hence resistance. Bacterial strains that have become resistant through this mechanism may exhibit cross-resistance to unrelated antibiotics which use the same porins.

Table 14.1 Mechanisms of action of antibiotics (Walters 1988, 1989, 1990, 1993)

Mechanism of action	*Examples*
Prevent formation of cell wall	Carbapenems, cephalosporins, penicillins, vancomycin
Alter permeability of cell membrane	Cyclic polypeptides, polyene antifungals
Interfere with protein synthesis	Aminoglycosides, chloramphenicol, erythromycin, tetracyclines
Interfere with nucleic acid synthesis	Rifampicins, quinolones
Interfere with cell metabolism	Sulphonamides, trimethoprim

Another highly topical example is methicillin-resistant *Staphylococcus aureus* (MRSA). These bacteria use enzymes termed 'penicillin binding proteins' (PBP), which are important in the final stages of cross-linking the building blocks of the bacterial cell wall. Antibiotics such as penicillin work by blocking these enzymes. Resistant species such as MRSA synthesise an additional penicillin binding protein that has a much lower affinity for the antibiotics than the normal enzyme. Consequently the bacteria are able to continue cell wall synthesis even when other penicillin binding proteins are inhibited (Mims et al., 1993).

Selecting for resistance

Once one bacterium has become resistant to an antibiotic, it will spread this resistance on to its offspring, as well as to other bacteria through plasmid transfer. However, the making of an abnormal protein is often costly to a bacterium and so in straight competition with other bacteria without the abnormal protein it will often not survive. However, if antibiotic is added to the environment the resistant bacteria will have a selective advantage. This means that the antibiotic will kill the surrounding non-resistant bacteria, while the resistant bacteria will be free to multiply, without competition for food and space. The resistant bacteria will then become common in the environment. It can thus be seen that the use of antibiotics can actually encourage the development of resistant bacteria.

The use of antibiotics has greatly increased in recent years particularly in intensive care units (Amyes and Thomson, 1995). This is because developments in medical procedures have been advancing at an unparalleled rate, and many of these procedures require the immunosuppression of the patient. Such patients must be protected against bacterial infection, so explaining the increased need for antibiotics. However, although there has been a genuine need to increase the antibiotics used, the problem of resistance has been aggravated by the misuse and overuse of antibiotics. For example, a survey in 1974 noted that 24% of patients given antibiotics had no evidence of infection (Cooke et al., 1980). Furthermore, researchers at the Centres for Disease Control and Prevention have estimated that some 50 million of the 150 million outpatient prescriptions for antibiotics each year are unneeded (Levy, 1998). The reasons for antibiotic abuse are varied and examples are given in Table 14.2.

Table 14.2 Examples of antibiotic abuse

- Use of potent broad-spectrum agents for prophylaxis and treatment of infections (Goldmann and Huskins, 1997)
- Unjustifiably prolonged courses of treatment and prophylaxis (Holzheimer et al. 1997; Sanderson, 1984)
- Needless treatment of colonization, e.g. acute bronchitis in otherwise healthy people (Cohen et al., 1997)
- Use of antibiotics such avoparcin, which is closely related to vancomycin, in treating livestock (Bonner, 1997; Coghlan, 1996)
- Treatment of viral infections with antibiotics (Levy, 1998)
- Topical use of systemic antibiotics (Lear, 1995)
- Partial treatments of infections due to non-compliance, or inadequate supplies of antibiotics, as are found in some third world countries (Jordan and Tait, 1999)

Antibiotics are not the only antimicrobial substances being overexploited today. Use of disinfectants and antiseptics has also rocketed, and resistance has developed to antiseptics such as chlorhexidine (Morgan, 1993) and the antimicrobial silver (Wright et al., 1998). Historically these substances have been used in hospitals for cleansing purposes, but more recently substances such as triclocarbon, triclosan and quaternary ammonium compounds such as benzalkonium chloride have been added to soaps, detergents and impregnated into such items as toys, mattress pads and cutting boards (Levy, 1998).

Prevention of bacterial resistance

Unfortunately the problem of antimicrobial resistance is not high on the strategic agenda of many hospitals, which is surprising given the costs and consequences of infectious diseases due to these microorganisms (Goldmann and Huskins, 1997). Furthermore, the Chief Medical Officer of Scotland predicts that we will have run out of antibiotics by the year 2020 (Kendell, 1994). Scientists are working hard to find new drugs to fight infection (Ellis and Pillay, 1996; Gavaghan, 1999), but as there are unlikely to be any completely novel antibiotics in the near future (Amyes and Thomson, 1995) solutions to the problem of bacterial resistance must be found.

The most effective and least expensive way to prevent and curb resistance is to use antibiotics appropriately and for as short a time as possible, thereby reducing their overall selective effects (Levy, 1991). The value of this approach is demonstrated by a hospital that reduced its usage of erythromycin from a total of 3.3 kg in 1958 to 0.3 kg in 1959. Due to the reduced antibiotic usage, the frequency of erythromycin resistance in *S. aureus* fell from 18% to 3% (Ridley et al., 1970). Equally important is the early detection of resistant organisms and prevention of their cross-infection. Cross-infection can be partly achieved by the dedicated use of non-critical-care items such as stethoscopes (Jones et al., 1995), electronic thermometers, and pens (French et al., 1998) for individual colonized or infected patients. In addition, barrier methods have a role to play, with a literature review identifying that the use of occlusive dressings, rather than conventional dressings, could reduce the wound infection rate from 7.1% to 2.6% (Hutchinson and McGuckin, 1990). There must also be increasing emphasis on good hygiene, especially handwashing, and on giving holistic client care so as to promote an active immune system, which will prevent infection and minimize the need to use antibiotics. Increased education of all members of the multidisciplinary team, including the patient, on how to prevent and treat infection correctly would also serve to ameliorate the problem (Freeman, 1997). Finally, there must be increased research and development into vaccines as these offer the best hope for reducing, on a world-wide basis, the appalling toll of death from infectious diseases, and they far outstrip antibiotics in cost-effectiveness (Beardsley, 1995).

Resistance to cytotoxics

Microorganisms are not alone in being resistant to drugs; cancers can also be resistant. Just as in the case of bacterial resistance, cancers cells may have primary resistance, i.e. the tumour has never been chemosensitive, e.g. melanoma, colorectal carcinoma; or secondary resistance, where the tumour is initially chemosensitive but subsequently becomes resistant, e.g. small cell lung carcinoma, ovarian cancer, metastatic breast cancer. Drug resistance can be caused by a variety of cellular mechanisms as indicated in Table 14.3.

Table 14.3 Mechanisms by which tumour cells become cytotoxic-resistant (Adapted from Vora, 1996)

Cellular changes	*Effect*
Altered cell membranes leading to impaired drug transport into the cell or to pumps for drug removal. Increased activity of enzymes that inactivate drug. Loss of drug activation enzymes.	Decreased intracellular drug accumulation
Increased production of drug target molecules. Alteration in target enzyme specificity. Production of non-essential competitors that bind and inactivate drug.	Altered drug targets
Alteration in biochemical pathways that bypass blocked enzymes. Increased DNA repair.	Repair of cytotoxic damage

To date the best understood form of resistance involves the multidrug resistance gene MDR1, which was identified ten years ago and found to encode a protein called phosphoglycoprotein (PGP). This is a plasma membrane protein that is found in many normal cells and fulfils a detoxifying function by pumping harmful substances (especially chemotherapeutic agents) out of the cell. It is particularly active against substances derived from plants, e.g. anthracyclines (doxorubicin, daunorubicin), epipodophyllotoxins (etoposide, teniposide), vinca alkaloids (vincristine, vinblastine), and taxanes (paclitaxel, docetaxel) (Rieger, 1997). The expression of PGP is increased in many cancer cells and may correlate with poor response to chemotherapy.

Research has shown that the PGP pump can be inhibited by a variety of structurally unrelated drugs including cyclosporin, nifedipine, verapamil and tamoxifen (Davidson, 1997). These drugs are being used in combinations with chemotherapy in order to block PGP and reverse this type of drug resistance. There have been encouraging effects in the case of blood cancers, but not that of solid tumours.

Other methods of minimizing drug resistance include starting cytotoxic treatment as early as effectively possible so that resistant tumour cell clones do not develop. In addition, the use of combination chemotherapy with a variety of cytotoxic drugs that have different killing modes will help to avoid selection of resistant clones.

References and further reading

Amyes SGB, Thomson CJ (1995) Antibiotic resistance in the ICU. The eve of destruction. British Journal of Intensive Care 5: 263-71

Beardsley T (1995) Better than a cure. Scientific American 272: 88-95

Bonner J (1997) Hooked on drugs. New Scientist 153: 24-27

Coghlan A (1996) Animal antibiotics 'threaten hospital epidemics'. New Scientist 151: 7

Cohen M, Rex JH, Anderson D (1997) Wise antibiotic use in the age of drug resistance. Patient Care 31: 165-78

Cohen FL, Tartasky D (1997) Microbial resistance to drug therapy: a review. American Journal of Infection Control 25: 51-64

Cooke D, Salter AJ, Phillips I (1980) Antimicrobial misuse, antibiotic policies and information resources. Journal of Antimicrobial Chemotherapy 6: 435-43

Davidson TG (1997) Modulation of P-glycoprotein-induced multidrug resistance in oncology. Cancer Practice 5: 58-61

Department of Health (1999). Resistance to antibiotics and other antimicrobial agents. Health Service Circular HSC 1999/049 5 March

Domin MA (1998) Highly virulent pathogens – a post antibiotic era? British Journal of Theatre Nursing 8: 14-18

Ellis R, Pillay D (1996) Antimicrobial therapy: towards the future. British Journal of Hospital Medicine 56: 145-50

Finland M (1955) Changing patterns of resistance of certain common pathogenic bacteria to antimicrobial agents. New England Journal of Medicine 252: 570-80

Freeman CD (1997) Antimicrobial resistance: implications for the clinician. Critical Care Nursing Quarterly 20: 21-35

French G, Rayner D, Branson M, Walsh M (1998) Contamination of doctors' and nurses' pens with nosocomial pathogens. Lancet 351: 213

Friedland IR, McCraken GH (1994) Management of infection caused by antibiotic-resistant Streptococcus pneumonia. New England Journal of Medicine 331: 377-82

Gavaghan H (1999) To kill a superbug. New Scientist 161: 34-7

Godfrey K (1997) The bugs they couldn't kill. Nursing Times 93: 24-37

Goldmann DA, Huskins WC (1997) Control of nosocomial antimicrobial-resistant bacteria: a strategic priority for hospitals worldwide. Clinical Infectious Diseases 24 (Suppl 1): 139-S145

Holzheimer RG, Haupt W, Thiede A, Schwarzkopf A (1997) The challenge of postoperative infections: does the surgeon make a difference? Infection Control and Hospital Epidemiology 18: 449-56

Hutchinson JJ, McGuckin M (1990) Occlusive dressings: a microbiologic and clinical review. American Journal of Infection Control 18: 257-68

Jones JS, Hoele D, Riekse R (1995) Stethoscopes: a potential vector of infection. Annals of Emergency Medicine 26: 296-9

Jordan S, Tait M (1999) Antibiotic therapy. Nursing Standard 13: 49-54

Kain KC (1993) Antimalarial chemotherapy in the age of drug resistance. Current Opinion in Infectious Diseases 6: 803-11

Kelly J, Chivers G (1996) Built-in resistance. Nursing Times 92: 50-4

Kendell R (1994) From the Chief Medical Officer. Health Bulletin 1994: 311-2

Lear J (1995) Properties and uses of topical antimicrobials. Prescriber 6: 21-37

Levy S (1998) The challenge of antibiotic resistance. Scientific American 278: 32-9

Levy S (1991) Antibiotic availability and use: consequences to man and his environment. Journal of Clinical Epidemiology 44 (Supp II): 83-7S

Mims C, Playfair J, Roitt I, Wakelin D, Williams R (1993) Medical Microbiology. London: Mosby

Morgan D (1993) Is there a role for antiseptics? Journal of Tissue Viability 3: 80-4

Neal MJ (1997) Medical Pharmacology at a Glance 3rd ed. Oxford: Blackwell

Rieger PT (1997) Emerging strategies in the management of cancer. Oncology Nursing Forum 24: 728-37

Ridley M, Lynn R, Barrie D, Stead KC (1970) Antibiotic-resistant Staphylococcus aureus and hospital antibiotic policies. Lancet i: 230-3

Rowe B, Ward LR, Threfall EJ (1997) Multidrug resistant Salmonella typhi: a worldwide epidemic. Clinical Infectious Diseases 24(suppl): 106-S109

Sanderson PJ (1984) Common bacterial pathogens and resistance to antibiotics. British Medical Journal 289: 638-9

Saunders JR (1984) Genetics and evolution of antibiotic resistance. Medical Bulletin 40: 54-60

Swartz MN (1997) Use of antimicrobial agents and drug resistance. New England Journal of Medicine 337: 491-2

Valigra L (1994) Engineering the future of antibiotics. New Scientist 142: 25-7

Vora AR (1996) Problems associated with treating cancer. Journal of Cancer Care 5: 141-9

Walters J (1988) How antibiotics work. Professional Nurse 3: 251-4

Walters J (1989) How antibiotics work: the cell membranes. Professional Nurse 4: 509-10

Walters J (1990) How antibiotics work: nucleic acid. Professional Nurse 5: 641-3

Walters J (1993) How antibiotics work: protein synthesis. Professional Nurse 8: 788-91

Wright JB, Lam K, Burrell RE (1998) Wound management in an era of increasing bacterial antibiotic resistance: a role for topical silver treatment. American Journal of Infection control 26: 572-7

Wuethrich B (1994) Migrating genes could spread resistance. New Scientist 144: 9

Part 2
The Art of Adverse Drug Effects

Chapter 15
Nurse administration and prescribing

Drug administration and errors

Medication errors can be defined as preventable prescribing, dispensing or administration mistakes (Cousins and Upton, 1993); they are frighteningly common events. In the community, drug errors are the commonest cause of negligence claims against GPs. A report issued in June 1996 by the Medical Defence Union found that a quarter of claims against its members were directly related to errors in prescribing, monitoring and administering medicines. In UK hospitals around 1 in 20 doses is given incorrectly or omitted (Table 15.1), and in one week in the North Thames Region, pharmacists intercepted over 900 prescribing errors that they thought could have resulted in severe morbidity or death (Barber and Dean, 1998). However, as few outcome studies have been carried out in this country it is hard to know how much harm would have actually occurred. Outcome studies are common in the USA. An examination of all US death certificates between 1983 and 1993 identified that there has been a 2.6-fold increase in deaths from medication errors (from 2876 in 1983 to 7391 in 1993), with 1195 of the deaths in 1993 being inpatient deaths (Phillips et al., 1998).

A review of coroner's records in Birmingham concluded that about a fifth of deaths relating to prescribing and administering drugs were due to errors, and that these are more easily prevented than deaths due to adverse drug reactions (Ferner and Whittington, 1994). In order to develop safer systems it is necessary to establish the risks of the current system, however, it is not known how many medication errors really occur within most hospitals in the UK as there is considerable under-detection and under-reporting (Cousins

Table 15.1 Observation-based studies of medication administration errors in UK hospitals

Study	*Doses observed*	*Error rate*
Dean et al., 1995	2756	3.0%
Ridge et al., 1995	3312	3.5%
Gethins, 1996	2000	3.2%
Cavell and Hughes, 1997	1206	5.7%
Ho et al., 1997	2170	5.5%
Ogden et al., 1997	2973	5.5%
Taxis et al., 1998	842	8.0%

and Upton, 1993). Methods for detecting medication errors include anonymous self-reports (questionnaires), incident reports, a critical incident technique (analysis of a large number of individual errors to identify common causal factors), and direct observation (including the disguised-observation and participant-observer techniques) (Allan and Barker, 1990). Of these methods, the most practical for day-to-day use is encouraging staff to complete incident forms to document errors and near misses. However, staff are not happy to admit to drug errors, as the response by management, particularly in the case of nurses, is often punitive (Bassett, 1998). This is not a helpful response as it means that errors are covered up, rather than reported (Arndt, 1994), and it is a response criticized by the UKCC (1996a). Thus a no-fault reporting system is required (Carlisle, 1996).

Nurses are held responsible for detecting prescription or dispensing errors made by doctors and pharmacists (Baker and Napthine, 1994). If they detect these mistakes then no medication error has occurred; if they fail to detect the mistake then the medication error is theirs for they have given the wrong medication to the patient. Why should a nurse be accountable for the errors of others? Research clearly identifies that medication errors occur as a result of the system, rather than the individual, hence analysis and correction of underlying systems faults is more likely to result in enduring changes and significant error reduction (Leape et al., 1995). For example, Ho et al. (1997) found that the predominant cause of medication administration error in their study, in common with many other studies, was omission of drugs. The solutions suggested evolved around matters of procedure, and included alteration in drug delivery times and restocking procedures.

It is time that hospitals recognize that human error is inevitable and must be anticipated, no matter how knowledgeable and careful health care workers are. A technique developed in the aerospace industry and known as 'failure mode and effects analysis' involves identifying mistakes that will happen before they happen, and determining whether the consequences of those mistakes would be tolerable or intolerable. Where potential effects are unacceptable actions are taken to eliminate the possibility of error, trap error before it reaches a patient or minimize the consequences of the error when potential errors cannot be eliminated. This approach could be applied to drug management in order to prevent errors (Cohen et al., 1994). For example, potassium chloride for injection concentrate in vials of 20 mEq/20 mL, has been involved in more fatal medication errors than any other drug (Davis, 1995). Failure mode and effects analysis identifies the answer to this problem as removal of the possibility of error. This is achieved by removing potassium chloride for injection concentrate from ward environments and stocking minibags of potassium chloride injection 20 mEq/100 mL instead.

Ten categories of medication errors have been defined by the American Society of Hospital Pharmacists (Table 15.2), while research has identified a variety of sources of serious medication errors (Table 15.3) and potential solutions have been sought (Table 15.4). Some of these solutions may be transferable from other institutions, but as we are dealing in human systems, beliefs and values, each institution will have to look at its own practices and identify ways forward. One potential method for improvement is the use of computers. If nothing else these should reduce errors by getting rid of mistakes resulting from doctors' illegible handwriting (Lyons et al., 1998), and if an 'intelligent' system is utilized then prescribing errors should also be reduced. However, in their study Cavell and Hughes (1997) showed only a 0.2% reduction in error of computerized over manual prescribing. This is perhaps not surprising, as the majority of the mistakes observed in their study were errors of omission.

As the main administrators of drugs, nurses have an important role to play in reducing errors. Cavell (1998) found that qualified nurses' knowledge of drugs and drug management was poor, but improved with educational input. Gladstone (1995) suggests that

Table 15.2 The American Society of Hospital Pharmacists' Categories of Medication Errors (ASHP, 1993)

Category	*Definition*
Prescribing	Errors in dose, dosage form, quantity, route, concentration, rate of administration, directions for use; incorrect drug selection based on indications, contraindications, known allergies, and existing drug therapy
Omission	The patient fails to receive medication by the time of the next scheduled dose. (A patient's refusal to take the medication is not considered an error of omission)
Wrong time	The patient does not receive his medication within a predefined time interval (this interval should be established by each individual health care facility)
Unordered drug	A patient receives a drug that has not been authorised for him by a legitimate prescriber, e.g. a dose for another patient, an incorrect drug
Improper dose	A patient receives a dose greater or less than the amount prescribed, or duplicate doses are administered to the patient
Wrong dosage-form	Administration of a drug to the patient in a form different from that prescribed, e.g. an intramuscular dose rather than an intravenous dose
Wrong drug preparation	Errors in preparation or manipulation of a drug prior to administration, including errors of reconstitution and dilution, combining drugs that are incompatible, failure to protect the drug from light
Wrong administration technique	Drugs administered via the wrong route, via the right route but wrong site, e.g. left eye instead of right eye, via the correct route but incorrectly administered, e.g. a bolus instead of a slow infusion
Deterioration of drug	The physical or chemical integrity of the medication has been compromised, including expired drugs and medications that require refrigeration that are stored at room temperature
Monitoring error	Failure to review a prescribed regimen for appropriateness, or failure to use appropriate clinical or laboratory data to instruct prescribing, e.g. treating infection with antibiotics without finding the causative organism

Table 15.3 Common causes of medication errors

- Look-alike packaging (Knowles, 1998)
- Similar drug names, e.g. carbimazole and carbamazepine (Boyce, 1998)
- Use of abbreviations, e.g. AZT – zidovudine or azathioprine (Ambrosini et al., 1992)
- Illegible handwriting (Lyons et al., 1998)
- Duplicate prescribing, e.g. drug prescribed both as a 'regular' and 'as required' (Gethins, 1996)
- Trailing zeros, e.g. writing 1.0 mg rather than 1 mg (Davis, 1994c)
- Inaccurate dosage calculations (Gladstone, 1995)
- Inadequately trained personnel (lack of knowledge about the drug and/or patient) (Leape, 1995)
- Single-handed drug administration (Cohen et al., 1994)
- Lapses in individual performance often due to interruptions during drug rounds (Davis, 1994b)
- Work load and poor skill mix (ASHP, 1993)
- Verbal orders (Fuqua and Stevens, 1988)

Table 15.4 Possible solutions of medication errors

- Encouragement of drug companies to avoid similar sounding names for their products and to avoid corporate packaging (ASHP, 1993)
- Intelligent computer system for drug prescribing (Cavell and Hughes, 1997)
- Participation of pharmacists in ward rounds (Leape et al., 1999)
- Computerised drug distribution systems (Davis, 1994a)
- Closer supervision of junior staff (Baldwin et al., 1998)
- No interruptions of staff giving out medications (Cooper, 1995)
- Not accepting verbal orders for drugs (UKCC, 1992c)
- Regular updating sessions on drug administration and calculation, including use of infusion pumps (Jeanes and Taylor, 1992)
- Clear guidelines for defining what constitutes a drug error and what specific action should be taken in the event (Cousins and Upton, 1993)
- Development of documentation which collects relevant and detailed information regarding the circumstances and effect of each drug error together with a data base of all drug incidents to enable continuous monitoring and the early identification of trends and variations (Cousins and Upton, 1993)

nurses lack mathematical skills and so make errors in calculating drug dosages. This suggests the need for nurses to attend regular update courses in drug calculations and other aspects of drug usage and administration. This may be achieved using computer-assisted instruction packages (Gee et al., 1998). Nurses also have to be prepared to admit when they cannot read prescriptions and seek clarification, otherwise they may find themselves being made the scapegoat of doctors' errors (Howell, 1996). However, nurses do not need to have an encyclopaedic knowledge of drugs, their doses, interactions and their adverse effects. What they do need is to use their common sense. This means utilizing the British National Formulary, or a similar resource, when they come across a drug with which they are not familiar, as well as using the drug information services provided by most hospital pharmacies. Nurses should also recognize that drug companies go to great lengths to package drugs in sizes that correspond to standard doses. Consequently, whenever a nurse has to use more than two dose packages to make a single dose, it should be a warning that the prescribed amount is out of the ordinary (Davis, 1994c). Recognizing this simple fact would prevent many errors of improper dosage.

Accountability

Although it is true that nurses should not be blamed for drug errors because it is the system that is usually at fault, this does not absolve nurses from all responsibility for drug errors. Nurses are professionals who are accountable for their actions, i.e. they are answerable and responsible for the outcome of what they do, or do not do. In practice, the nurse is accountable in four ways. Firstly, because of common or civil law, the nurse is accountable to the patient and has to be able to justify her actions. Failure to do so may result in a claim of negligence. Secondly, the nurse is accountable to the state in case of a criminal charge. This is clearly illustrated by the case of Beverly Allitt who was convicted of murder, attempted murder and causing grievous bodily harm, as a result of inappropriate administration of drugs to a number of children at Grantham Hospital (DoH, 1991). Her case may appear extreme, but in America nurses who have made errors of judgement in giving medication have also had criminal charges brought against them (Ventura, 1997). Thirdly, through contract law, the nurse is answerable to his employer. This arises because every contract has the implied term that the nurse will first use 'all care and skill' in his work and, second, 'obey' his employer by working within hospital policies (Elliot Pennels, 1997c). Finally, the nurse is accountable to the UKCC for breaches in professional conduct as laid down in the Code of Professional Conduct (UKCC, 1992a).

Negligence is defined as causing harm to a person to whom a duty is owed, either by doing some act that a reasonable person would not have done, or not doing what a reasonable person would have done. There are six 'tests' applied to any claim against a health care professional (Table 15.5). If the person is to be found negligent then the first five items must apply. The sixth test is an additional consideration, but is not conditional.

The Health and Safety at Work Act (1974) makes it clear that employees must be properly trained in the use of any equipment which they are required to operate, and this includes the multitude of pumps used to administer drugs. Thus for example, if a nurse is caring for a patient who has a syringe-driver administering heparin, and the patient suffers a haemorrhage as a result of a heparin overdose due to the nurse setting up the pump incorrectly, then the patient or their relatives can sue for negligence (Grant, 1998). Although it can be argued that ensuring staff are better trained is down to managers, it is also a requisite that the nurse acknowledges her limitations in her knowledge and competence and declines any duties or responsibilities unless able to perform them in a safe and skilled manner (UKCC, 1992b).

Table 15.5 Six 'tests' for negligence

1	Did the nurse owe a duty of care to the injured person?	Yes	No
2	Did the nurse provide an inappropriate standard of care in the circumstances, i.e. did she not do what a reasonable nurse would have done	Yes	No
3	Did a breach in the standard of care cause the person's injuries?	Yes	No
4	Were the injuries sustained reasonably foreseeable?	Yes	No
5	Are the injuries of a kind that the court can compensate?	Yes	No
6	Did the injured person contribute to the occurrence of, or extent of, the injuries?	Yes	No

Competence in nursing relates to the expectation that on completion of basic training the knowledge gained will enable the nurse to function safely and take responsibility for her personal professional development. Thus, the patient can be confident that the nurse's position and registration means that she is competent to care for him. Case law helps to clarify the concept of competence as Bolam v. Friern Hospital Management Committee (1957) identifies that a competent standard of care is that expected of a 'reasonably skilled and competent nurse' and that it is sufficient to exercise an 'ordinary level of skill'. Wilsher v. Essex Area Health Authority (1986) makes it clear that the level of competence is what is needed for the job, not what the nurse can offer, while Nettleship v. Weston (1971) identifies that to be inexperienced and of insufficient competence is never a defence if an accident happens.

In order to be competent in the management of drugs nurses need be familiar with the procedures and policies that govern:

- drug ordering and transport
- drug storage and security
- drug prescription
- drug administration and disposal
- record-keeping
- self-medication by patients
- delegation of duties (Dimond, 1990).

The main legislation controlling the supply, storage and administration of medicines is the Medicines Act 1968 and the Misuse of Drugs Act 1971, together with the Misuse of Drugs Regulations of 1985. The Medicines Act classifies drugs into categories for the purposes of supply to the public (Table 15.6), while the Misuse of Drugs Act and the 1985 Regulations make provision for the classification of controlled drugs and their possession, supply and manufacture (see British National Formulary).

Self-administration of drugs by patients is becoming increasingly popular as a form of rehabilitation and as an aid to compliance (Hancock, 1994; Collingsworth et al., 1997), and is recommended by the UKCC (1992c) for this reason. Reynolds (1998) found that such a scheme allowed substantial financial savings to be made, while Jones

Table 15.6 Classification of drugs according to the Medicines Act 1968

General sales list	Medicinal products which may be sold other than from a retail pharmacy, e.g. newsagents selling aspirin
Pharmacy-only products	Medicinal products that can only be sold or supplied by a retail pharmacy when the product must be sold under the supervision of a registered pharmacist, e.g. domperidone (Nathan, 1998)
Prescription-only products	Medicinal products that are only available on a practitioner's prescription, e.g. oral contraceptive

et al. (1996) also found that the unexpected outcome of self-medication was the detection of errors in dispensing in drugs brought into hospital such as incorrect doses or drugs in wrongly labelled bottles. However, the retention by the patient of medication in his bedside locker puts additional responsibilities on the nurse. He or she needs to ensure that there is a clear policy in relation to the safety of the medicines, especially from other patients and visitors, and in relation to the training and supervision of the patient himself, and that these policies are implemented.

Nurses are being increasingly aided by a variety of staff including students, health care assistants, auxiliaries and support workers. However, it must be appreciated that the registered nurse retains accountability for assessing, planning, implementing, and maintaining standards of care (UKCC, 1996b). Consequently, where care is delegated, the person delegating will be held accountable for giving a task to an inappropriately trained colleague (Elliott Pennels, 1997a). Thus for example, if a staff nurse sends a junior student nurse unsupervised to give a patient an injection and the patient suffers as a result, the staff nurse as well as the student actually giving the injection could be sued for negligence (Young, 1981).

Protocols and nursing formulary

Until recently the main role of the nurse was in the administration of drugs, now however prescribing drugs is becoming part of the nurse's role. Recommendations for nurse prescribing were first made in the Cumberlege report (DHSS, 1986) when it was recommended that community nurses should be able to prescribe 'prescription-only medicines' from a limited list. This was reinforced by the Crown report (DoH, 1989) which recommended that 'suitably qualified nurses working in the community should be able – in clearly defined circumstances – to prescribe from a limited list of items and to adjust timing, and dosage of medicine within a set protocol'. In 1992 the Medicinal Products: Prescribing by Nurses Act was passed enabling nurses in the community to prescribe by identifying them as 'appropriate practitioners'. The Pharmaceutical Services Regulations were later passed in 1994 to allow pharmacists in the community to dispense medicines prescribed by nurses. Finally, the Medicines Order 1994 sets the limitations of the prescribing powers of nurses. Thus, community nurses can prescribe a limited range of drugs from the Nurse Prescribers' Formulary (Table 15.7) provided the nurse:

- Is a first-level registered nurse with a district nurse, midwifery or health visitor qualification
- Works within a primary care setting
- Has successfully completed a nurse prescribing programme
- Is registered with the UKCC as a nurse prescriber
- Is authorized/required by his or her employer to prescribe.

Table 15.7 Types of items included in the Nurse Prescribers' Formulary (NPF)

Laxatives	Mild analgesics
Local anaesthetics	Drugs for the mouth
Drugs for threadworms	Drugs for scabies and head lice
Skin preparations	Disinfection and cleansing agents
Wound management products	Elastic hosiery
Urinary catheters and appliances	Stoma care products
Appliances and reagents for diabetes	Fertility and gynaecological products

Full implementation of nurse prescribing was promised by April 1998 (DoH, 1996) and every Trust and health authority in England has been commissioning training programmes, changing nurses' job descriptions and negotiating protocols, so that by March 2001, 26 000 district nurses and health visitors will have prescribing authority (Gooch, 1999). The publication of the second Crown report (DoH, 1999) has added impetus to the drive for nurse prescribing by concluding that doctors are not the only health professionals who take legitimate responsibility for making clinical assessments leading to a diagnosis. Crown recommended a two-tier approach with independent prescribers who would diagnose and prescribe and dependent prescribers who would meet the needs of patients with a known diagnosis. The government is presently reviewing these recommendations.

There is no provision at the moment in the nurse prescribing legislation that allows RGNs without a district nurse, midwife or health visitor qualification to prescribe, nor does the legislation allow hospital nurses to do so. This has resulted in 'the emplacement of imaginative, interpretative and potentially unlawful practices within hospitals, typified by the increased use of protocols – developed as a means of circumventing the clear legal rules regulating who is an appropriate practitioner to prescribe' (Elliott Pennels, 1997b). The use of protocols is based on an imaginative interpretation of section 58 of the 1968 Medicines Act (Elliott Pennels, 1997c), which is endorsed in paragraphs 35 and 36 of Standards for the Administration of Medicines (UKCC, 1992c). The Crown report on group protocols (DoH, 1998) recommended that the law be clarified, and set a new high standard for protocols.

In order to comply as closely as possible with the current law, a drug protocol should be a detailed written document, as oral protocols are not safe and should not be used. The protocol is a substitute for a prescription, and so it must comply with all the details expected of a prescription, i.e. it should identify all the drugs that can be considered for each patient, together with a clear description of the dosage, frequency of administration and route. It should also provide clinically relevant information on indications for use, contra-indications and side-effects, together with an indication of when to give to the drug, when to withhold it, and when to refer to a doctor. The protocol should be designed for a specific clinical environment, it should ideally be specific to an individual named nurse and used only by her, and it should be reviewed and updated at least yearly. The protocol should be formalized by being signed by all those involved including the doctor, nurse and hospital management. Finally, it must be remembered that a protocol must be under the control of a doctor who has overall accountability for the protocol, whilst the nurse administering the drug should be suitably qualified and competent and has complete accountability for all actions she undertakes while using the protocol.

References and further reading

Allan EL, Barker KN (1990) Fundamentals of medication error research. American Journal of Hospital Pharmacy 47: 555-71

Ambrosini MT, Mandler HD, Wood CA (1992) AZT: zidovudine or azathioprine? Lancet 339: 935

American Society of Hospital Pharmacists (1993) ASHP guidelines on preventing medication errors in hospitals. American Journal of Hospital Pharmacy 50: 305-14

Arndt M (1994) Nurses' medication errors. Journal of Advanced Nursing 19: 519-26

Baker H, Napthine R (1994) Ritual + workloads = medication error. Australian Nursing Journal 2:34-6

Baldwin PJ, Dodd M, Wrate RM (1998) Junior doctors making mistakes. Lancet 351: 804

Barber N, Dean B (1998) The incidence of medication errors and ways to reduce them. Clinical Risk 4: 103-6

Bassett S (1998) The carrot beats the stick. Nursing Management 5: 6-7

Bolam v. Friern Hospital Management Committee (1957) 2 All England Law Reports 118

Boyce N (1998) It sounds like a prescription chaos. New Scientist 160: 28

British Medical Association and Royal Pharmaceutical Society of Great Britain (1997) British National Formulary. London: Pharmaceutical Press

Carlisle D (1996) An injection of danger. Nursing Times 92: 26-8

Cavell GF, Hughes DK (1997) Does computerised prescribing improve the accuracy of drug administration? The Pharmaceutical Journal 259:782-4

Cavell GF (1998) System improvement by competancy assessment – the King's College Hospital's perspective. Paper presented at course on Medication Errors – Managing the Risk, 5 November at Harrow, London

Cohen MR, Senders J, Davis NM (1994) Failure mode and effects analysis: a novel approach to avoiding dangerous medication errors and accidents. Hospital Pharmacy 29: 319-30

Collingsworth S, Gould D, Wainwright SP (1997) Patient self-administration of medication: a review of the literature. International Journal of Nursing Studies 34: 256-69

Cooper M (1995) Can a zero defects philosophy be applied to drug errors? Journal of Advanced Nursing 21: 487-91

Cousins DH, Upton DR (1993) Do you report medication errors? Hospital Pharmacy Practice 3: 376-8

Davis N (1994a) Can computers stop errors. American Journal Nursing 94: 14

Davis N (1994b) Concentrating on interruptions. American Journal Nursing 94: 14

Davis N (1994c) Beware of trailing zeros. American Journal Nursing 94: 17

Davis N (1995) Potassium perils. American Journal Nursing 95: 14

Dean BS, Allan EL, Barber ND, Barker KN (1995) Comparison of medication errors in an American and a British hospital. American Journal of Health-System Pharmacy 52: 2543-9

Department of Health (1989) Report of the Advisory Group on Nursing Prescribing (Crown Report). London: Department of Health

Department of Health (1991) Report of the independent inquiry relating to the deaths and injuries on the children's ward of Grantham and Kestevin General Hospital during the period February to April 1991. London: HMSO

Department of Health (1996) Primary Care: Delivering the Future. London: HMSO
Department of Health (1998) Review of Prescribing and Administration of Medicines: A report on the supply and administration of medicines under group protocols. London: Department of Health
Department of Health (1999) Review of Prescribing, Supply and Administration of Medicines (Crown Report II). London: Department of Health
Department of Health and Social Services (1986) Neighbourhood Nursing: a focus for care (Cumberlege report). London: DHSS
Dimond B (1990) Legal aspects of nursing. London: Prentice Hall. Chapter 28
Elliott Pennels CJ (1997a) Clinical responsibility. Professional Nurse 13: 162-4
Elliott Pennels CJ (1997b) Nurse prescribing. Professional Nurse 13: 114-15
Elliott Pennels CJ (1997c) Protocols. Professional Nurse 13: 115-17
Ferner RE, Whittington RM (1994) Coroner cases of death due to errors of prescribing or giving medicines or to adverse drug reactions: Birmingham 1986-1991. Journal of the Royal Society of Medicine 87: 145-8
Fuqua RA, Stevens KR (1988) What we know about medication errors: a literature review. Journal of Nursing Quality Assurance 3: 1-17
Gee P, Peterson GM, Martin JLS, Reeve JF (1998) Development and evaluation of a computer-assisted instruction package in clinical pharmacology for nursing students. Computers in Nursing 16: 37-44
Gethins B (1996) Wise up to medication errors. Pharmacy in Practice 6: 323-8
Gladstone J (1995) Drug administration errors: a study into the factors underlying the occurrence and reporting of drug errors in a district general hospital. Journal of Advanced Nursing 22: 628-37
Gooch S (1999) Nurse prescribing and the Crown review. Professional Nurse 14: 678-80
Grant L (1998) Devices and desires. Health Service Journal 108: 34-5
Hancock B (1994) Self-administration of medicines. British Journal of Nursing 3: 996-999
HMSO (1974) Health and Safety at Work Act. London: HMSO
Ho CYW, Dean BS, Barber ND (1997) When do medication errors happen to hospital inpatients? International Journal of Pharmacy Practice 5: 91-6
Howell M (1996) Prescription for disaster. Nursing Times 92: 30-1
Jeanes A, Taylor D (1992) Stopping the drugs trolley. Nursing Times 88: 27-9
Jones L, Arthurs GJ, Sturman E, Bellis L (1996) Self-medication in acute surgical wards. Journal of Clinical Nursing 5: 229-32
Knowles DR (1998) Supplying medicines safely. Clinical Risk 4: 107-9
Leape LL, Bates DW, Cullen DJ, Cooper J, Demonaco HJ, Gallivan T, Hallisey R, Ives J, Laird N, Laffel G (1995) Systems analysis of adverse drug events. Journal of the American Medical Association 274: 35-43
Leape L, Cullen DJ, Clapp MD, Burdick E, Demonaco HJ, Erickson JI, Bates DW (1999) Pharmacist participation on physician rounds and adverse drug events in the intensive care unit. Journal of the American Medical Association 282: 267-70
Lyons R, Payne C, McCabe M, Fielder C (1998) Legibility of doctors' handwriting: quantitative comparative study. British Medical Journal 317: 863-4
Nathan A (1998) Non-prescription Medicines. London: Pharmaceutical Press
Nettleship v. Weston (1971) All England Law Reports 581
Ogden DA, Kinnear M, McArthur DM (1997) A quantitative and qualitative evaluation of medication errors in hospital inpatients. Pharmacy Practice Research. Supplement to Pharmaceutical Journal 259: R19

Phillips DP, Christenfeld N, Glynn LM (1998) Increase in US medication-error deaths between 1983 and 1993. Lancet 351: 643-4
Reynolds N (1998) A special dispensation. Health Service Journal 108: 30-1
Ridge KW, Jenkins DB, Noyce PR, Barber ND (1995) Medication errors during hospital drug rounds. Quality in Health Care 4: 240-3
Taxis K, Dean BS, Barber ND (1998) Hospital drug distribution systems in the UK and Germany – a study of medication errors. Pharmacy World and Science 21: 25-31
UKCC (1992a) Code of Professional Conduct 3rd ed. London: UKCC
UKCC (1992b) Scope of Professional Practice. London: UKCC
UKCC (1992c) Standards for the Administration of Medicines. London: UKCC
UKCC (1996a) Issues arising from professional conduct complaints. London: UKCC
UKCC (1996b) Position statement on Clinical Supervision for Nursing and Health Visiting. London: UKCC
Ventura MJ (1997) Are these nurses criminals? RN 60: 27-9
Wilsher v. Essex Area Health authority CA (1986) All England Law Reports 801
Young AP (1981) Legal problems in Nursing Practice. London: Harper and Row.

Chapter 16
Ethics of drug development and testing

Drug development

The search for new and better drugs is continuous but expensive, with the cost of developing one drug being in the region of £100–£200 million (Chaplin, 1996). This is because less than five out of every 10000 potential medicines screened ever become licensed. This is not surprising as the drug produced must be non-toxic, potent *in vitro* and *in vivo* and ideally have a good half-life, be orally bioavailable, and have minimal drug-drug interactions (Houston, 1996).

New drugs are usually developed by screening chemicals obtained from microbes, plants, animals, and the chemical industry for interesting properties. In the process a huge number of chemicals are tested against a wide range of targets, such as enzymes and receptors, that have been identified or implicated in a disease state. Although huge numbers of samples can be screened by utilizing fully automated robot-driven screening, the process is rather 'hit and miss'. However, with increasing knowledge of molecular biology, X-ray crystallography and computer techniques drug development is becoming more rational as drugs can be designed to interact with a known target in a specific manner. For example, in 1989 crystallographers solved the structure of human immunodeficiency virus (HIV) protease, an enzyme used by the virus to process the proteins it needs to infect new cells. The active site of the enzyme contained a cavity, which, if blocked by the correct shaped molecule, would prevent the enzyme fulfilling its function and interrupt the life cycle of the virus. In 1990, a molecule that fitted the description was found by Rene DesJarlais and her team at the University of California

(Aldridge, 1998). Although the compound found, bromoperidol, failed at the next stage of drug development, it sparked off the search for similar compounds and led to the protease inhibitors, indinavir, ritonavir and saquinavir.

Once a potential new drug has been identified, it undergoes both *in vitro* and *in vivo* studies in the laboratory. The *in vitro* studies set out to examine if the potential drug has useful therapeutic activity, and to identify how potent and selective it is in its action compared with available drugs. The *in vivo* studies utilize laboratory animals that are thought to give responses representative of humans, although the validity of animal models is open to question. In addition, as well as being expensive, animal experiments turn public opinion against medical research and pharmaceutical companies, especially when higher animals like monkeys are used; the industry would prefer not to have to do them (Aldhous et al., 1999). However, whilst the necessity still exists, the Animals Act (1986) endeavours to ensure the well being of the animals being utilized in research by requiring that people doing animal experiments are competent and that the premises are correctly equipped. To be honest most animal studies do involve a degree of suffering, although analgesics and anaesthetics are used where possible to minimize this (Aldridge, 1998). To ensure that the requirements of the Act are adhered to, Home Office inspectors visit laboratories unannounced and require evidence that the benefits of the research outweigh the distress to the animals. There is also pressure to develop new techniques of drug testing to minimize animal use. Burch and Russell in 1959 suggested the three Rs approach, i.e. reduction, refinement and replacement. Reduction means minimizing the number of animals used by, for example harmonizing the licensing regulations between countries so that animal testing does not have to be repeated when a licence is sought in a new country. Refinement means extracting the maximum amount of information from any one experiment, whilst replacement looks for alternatives to animals in the form of cells, tissues, organ slices and computer models.

The *in vivo* studies examine the pharmokinetic effects of the drug and evaluate its safety, including acute, chronic and reproductive toxicity, and its potential for causing cancer (Nials et al., 1996). If the potential drug is showing promise, the company will take out a patent that prevents any other company copying its idea and gives it a monopoly on production. Patents last for twenty years, but as new pharmaceuticals take 10–12 years to bring to the market, the company only has only 8–10 years to recoup its research and development costs and make a suitable profit. Once the patent has expired, generic manufacturers can make the drug and prices come down with the consequent competition.

At the same time as the preclinical studies are going on, the pharmaceutical chemists are also looking at developing the most efficacious and safe formulation, and researching how the production of the drug can be scaled up for commercial manufacture. Modern drugs may involve up to 15 different synthetic stages, and several chemical pathways can often be used to obtain one drug. The chemists have to decide which route to use based on the availability and expense of raw materials, the safety and expense of the process, and the purity and yield of the final product. Once the *in vivo* and *in vitro* studies are complete, the company applies for a clinical trial certificate from the Medicines Control Agency. If the Committee is satisfied with the results of the animal studies, they will allow clinical trials to go ahead.

Clinical trials

These start with Phase I trials where the drug is administered to young male volunteers in very small doses. The doses are slowly escalated until there is a detectable effect, whilst metabolic and pharmokinetic studies are carried out. The dose ranges derived from Phase I studies are used in Phase II trials in which the potential therapeutic and toxicity effects of the drug are evaluated by administration for a limited period of time to small numbers of patients. The study population is as homogenous as possible, and usually involves between 100 and 500 patients. The aim of Phase II trials is to answer the question 'Does this new drug work under tightly controlled conditions?' Ideally, Phase II trials do this by comparing the effects of the new drug with a placebo. This is a pharmacologically inert substance prepared to be identical in appearance to the new treatment. Although this is the 'gold standard' there are times when it is not ethically acceptable nor appropriate to deprive the patient of a known effective treatment, so the comparison has to be made between the established drug plus placebo and an established drug plus treatment. It might be asked why not just compare the new drug with the standard treatment, but this is unlikely to show a difference in efficacy unless the new drug represents a substantial advance in treatment, or unless large numbers of patients are studied (Williams, 1996).

As well as using a placebo, Phase II trials are also ideally randomized, double-blind, and cross-over. Randomization means that computer generated random numbers, or a similar selection process is used, which ensures that all patients have an equal chance of receiving the new treatment. This is done in order to reduce selection bias, as clinicians will tend to choose the best treatment for an individual patient, and consequently this may result in significant differences between the treatment and placebo groups. Similarly, bias can occur due to health care professionals' and patients' expectations of the effect of treatment. To prevent this trials are double-blinded so that neither the patient nor the clinician knows which treatment the patient is receiving, or single-blinded where only the doctor knows. It is suggested that because drug companies fund much of the research into drugs and make presents to universities, there is a conflict of interests for the researcher, which may again result in bias (Day, 1998). In order to be seen to maintain their impartiality and professional credibility researchers naturally favour the double-blind approach themselves. Phase II trials last for between two and three years depending on the nature of the target disease, and about one third of new drugs that enter this phase will fail (Williams, 1996).

The use of a crossover approach means that the patients switch groups half way through the trial. This procedure allows each patient to act as their own control, so twice as much data is generated and less people need to be recruited for the study. This approach is also more ethically acceptable as every patient receives the new drug. It also minimizes the risk of patients manipulating the programme for their own ends. For example, during the trial of AZT some of those taking part objected to the use of placebos and got together and shared out their drugs. Thus, every member of the group got some AZT although it was at a lower dose than the treatment group would have got. This activity makes clinical trials meaningless.

Phase III trials move to a larger, more varied population, who are treated for up to six months or a year. As well as the safety and efficacy studies demanded by the Medicines Control Agency, companies increasingly carry out quality of life and cost-effectiveness studies, during this part of the clinical trial (Bryan, 1996). The results of these studies help support the marketing arguments for the drug when it is finally launched, especially when there is little to choose between the new product and those already on the market in terms of efficacy and side-effects.

Although a more varied population is involved in Phase III trials, there are complaints that they are still not representative of the population who will be using the drug in the future (Manning, 1998). Thus, there are often exclusion criteria which can bar people who drink, smoke, have coexisting diseases and take other medicines. McEnany (1998) also maintains that there is an inclination amongst researchers in many areas of science to give preferential regard to men in study protocols over women. In many instances, the assumption that data from men are easily applicable to women is not only erroneous but yields information that leads to poor practice.

One client group frequently excluded from drug trials is children. Consequently, doctors are forced to prescribe drugs 'off label', i.e. outside the conditions for which they have been licensed, and to gamble on a child being able to cope with the dosage they prescribe (Fricker, 1999). Accordingly, liability for outcomes rests with the doctor or the health authority rather than with the drug company. In the US, an estimated 80% of prescription drugs are not licensed for use in children (Cote et al., 1996). Reasons given for not testing drugs on children are the relatively small market share, fear of legal liability, potential long-term adverse effects, the reluctance of parents to give permission to allow their children to be research subjects, and the lack of adequate funding from government, industry and health care providers (Asbury, 1991). However, the situation is set to change with the Food and Drug Administration's 1997 Modernization Act, which came into force in April 1999. This will force drug companies to provide the FDA with information on the paediatric use of any medicines that may offer children better treatment than existing therapies or will be widely used by children. It is hoped that similar legislation will follow in Europe.

Clinical trials may also be supported by the use of laboratory work and more up-to-date techniques like computer modelling. In 1997, for example, clinical trials of the new antihypertensive mibefradil found that it produced unusual electrocardiograms in those taking it, which clinicians claimed were dangerous. Ordinarily Hoffman-LaRoche, the manufacturers of the drug, would have scrapped the drug or started more costly clinical trials. Instead they applied the drug to a virtual heart which allowed them to get inside the cardiac cells and demonstrate to the satisfaction of the US Food and Drug Administration that the ECG abnormalities were not the result of a major abnormality, and consequently the drug was approved (Buchannan, 1999).

Licensing

For a major new drug application, evidence of efficacy from around 150 patients and safety data from perhaps 2000–3000 patients is required before licensing will be considered. The data will be scrutinized and a licence granted if satisfactory. In an average year the Medicines Control Agency will receive approximately 40 new drug applications and about 1 000 abridged applications (Jefferys, 1996). The abridged application will range from the development of a major new indication for an already licensed drug, to the introduction of a new formulation such as an aerosol, sustained-release, parenteral or topical preparation through to a generic drug and an over-the-counter formulation.

Phase IV trials and the yellow card scheme

In order to observe for long-term and low incidence side-effects, drug monitoring continues after the drug has become commercially available. This initially involves Phase IV studies in which the drug company recruits a number of doctors and requests them to report back on their experiences on the first 100 or so patients to whom they prescribe the new drug. After this, long-term surveillance is carried out with the yellow card scheme, which was set up in 1964 in response to the thalidomide disaster. It is run jointly by the Committee on Safety of Medicines (CSM) and the Medicines Control Agency (MCA). Doctors, dentists and coroners are asked to report suspected adverse drug reactions as described in Table 16.1.

Table 16.1 Adverse drug reactions that should be reported on the yellow card scheme

- Report all reactions to new products, including minor ones that could conceivably be attributed to the drug. 'New' drugs refer to those marketed in the past two years and are indicated in prescribing literature by an inverted triangle thus (▼)
- Report any reactions to vaccines
- Report suspected drug interactions
- Report serious or unusual suspected reactions to established products. Include reactions that are fatal, life-threatening, disabling, incapacitating or that result in or prolong hospitalization. Do not include minor reactions

The yellow card system has four main functions (Table 16.2), the main purpose being to allow unrecognized adverse reactions, particularly to new drugs, to be identified as quickly as possible, so that appropriate action can be taken. This is necessary because by the time a medicine is granted a product licence, on average only about 1 500–3 000 people will have taken it, and clinical trials will only have identified the most common adverse effects (Lee and Beard, 1997). Type B reactions, particularly those with an incidence of 1 in 500 or less, are unlikely to have been identified. The scheme has been very successful in this part of its role. For example, in 1990 Chloraseptic throat spray was reformulated when it was noted that the phenol in it caused oedema of the epiglottis and pharynx, and in 1993 remoxipride (Roxiam) was withdrawn as it was found to cause aplastic anaemia.

As to its other functions, the yellow card scheme has enabled predisposing factors to be identified, e.g. dose and age, and it has allowed the frequency of adverse drug reactions between similar products to be identified, both of which can aid doctors in their drug choice when prescribing. Thus for example, the scheme has identified that azapropazone (Rheumox) is more toxic to the upper gastro-intestinal tract than other NSAIDs, and it has identified the differing adverse drug reaction profiles of fluvoxamine and fluoxetine (Price et al., 1992).

Table 16.2 Main functions of the yellow card system (Rawlins, 1996)

- To give early warning of adverse reactions
- To identify predisposing factors
- To examine comparative toxicity
- To allow long-term monitoring

The fourth role of the yellow card scheme, long-term monitoring of drugs, is necessary because previously unrecognized hazards may emerge with drugs even when they have been available for many years. Thus unsuspected adverse reactions may become apparent, e.g. Reye's syndrome with aspirin, and arrhythmias with terfenadine, or novel interactions with newer drugs may be manifested, e.g. fluvoxamine and theophylline (CSM and MCA, 1994).

The yellow card system has much to its credit, but it is only as good as the doctors who use it, and a current criticism is that doctors do not complete yellow cards as often as they should. Consequently, harmful drugs are not being withdrawn as rapidly as they could be. For example, two popular slimming drugs, fenfluramine and dexfenfluramine, remained on the market for 10 years, despite the fact that they were known to cause heart valve problems. It has been suggested that nurses and pharmacists should also be enabled to complete yellow cards in order to increase the data available to the scheme.

The nurse's role

The nurse is involved in the process of drug development, once the clinical trials start, particularly Phases II and III. Nurses have an important role to play in noting and reporting any unusual or unanticipated response to either new or established drugs, as they often spend much more time with the patient than the investigating doctor. Furthermore, it is common for doctors to employ research nurses to help them carry out their studies into new drugs. It must be appreciated by staff conducting drug trials involving the general public, that patients seek medical help when they are ill and place their trust in the professionals to do their best to help them and to prevent unavoidable suffering. To do otherwise is to betray the patient's trust (Rumbold, 1993). Consequently, it is crucial in any experimentation involving patients, whether it is for their own benefit or that of another, that it is carried out with their consent. This consent has to be freely given and informed, as is required by the Declaration of Helsinki (1975; Table 16.3).

As the patient's advocate the nurse must be sure that the patient has given informed consent to taking part in any drug trials, preferably in writing. Before any drug trial starts in a clinical area a

Table 16.3 The Declaration of Helsinki (1975)

In any research on human beings, each potential subject must be adequately informed of the aims, methods, anticipated benefits and potential hazards of the study and the discomfort it may entail. He or she should be informed that he or she is at liberty to abstain from participation in the study and that he or she is free to withdraw his or her consent to participation at any time.

Research Ethics Committee will have vetted it to ensure that protocols are set up to protect the patient and ensure that informed consent is gained. These committees exist to ensure that research involving human subjects is not only conducted ethically, but also seen to be ethical (Parker, 1994). However, the ethical committee does not closely monitor the study, and clinicians are responsible for ensuring that the protocols set are followed. There is considerable concern that patients, particularly the elderly and psychiatric patients, may agree to take part in clinical trials without realising what they are letting themselves in for (Boyce, 1998). It must also be questioned whether they can give informed consent to take part in a drug trial when their illness may prevent them from making a sensible decision. In such cases consent should be sought from an appropriate advocate or significant other person (RCN, 1993).

The members of the research team are both clinicians and researchers and conflict of interests may arise (Raybuck, 1997). The research team must carefully weigh up the benefits of their research to society and the subject, evaluating the risk/benefit ratio. They must not let teleological arguments; i.e. the end justifies the means, overpower their deontological principles, i.e. the duty to give patients best care. The principles of beneficence (do good) and nonmaleficence (do no harm) should be considered in relation to the research team's obligations to the study participants. Participants are free to withdraw consent at any time during the study, either electing to withdraw prematurely for reasons of their own, or by failing to adhere to the required protocol. The research team must not pressurize participants to remain in the trial against their better judgement and should offer them alternative treatments. The researchers must also make every attempt to contact participants who withdraw in order to carry out an exit interview so that this data is available to be included in the final research report.

Another potential dilemma regarding clinical trials relates to further treatment options for subjects who complete the protocol and show marked improvement in their condition on the trial drug, which is yet to be available to the general public. These subjects should be offered some form of follow up treatment, either by the research team or by referrals elsewhere. Conversely if a client's condition deteriorates during the trial and early discontinuation from the protocol is warranted some mechanism should be in place to offer treatment to stabilize the patient's condition.

Another possible area of conflict of interests occurs when practitioners receive financial support or sponsorship from drug companies. Stelfox et al. (1998) examined the effect of financial conflict of interests, by reviewing articles published on the controversial calcium-channel antagonists and classifying the papers as being supportive, neutral or critical with respect to the use of these drugs. They found that authors who supported the use of calcium-channel antagonists were significantly more likely than neutral or critical authors to have financial relationships with manufacturers of calcium-channel antagonists. Although this study relates to the medical profession, it has implications for nurses who carry out research into wound care and stoma products, as well as those who support their medical colleagues in carrying out drug-related research. Health care professional may claim to be able to carry out unbiased research whilst receiving financial support from a drug company, and perhaps they can. However, it is not sufficient to be impartial, it is necessary to be seen to be so. This is achieved by authors disclosing in published studies their relationship with the pharmaceutical company, in order to affirm the integrity of the profession and maintain public confidence.

References and further reading

Aldhous P, Coglan A, Copley J (1999) Animal experiments. Let the people speak. New Scientist 162: 26-31

Aldridge S (1998) Magic Molecules: how drugs work. Cambridge: Cambridge University Press

Animals (Scientific Procedures) Act 1986: Elizabeth II. Chapter 1

Asbury CH (1991) The Orphan Drug Act. The first 7 years. Journal of the American Medical Association 265: 893-7

Boyce N (1998) Knowing their own minds. New Scientist 158: 20-1

Bryan J (1996) Marketing: the key to a successful drug launch. Prescriber 7: 110-3

Buchanan M (1999) The heart just won't die. New Scientist 161: 24-8
Burch R, Russell W (1959) The Principles of Humane Experimental Technique. London: Methuen and Co.
Chaplin S (1996) The final stage: gaining protection for the product. Prescriber 7: 28-31
Committee on Safety of Medicines and Medicines Control Agency (1994) Fluvoxamine increases plasma theophylline levels. Current Problems in Pharmacovigilance 20: 12
Cote CJ, Kauffman RE, Troendle GJ, Lambert GH (1996) Is the 'therapeutic orphan' about to be adopted? Pediatrics 98: 118-23
Day M (1998) He who pays the piper. New Scientist 158: 18-19
Declaration of Helsinki, adopted by the 18th World Medical Assembly in 1964 in Helsinki, and revised by the 29th World Medical Assembly in Tokyo 1975
Fricker J (1999) Too much too young. New Scientist 161: 18-19
Houston J (1996) Drug discovery: turning serendipity into certainty. Prescriber 7: 58-61
Jefferys D (1996) The registration and licensing of new drugs. Prescriber 7: 29-34
Lee A, Beard K (1997) Adverse drug reactions. (1) Pharmacovigilance and the pharmacist. The Pharmaceutical Journal 258: 592-5
Manning C (1998) Drug trials: time to include typical patients. Prescriber 9: 13
McEnany G (1998) Sexual dysfunction in the pharmacological treatment of depression: when 'don't ask, don't tell' is an unsuitable approach to care. Journal of the American Psychiatric Nurses Association 4: 24-9
Nials T, Whelan C, Wilding Y, Strong P (1996) Ensuring the safety and efficacy of new medicines. Prescriber 7: 19-23
Parker B (1994) Research Ethics Committees. In Tschudin V Ethics. Education and Research. London: Scutari Press. Chapter 3
Price J, Waller P, Wood S, Mackay A (1992) Safety of fluoxetine: comparison with fluvoxamine. Pharmacoepidemiology and Drug Safety 1: 111-17
Raybuck JA (1997) The clinical nurse specialist as research coordinator in clinical drug trials. Clinical Nurse Specialist 11: 15-18
Stelfox HT, Chua G, O'Rourke K, Detsky A (1998) Conflict of interest in the debate over calcium-channel antagonists. The New England Journal of Medicine 338: 101-6
Rawlins M (1996) The yellow card scheme: monitoring drug safety. Prescriber 7: 101-4
Royal College of Nursing (1993) Ethics Related to Research 2nd edn. London: Royal College of Nursing
Rumbold G (1993) Ethics in Nursing Practice 2nd edn. London: Bailliere Tindall. p114-7
Williams P (1996) From the guinea-pigs to the patients: phase II and III. Prescriber 7: 33-7

Chapter 17 Compliance, patient education and empowerment

What is compliance?

Compliance and non-compliance are two terms frequently associated with drug therapy. The definition of compliance most frequently used is 'the extent to which a person's behaviour, in terms of taking medications, following diets, or executing lifestyle changes, coincides with medical health advice' (Haynes, 1979). Despite its frequent use however, compliance is not the ideal term to use as it is value-laden and implies a paternalistic relationship in which the patient's role is one of submission. This does not fit with the modern ethos of nursing which aims to promote patient autonomy, and views the nurse-patient relationship as a partnership (UKCC, 1992).

It has been argued that because health care professionals have special knowledge and expertise they have the right to be the decision-maker, rather than the patient. This may occasionally be the case, but usually, although the health care professional may be the expert on the disease in general, the patient is the expert on *his* disease and its specific manifestations (Holm, 1993). The patient may know that strict adherence to the regime prescribed by the health care professional will lead to severe and incapacitating side-effects and it seems ludicrous to talk of 'non-compliance' if the patient alters the regime to gain a tolerable life. Health care professionals do not treat diabetics to keep their glucose levels low or epileptics to maintain a steady phenytoin level, but to enable them to have a good quality of life.

A further problem is that the diagnosis of some disorders, for example hypertension, is difficult and the choice of the best treatment is open to debate. Sometimes we get it wrong and for this eventuality Weintraub (1981) coined the term 'intelligent non-compliance'.

He quotes studies on digoxin, antihypertensives and anti-epileptics where non-compliant patients fared as well as compliant patients because the prescribed dose was too high or therapy was unnecessary. If we are not positive of our diagnosis and the best form of treatment has not been agreed upon, can we insist upon compliance?

In line with the modern market economy, it can be argued that it is not the patients who should comply with the health care professionals' demands, but rather health care professionals who should comply with their patients' informed and considered desires. This is accepted by Moore (1995) who defines non-compliance as 'a lack of recognition by the health care professional of the meaning of the regimen to the patient'.

Despite all the problems with the terms compliance and non-compliance, as discussed above, in keeping with other literature on the subject, they will both be used in this book, but the reader must bear in mind that they are not ideal.

Why are patients non-compliant?

The five most common forms of non-compliance are:

- not having the prescription filled
- taking the incorrect dose
- taking the medicine at the wrong times
- forgetting to take the medicine
- stopping the medicine too soon (Hughes, 1998)

This non-compliance can involve under-use and over-use of medication, and may be deliberate or unintentional (Table 17.1).

Table 17.1 Reasons for non-compliance

Deliberate	*Unintentional*
• Fear of adverse effects	• Cannot fit regimen into lifestyle
• Low trust in health care personnel	• Forgetfulness
• Misinformed	• Insufficient information
• Misunderstanding	
• Perceive drugs as unnecessary	
• Poverty	
• Vested interest in keeping symptoms	

Deliberate non-compliance

Patients may choose to be deliberately non-compliant for a variety of reasons. Firstly, they may be misinformed and thus for example believe that a larger dosage of a drug will be more therapeutic, or alternatively they may perceive the drugs as unnecessary. Secondly, they may misunderstand what they have been told. This is illustrated by the elderly gentleman who was prescribed the vasodilator glyceryl trinitrate for his chest pain. He incorrectly believed that the tablet was a general painkiller, and consequently he took it whenever he had any form of pain. Thirdly, the patient may have a low trust in health care personnel. This is not surprising as the media frequently highlight the misjudgements of the health care professions, and society no longer regards doctors and nurses with the respect that it once did. An example of the development of this lack of trust occurred with a lady who was prescribed amitriptyline for her post-herpetic neuralgia. When she went home and read up on the drug in her reference book she found that it was an antidepressant. She was consequently very angry as she concluded that her doctor did not believe that she was in pain and had 'fobbed her off with antidepressants'. She did not take the prescribed drug, being unaware of its value in neuralgia-type pain, nor did she revisit her doctor. Instead she attempted to control her pain with large quantities of ibuprofen.

Deliberate non-compliance may occur because of poverty. A recent survey found that up to a third of the 300 respondents were failing to get a doctor's prescription because of the high cost, while more worrying, 21% said they had made a decision not to consult their GP because they feared the prescription charges (Anon, 1995). Another reason is that the patient may have a personal stake in keeping his symptoms. It is a sad reflection on modern society that the only company some elderly people receive is the Community Nurse visiting them in order to give them their insulin injections or dress their leg ulcers.

The main reason for deliberate non-compliance however is the fear of side-effects or dependency. A survey of 540 London patients found that 30% of patients had serious worries about their medication, much of which was unwarranted. Diabetics for example worried that they might become addicted to their insulin, while asthmatics were concerned about the long-term effects of using steroid inhalants (Horne, 1997; Kiernan, 1996). As Tettersell (1993) found in her study, the side-effects that discourage patients from taking their drugs, are not just the pharmacological ones. Forty-eight per cent of the asthmatics in her study stated that they were reluctant to use their inhalers in public due to the stigma and embarrassment of doing so, and they indicated that they would prefer to take tablets.

Donovan and Blake (1992) in their study of compliance in patients with inflammatory arthropathy concluded 'patients carry out their own cost-benefit analysis for each treatment they are offered. They weigh up the expected benefits (usually symptomatic relief) against the severity of their symptoms and the perceived risks of treatment (side-effects, dependence, time and effort involved, stigma, etc.) according to their lay beliefs and the information at their disposal'.

Unintentional non-compliance

Forgetfulness has been cited as the commonest cause of failing to take medication, and is particularly prevalent in the elderly (Col et al., 1990). It can take the form of forgetting to take individual doses or forgetting to order repeat prescriptions from the chemist, both of which result in under-use of medication. Conversely patients may forget that they have already taken their medication resulting in repeat dosing, and possible toxicity reactions. The problem can be increased by the prescription of drugs like benzodiazepines and anticholinergics which may themselves result in impaired memory (Hughes, 1998).

In the case of chronic diseases, particularly ones like diabetes, asthma and renal failure, the prescribed regime may be too complicated to adhere to. This again may be partially due to forgetfulness. Poulton (1991) identifies that immediately after a consultation roughly 40% of what is said is forgotten. This forgetfulness will become increasingly problematic as the health care advice becomes more detailed and complex. Sometimes the client cannot fit the complex regimen into his busy lifestyle, or in the case of some of the elderly, cannot get into the blister pack that holds her tablets (Chesterman, 1999)!

In some cases the patient may not have enough information to comply (Table 17.2). The problem may be that the health care professional has given the requisite information but that the patient has not taken it in for a variety of reasons. Alternatively the staff may not have given the patient all the information he needs due to time constraints or incorrect beliefs that patients do not want to know. It is frequently assumed that nurses make good health educators, but Tettersell (1993) maintains that this is not necessarily the case as 25% of the patients she studied who had had an explanation about asthma from a nurse claimed to not have understood all that they were told.

Table 17.2 Reasons why patients may have insufficient information to comply

Patient does not take in the information because of:	*Patient is not given the information they want because:*
• Poor attention due to over anxious state	• Staff do not have the knowledge or skills to provide the information clearly
• Organic difficulty, e.g. deafness blindness	• Staff have insufficient time to communicate
• Toxic confusional states	• Staff believe that patients do not want to know
• Language barriers	• Staff believe that someone else has told the patient what they need to know
• Abstract nature of the information	• Patient is reticent in asking questions

Health care workers frequently assume that lack of knowledge is the main explanation for patient non-compliance. However, Brown (1996) maintains that in over 220 studies lack of knowledge was not the primary reason for patient non-compliance, although she does not say what was. This means that although giving patients information about their disease and its management is important, nurses are unlikely to be able to increase patient compliance *just* by giving more information, especially as overloading a patient with information can demotivate them (Parkin, 1997).

The size of the problem

Haynes et al. (1979) compiled the only comprehensive and critically rigorous review of compliance studies. Their review of 537 original studies found less than 40 that satisfied strict methodological requirements concerning study design, sample selection, completeness of definition of compliance and adequacy of measurement of compliance. Analysis of the studies which satisfied the requirements, led the authors to conclude that with long-term medication, compliance was around the 50% mark. Even where there are grave consequences of non-compliance as in the case of glaucoma and blindness, renal transplant and organ rejection, and the patient understands this, significant non-compliance has been reported in as many as 20% of patients (Laurence et al., 1997).

Measuring non-compliance

A statistic of 50% non-compliance sounds quite drastic, but it needs to be put into context. Compliance is very difficult to measure and usually indirect methods are used for the purpose (Table 17.3).

Table 17.3 Limitations of traditional methods for measuring compliance

Method	*Limitations*
• Patient's self-reports	• Patient may believe that they are being compliant when they are not • Patients tend to tell professionals what they think they want to hear (Kyngas and Barlow, 1995)
• Pill and bottle counts	• Does not allow for the use of 'tablet diaries' • Tablets may be removed but not taken • Does not detect whether the correct dosing schedule is being followed
• Mechanical devices which record each time the bottle is opened	• Does not allow for the use of 'tablet diaries' • Tablets may be removed but not taken
• Blood and urine tests for drug, metabolite or marker	• Drugs with a short half-life only need to be taken for a few days before the scheduled blood/urine test to achieve therapeutic levels • Tests may be unacceptable to patients
• Outcome of treatment, i.e. the progress of the illness or condition	• Ignores individual differences in response to treatment • Outcome variable might not be very responsive to changes in compliance or affected by factors other than compliance with prescribed treatment
• Clinician's judgement as to whether patient is compliant	• Generally believed to be of low validity (Ley, 1988; Gordis, 1979)

These methods are all open to inaccuracy and frequently tend to overestimate non-compliance. Thus when reading studies which measure compliance it is important to consider the methods used, together with their limitations.

The cost of non-compliance

Does it matter that patients are non-compliant? The answer is yes, as non-compliance puts a heavy burden on society in terms of health, social and economic costs (Higgins and Morlidge, 1998; Hughes, 1998). Failure to take adequate medication may result in disease breakthrough, and in conditions like infection with human immunodeficiency virus for example, the patient cannot 'start afresh' with the same treatment plan once they have been non-compliant because the virus becomes resistant to the drugs. Conversely, patients taking larger or more frequent doses than prescribed may suffer toxic effects. Either of these may be severe enough to warrant further medical attention or even hospital admission. Ausburn (1981) assessed reasons for admission to medical wards among 205 patients and found that 20% of admissions were probably, and a further 5% were possibly, the result of medication non-compliance. Similarly Col et al. (1990) interviewed 315 elderly patients admitted consecutively to acute hospital care and found that 11.4% of the admissions were due to non-compliance. Even more worrying is the suggestion by Bartlett and Moore (1998) that incomplete adherence to HIV therapy accounts for about half of treatment failures. Based on these findings between a tenth and a quarter of medical inpatient beds may be occupied by patients who are in hospital due to non-compliance (Ley, 1988). This makes non-compliance very expensive. This conclusion is supported by the US Department of Health and Human Services, which estimated that the financial cost of non-compliance with 10 common prescription drugs was $396–$792 million (Ley, 1988). On top of these financial costs there are also the costs to the patient and his family in terms of suffering and inconvenience.

Improving compliance – how can this be achieved?

As the introduction suggests, we do not particularly want to promote compliance and have patients submit to our wishes. What we actually want is to empower them. Funnell et al. (1991) suggest 'patients are empowered when they have the knowledge, skills, attitudes and self-awareness necessary to influence their own behaviour and that of others in order to improve the quality of their lives'. An important focus of this definition is on quality rather than quantity. Health care personnel frequently concentrate on the latter, while the former is more important to patients. Cameron and Gregor (1987) suggest that whereas physical health is the priority for health care personnel, this is of secondary importance to patients whose priority is the pursuit of their own personal goals. Thus, health care professionals may prescribe drugs with the intention of maintaining or improving the patient's health, but the individual will not evaluate his regimen for whether or not it allows him to maintain a state of health. Instead, the patient will judge the regimen on a social basis. Thus for example the patient prescribed metronidazole for an infection may choose not to take it if it interferes (through its emetic effect when combined with alcohol) with his nightly trips to the pub with his friends.

Assessment

In order to prevent the nurse and patient from looking at health care problems from very different perspectives it is vital to carry out a comprehensive, holistic assessment with the patient. This will only be achieved if the nurse can develop a good nurse-patient relationship (Brown 1997). This requires the nurse to have a non-judgemental attitude and to have a genuine concern for the patient. The nurse must also be prepared to compromise and to be honest. Without these traits a trusting relationship cannot develop, allowing the health care professional and client to work together in partnership to deal with the health problem and identify the most appropriate medication.

The depth of the assessment will depend on the health problem that is being dealt with. The more complex and chronic the problem, the more detailed the assessment. Areas to be considered for assessment include the patient's usual self-care parameters and his knowledge base, i.e. what he knows about his disease. If the patient is confused or misinformed about his disease process, then he is not in a position to make an intelligent decision about whether to comply with his treatment. As drug side-effects are a significant reason for non-compliance, these should be asked about. Bennet (1999) identifies some tools that may be used by the psychiatric nurse to help in this process.

The third major area for assessment is the patient's attitudes and beliefs about his disease. These are very difficult to assess, but are vital areas for consideration, as a patient will rarely follow advice that is incongruous with his existing beliefs (King, 1984b). Furthermore, King (1984a) identifies that for some physically dependent patients the only things they have left are their attitudes and it can therefore be highly distressing to have them dismissed. Thus beliefs and attitudes need to be explored with great care.

A detailed assessment of the patient's beliefs can be carried out utilizing the concepts of the Health Belief Model (Becker and Maiman, 1975). The Health Belief Model suggests that people are most likely to take preventive actions or comply with medical advice if they:

- feel concerned about their health and motivated to protect it
- feel threatened by their current behaviour
- feel change would be beneficial/have few adverse consequences
- feel competent to carry out change (Naidoo and Willis, 1995).

By eliciting information about the patient's health beliefs, the nurse can reinforce positive attitudes to health and counter myths and negative attitudes.

As well as the interview part of the assessment, measurements will need to be made, e.g. blood pressure, weight, and tidal volume, to provide a baseline to monitor progress. The patient's present health behaviour can be also assessed using a diary in which he records relevant information, e.g. diet, blood sugar levels, number of cigarettes. This again will provide a baseline in order to monitor progress and evaluate the medication, but more importantly it will provide the basis from which to give specific health care advice later.

Having completed the assessment and before compliance by the patient is actively negotiated, three points must be considered by the health care professional:

- is the diagnosis correct
- is the treatment being considered appropriate

- is the treatment going to do the patient more good than harm (Raynor, 1992)?

If the answer to any of these questions is no, then compliance should not be expected.

Patient education

One of the main strategies aimed at improving compliance involves educating and informing the patient. Information will particularly benefit two types of patient who are non-compliant:

- those who want to comply but need more information to allow them to do so
- those with fears and misconceptions which can be dispelled by providing information.

In order to educate the patient the nurse herself needs a good knowledge of the drugs that her patients are taking. Table 17.4 shows the type of information that patients need about their drugs, and which the nurse should therefore be able to provide.

Table 17.4 Information required by patients about their drugs

- The names of the medication, i.e. both the generic and proprietary
- The objective, i.e. is the medicine being used to relieve symptoms or treat the disease
- The length of time before the effect of the medicine is noticeable
- How and when to take the medicine
- Whether it matters if a dose is missed, and what action to take
- The length of time the medicine is likely to be needed for
- The side-effects of the drug, how can they be recognized, and what action should be taken if they occur
- Whether the medication interacts with alcohol, food or other drugs, and what action should be taken

This information can be provided verbally, but bearing in mind how little is retained, the use of general information leaflets can be helpful, and have been shown to increase both knowledge and compliance significantly (Dodds, 1986). It is vital that these leaflets are written clearly and in plain English. Alternatively, the use of individualized leaflets can increase patient satisfaction (Raynor 1992), and promote compliance, by tailoring doses to the patient's lifestyle, or linking dosages with the patient's daily activities, e.g. meal times.

Other simple methods of improving compliance are shown in Table 17.5. Particularly helpful are tablet diaries that allow the patient or an aide to lay out a week's supply of drugs. There are problems in that the containers are not childproof, airtight, and do not hold liquid formulations, but they can be particularly useful where memory impairment is a problem.

Table 17.5 Simple methods of improving compliance

- Verbal information giving
- Information leaflets
- Individualized leaflets with tailoring or cueing
- Packaging – calendar pack; multi-compartment containers, e.g. Dosett, Medidos, Redidose
- Simplification of medicine regimen
- Self-administration of drugs

Simplification of the medicine regime makes it easier to understand, easier to remember and increases the chances of it fitting into the patient's lifestyle (Raynor, 1992). It involves discontinuing drugs that are not really needed, the use of drug combinations, e.g. a formulation combining metoclopramide and paracetamol to treat migraine rather than two separate drugs, and wherever possible single daily doses.

Self-administration of drugs in hospitals is argued to improve compliance, but most studies have been too small to allow firm conclusions, and few trials have followed up the patient's progress after self-administration has been employed on the wards (Collingsworth et al., 1997). A study which did follow up 88 patients 10 days after discharge found a mean compliance score for self-medicated patients of 95% compared with 83% in the control group. Furthermore, 90% of the patients in the self-medication group knew the purpose of their drugs compared with 46% of the control (Lowe et al., 1995). Possible advantages and disadvantages of self-medication are listed in Table 17.6.

Self-concept

Information giving is only one aspect of promoting compliance, as Mazzuca (1982) found when he examined 30 studies of patient

Table 17.6 The advantages and disadvantages of self-medication in hospital (Bird and Hassall 1993)

Advantages	*Disadvantages*
• Compliance	• Accidental or intentional overdose
• Customized care	• Accidental or intentional underdosage
• Independence	• Added stress of drug management
• Improved patient education	• Non-compliance
• Partnership in care	• No partnership in care
• Patient empowerment	
• Reduced readmission rates	
• Safety	
• Simplified regimens	
• Trust	

education in chronic disease. He identified that increasing patient knowledge alone was rarely successful in improving compliance and that behaviourally orientated programmes were consistently more successful at improving the clinical course of chronic disease. However, Pfister-Minogue (1983) argues that before a plan of care can be developed, the patient must have accepted his disease and have a positive self-concept. In listening to the patient's story the nurse may become aware that the patient is expressing, verbally or non-verbally, strong feelings such as anger, confusion, embarrassment, or despair in relation to living with his disease. Reflecting on these feelings can be essential in encouraging patients to come to terms with their condition. If the patient is still in denial over his diagnosis, of for example diabetes, then it is impossible to produce a plan of care in partnership. You as the nurse may be able to do things to the patient, but not with the patient. It may be necessary to act in this way in the short term, e.g. administering the patient's insulin injections, but it is not a satisfactory solution, and must be viewed as only temporary. In the case of tuberculosis the World Health Organization/International Union Against Tuberculosis and Lung Disease (1997) recommends that patients be observed taking their medication correctly in order to ensure compliance and reduce the risk of multi-drug resistance tuberculosis.

The patient can be helped to accept his disease and develop a positive self-concept, i.e. a belief that he can become master of his disease, through a variety of supportive strategies on the part of the nurse. The nurse can encourage the patient to verbalize his feelings and so can assist him to appreciate that his feelings of anger, depression and frustration are normal. Putting him in contact with a self-support group may help this process. The patient may also be helped if the rest of the family can be encouraged to rally round and for a short time decrease the demands made on the patient, so that he has the energy to deal with his disease and the problems it entails. The patient should also be encouraged to focus on his strengths in order to promote a positive self-esteem.

Setting achievable goals

Once the patient is ready, the nurse can then work with the patient to develop the self-care behaviours to allow him to deal with his health problems in a positive way. The use of self-medication programmes in hospital is seen as an important method of aiding empowerment and of giving patients the skills to manage their own medication. In the study by Lowe et al. (1995) over 40% of the patients felt more confident about taking their medicines when at home, and the same number thought that the self-medication programme had increased their understanding of their drug regimen.

One of the essential elements to setting achievable goals is to be specific. Thus the diabetic patient for example, should not simply be advised to take his insulin three times a day. Instead, the advice must be individualized and related to the other aspects of his lifestyle, in particular diet and exercise. The use of a dietary and exercise diary made during the assessment stage, will help to tailor the advice given and allow it to be put in context of the other lifestyle changes he is likely to have to make in order to adjust to his diabetes. The goals set must be achievable so that the patient can succeed, as success is the best form of reinforcement. The use of reinforcement and positive feedback will help, especially in the initial stages, to promote behaviour change. The nurse can give this feedback by perhaps monitoring the patient's progress through weekly blood sugar levels or monthly glycosylated haemoglobin levels, and by displaying the results visually on a graph to enable him to see his progress. His family and friends may also be able to help to encourage and motivate him by giving him praise, or more concrete reinforcements may be used in the form of trips out or the purchase of gifts. Again as part of the negotiation process the patient's personality should be taken into account, as some people progress better alone, and others do better by joining patient support groups. The use of treatment contracts may allow goals to be formalized more clearly and enable the patient to have a sense of empowerment (Papadopoulos and Jukes, 1999).

Success?

The result of the developed action plan may be that the patient changes his behaviour and adjusts positively to coping with his disease. Alternatively the patient verbally states that he wants to change his behaviour, but he does not seem to be able to be successful. In that case it is necessary to employ alternative or additional change strategies to achieve success. The third possibility is that the patient refuses to change his behaviour and to comply with the recommended health and medication strategies. If he understands his health problem, recognizes that changing his behaviour and taking his medication might benefit his health, and recognizes and accepts the implications of not doing so then the nurse must respect his choice. As a professional charged by your Code of Conduct (UKCC, 1992) to recognize the rights of the individual, you have to respect his decision.

Follow-up

This however is not the end of compliance promotion, or empowerment. It is common to start out with good intentions and then to falter along the way. By maintaining frequent follow up appointments the nurse can help the patient with problems as they materialize, especially when there are lifestyle changes such as changing schools or job, getting married or having a baby. Also follow up should not just be made available to patients who progress well or not so well, it should also be offered to patients who initially refused to change. As their life situation changes they may well be prepared to reconsider health changes, and the nurse needs to be prepared to help them as and when appropriate. A clear example of this is the hypertensive patient who refuses antihypertensives as she feels well and is not prepared to tolerate the adverse effects of the drugs. The development of chest pain and fears of a heart attack may mean that she reconsiders the treatment offered.

Conclusion

The subject of compliance is a difficult one as the nurse is left with the dilemma of respecting patients' autonomy while ensuring that limited health resources are not wasted on clients who put themselves at risk of increased morbidity through non-compliance. However, at the end of the day all nurses, together with other health professionals, can do is discover what patients are really doing with their medication and other aspects of their therapy. Using this information practitioners can advise against any dangerous practices, and in the spirit of creative, cooperative compliance this information can be used to devise more effective and therapeutic regimens (Weintraub, 1981).

References and further reading:-

Anon (1995) Prescription cost deters drug uptake. Nursing Times 91: 8

Ausburn L (1981) Patient compliance with medication regimes. In: Sheppard JL (ed.) Advances in Behavioural Medicine: Volume 1. Sydney: Cumberland College

Bartlett JG, Moore RD (1998) Improving HIV therapy. Scientific American 279: 64-73

Becker MH, Maiman LA (1975) Sociobehavioural determinants of compliance with health and medical care recommendations. Medical Care 13: 10-24

Bennett J (1999) Antipsychotic drug treatment. Nursing Standard 13: 49-53

Bird C, Hassall J (1993) Self Administration of Drugs – A Guide to Implementation. London: Scutari Press. Chapter 5

Brown F (1996) Improving compliance with asthma therapy. Community Nurse 1: 30-1

Brown F (1997) Patient empowerment through education. Professional Nurse Study Supplement 13: 4-S6

Cameron K, Gregor F (1987) Chronic illness and compliance. Journal of Advanced Nursing 12: 671-6

Chesterman L (1999) Blistering attack. Nursing Standard 14: 24

Col N, Fanale JE, Kronholm P (1990) The role of medication noncompliance and adverse drug reactions in hospitalizations of the elderly. Archives of International Medicine 150: 841-5

Collingsworth S, Gould D, Wainwright SP (1997) Patient self-administration of medication: a review of the literature. International Journal of Nursing Studies 34: 256-69

Dodds LJ (1986) Effect of information leaflets on compliance with antibiotic therapy. Pharmaceutical Journal 236: 48-51

Donovan JL, Blake DR (1992) Patient non-compliance: deviance or reasoned decision making? Social Science Medicine 34: 507-13

Funnell MM, Anderson RM, Arnold MS, Barr PA, Donnelly M, Johnson PD, Taylor-Moon D, White NH (1991) Empowerment: an idea whose time has come in diabetes education. Diabetes Educator 17: 37-41

Gordis L (1979). Conceptual and methodological problems in measuring patient compliance. In: Haynes RB, Taylor DW, and Sackett DL (eds.). Compliance in Health Care. Baltimore: John Hopkins University Press

Haynes RB (1979) Introduction. In: Haynes RB, Taylor DW, Sackett DL (eds.). Compliance in Health Care. Baltimore: John Hopkins University Press

Haynes RB, Taylor DW, and Sackett DL (1979) (eds.). Compliance in Health Care. Baltimore: John Hopkins University Press

Higgins R, Morlidge C (1998) Causes of non-compliance after transplantation. British Journal of Renal Medicine 3: 9-11

Holm S (1993) What is wrong with compliance? Journal of Medical Ethics 19: 108-10

Horne R (1997) Representations of medication and treatment advances in theory and measurement. In: Petrie JK, Weinman J (eds.) Perceptions of Health and Illness: Current Research and Applications. London: Harwood Academic

Hughes S (1998) Compliance with drug treatment in the elderly. Prescriber 9: 45-54

Kiernan V (1996) Misplaced fears put patients off their pills. New Scientist 149: 10

King J (1984a) Psychology in nursing: striking it right. Part 1. Nursing Times 80: 29-31

King J (1984b) Psychology in nursing: the health belief model. Nursing Times 80: 53-55

Kyngas H, Barlow J (1995) Diabetes: an adolescent's perspective. Journal of Advanced Nursing 22: 941-7

Laurence DR, Bennett PN, Brown MJ (1997) Clinical Pharmacology 8th edn. Edinburgh: Churchill Livingstone

Ley P (1988) The problem of patients' non-compliance. In: Ley P Communicating with Patients - Improving Communication Satisfaction and Compliance. London: Chapman and Hall

Lowe CJ, Raynor DK, Courtney EA, Purvis J, Teale C (1995) Effects of self medication programme on knowledge of drugs and compliance with treatment in elderly patients. British Medical Journal 310: 1229-31

Mazzuca SA (1982) Does patient education in chronic disease have therapeutic value? Journal of Chronic Diseases 35: 521-9

Moore KN (1995) Compliance or collaboration? The meaning for the patient. Nursing Ethics: An International Journal for Health Care Professionals 2: 71-7

Naidoo J, Willis J (1995) Health promotion: foundation for practice. London: Souton

Papadopoulos A, Jukes R (999) Motivation and compliance in wound management. Journal of Wound Care 8: 467-9

Pfister-Minogue K (1993) Enhancing patient compliance: a guide for nurses. Geriatric Nursing 14: 124-32

Poulton B (1991) Factors influencing patient compliance. Nursing Standard 5: 3-5

Raynor DK (1992) Patient compliance: the pharmacist's role. The International Journal of Pharmacy Practice 1: 126-35

Tettersell MJ (1993) Asthma patients' knowledge in relation to compliance with drug therapy. Journal of Advanced Nursing 18: 103-13

UKCC (1992) Code of Professional Conduct. London: UKCC

Weintraub M (1981) Intelligent noncompliance with special emphasis on the elderly. Contemporary Pharmacy Practice 4: 8-11

Chapter 18
Complementary therapy

DEBRAE WARD-WALSH

The diversity of healing methods probably predates human history. Approximately 500 years ago a subset of medical practices arose and health care first split into conventional and unconventional practices (Vickers 1996). The concept of 'complementary medicine' remains heavily affected by this split, often classed as a 'non-conventional therapy', mainly because they stand outside the limits of health care traditionally available on the NHS (British Medical Association, 1993).

This classification may have to be reviewed in future as many complementary therapies are becoming available in both acute and community NHS care (Lundie, 1994), particularly within care of the elderly (Hudson, 1996; Millar, 1996; Cannard, 1996), palliative care (Horrigan, 1991; Machin, 1989), and intensive and coronary care (Rowe, 1989; Stevenson, 1994a). However, therapies which are complementary and those which are alternative are often wrongly used interchangeably, which weakens their overall value and worth.

Defining complementary and alternative therapies

- Complementary therapies are therapies which can work alongside and in conjunction with orthodox medical treatment (BMA, 1993). Examples include: Alexander technique, massage, aromatherapy, acupuncture, osteopathy, chiropractic and homeopathy
- Alternative therapies are those given in place of orthodox medicine and whose effects may be negated by orthodox medicines.

For example, herbal medicine is often given as an alternative to allopathic drugs (BMA, 1993).

The range of complementary therapies

In 1993 the BMA stated that approximately 180 different therapies are practised in the UK. To date only osteopathy has gained legislative power to sanction individuals guilty of malpractice (Rankin-Box, 1995). Types of therapy involving ingestion, inhalation or application only will be considered here, in line with the ethos of this book's overall aims. Aromatherapy will form the main focus of this chapter; the therapy that the writer is both qualified and practices within.

Herbal medicine

Qualified, experienced herbalists treat a wide range of conditions in patients including both the young and pregnant (Rankin-Box, 1995). Herbal medicines aim to use the patient's natural resistance to restore the balance of health. They are commonly used in treating chronic disorders including arthritis, back pain, stress and anxiety concerns, and sometimes malignant diseases.

Safety and efficacy

Many plants used in herbal medicine contain principles whose effects can be demonstrated pharmacologically; the action of the whole plant extract can usually be related to that of the isolated constituent (Trounce, 1997). A commonly held belief that herbal remedies, being natural products, are 'safer' than the synthetic drugs of orthodox medicine, which occasionally produce undesirable side-effects, is a myth.

Toxicity does occur, yet it is rarely an acute episode as a result of accidental consumption of an overdose. Reading the instructions and acting upon them is just as important as with orthodox medicine (Trounce, 1997). Herbal medicines are often taken over a long period of time and the appearance of toxicity may be delayed or may even appear after the remedy has been discontinued (Trounce, 1997).

The uncontrolled supply and administration of these herbal remedies has led the Committee on the Safety of Medicines (CSM) to remind doctors that the yellow card scheme applies in the same manner as it does for orthodox medicines. However, the CSM can take little action as these types of medicines do not have a product licence (Trounce, 1997).

Proven or suspended toxicity of herbal products

Comfrey has traditionally been used as a demulcent in chronic catarrhs, treatment of gastro-intestinal disorders and sometimes as a tonic. Herbalists in the UK use comfrey as a demulcent, an anti-haemorrhagic and anti-rheumatic agent and as an anti-inflammatory agent. Safety concerns centre on its content of pyrrolizoline alkaloids, which cause liver cell necrosis when metabolized in the liver leading the liver to produce toxic metabolites. Hepatotoxicity of comfrey in humans has been characterized by veno-occlusive lesions with hepatomegaly and inhibition of mitosis (Trounce, 1997).

A 'babchi' herbal tea has been associated with photosensitivity (Trounce, 1997). Herbs such as kavakava, khat, thornapple, valerian and skullcap have been linked to intoxication. In the UK hepatotoxicity has been reported in patients taking 'kalms' or 'neurelax' for relieving stress. The most hepatotoxic component was thought to be valerian but this has always been disputed (Trounce, 1997). More recently concern has been expressed about the safety of St John's wort (*Hypericum perforatum*) which has been phenomenally successful as a herbal antidepressant. There are few doubts about the efficacy of hypericum extracts, which are thought to act similarly to conventional serotonin-reuptake inhibitors, or that they are associated with substantially fewer adverse effects than synthetic antidepressants. However, at least eight cases have been reported that suggest that hypericum extracts are potent inducers of hepatic enzymes. This can result in increased metabolism of concomitant drugs and various adverse effects depending on the concomitant drug (Ernst, 1999). Furthermore, the combined use of prescribed serotonin reuptake inhibitors with over-the-counter St John's wort has resulted in symptoms characteristic of central serotonin excess. The possible adverse effects of herbal medicines are shown in Table 18.1.

Homeopathy

Homeopathy is a 200-year-old system of medicine (Haehl, 1995 cited in Rankin-Box, 1995) and is based on the law of similars (let

Table 18.1 Possible adverse effects of herbal medicines

Herbal preparation	*Indication*	*Adverse effect*
Alfalfa seeds	Lowers cholesterol	Pancytopenia, reactivation of systemic lupus erythematosus
Aristolochic acid (tincture infusion)	Anti-inflammatory	Carcinogenic, renal damage
Herbal preparation	Anti-carcinogenic	Hypokalaemia
Ginseng	Anti-fatigue, anti-stress	Oestrogen like effects. Hypertension
Honey (rhododendron)	Food supplement	Intoxication, nausea, vomiting, hypotension, bradycardia, reduces consciousness
Margosa oil (Neem tree extract)	Insecticide, spermicide	Hepatotoxicty
Mistletoe	Antispasmodic, diuretic, hypotensive	Hepatotoxicity (hepatitis) Diarrhoea
Zemaphyte (Chinese herbs)	Eczema	Hepatotoxicity, hepatitis

like be cured by like). Production of homeopathic medicines is from a variety of sources including plants, minerals, stings, venom, metals and even bacteria. The effectiveness of the medicines is the result of how the remedies are made. The original substances are diluted many times in a water and alcohol base. The mixture is shaken at each dilution a process known as 'succession' which homeopaths believe gives the medicine its power to heal (Livingston, 1991).

Accepted pharmaceutical principles are applied to devising different potencies. The two forms of dilution are decimal and centesimal, successive methods of reduction are in stages of 1/10 and 1/100. The number of stages determines the potency of the dilution or trituration (Rankin-Box, 1995).

Prescriptions are dispensed in four forms depending on the need, i.e. powders, tablets, granules, and liquids. Prescribing methods differ so that a low potency may be given over a period of weeks or months. Tablets may be used here which consist of lactose with added pure sugar. The desired potency of the homeopathic medicine is added and absorbed into the tablets (Rankin-Box, 1995).

Patients are often advised to avoid peppermint, menthol and coffee as they can counteract the effect of the remedies. Some homeopaths even recommend avoiding peppermint toothpaste for the same reasons. Chemists and health food shops often sell these medicines over-the-counter for self-help, for example Rhus Tox 6C for rheumatism or chammomilla 6C for teething problems (Rankin-Box, 1995). Self-help in many chronic illnesses is not enough and consultation with a qualified homeopath is essential for assessment and prescription of medicines at the correct potency.

Critics of this therapy have often linked the effects to little more than a 'placebo effect', and despite research being available, it is concentrated mainly on animals, a drawback in which many complementary therapies find themselves. However, to date, homeopathy is complementary to conventional medicine and may be useful in combating chronic illness without the risks of side-effects (Koehler, 1986 cited in Rankin Box, 1995).

Homeopaths may be non-medically qualified people, who have trained on courses extending over five years on a part-time basis, awarded a qualification which to date has no statutory recognition despite many colleagues promoting high training standards (Rankin-Box 1995). This drawback has the potential risk that with a non-medical/nursing background homeopaths may be less likely to know when to refer a patient for conventional medical assessment (Faculty of Homeopathy, 1993). The only statutory recognized training body is the faculty of homeopathy at the Royal London Homeopaths Hospital, Great Ormond Street, London; in 1993 it became the first professional training body to have a MSc degree in homeopathic medicine associated with a British university. This course which began in the autumn of 1994 is presently only open to medical doctors but trained nurses, midwives and pharmacists may complete the first module and be awarded a certificate in homeopathic medicine.

Homeopathy may be used to treat both minor and serious conditions. Rankin-Box (1995) highlighted that in advanced stages of terminal illness substantial pain relief and comfort may be attained. No two people presenting with the same symptoms receive the same prescription. A full assessment of that person's health, lifestyle, illness and factors influencing the onset of the symptoms are taken. Having taken this information, the prescription is always based on the overall presentation of the symptoms (Livingston, 1991). Some of the homeopathic medicines used in the treatment of symptoms of illness, are shown in Table 18.2.

Table 18.2 Some homeopathic medicines used in the treatment of symptoms of illness (Rankin-Box, 1995)

Symptoms	*Treatment*
General	
Bites and stings, e.g. bees or wasps	Apis mel, Urtica urens, Ledum
Insomnia	Coffee
Coughs, colds, sore throats and influenza	Gelsemium, Aconite
Fever	Belladonna
Coughs	Bryonia
Hayfever and simple allergies	Homeopathic grass pollen, Allium cepa
Hyperactive children	Belladonna, Agaricus
Burns and scolds, severe blistering	Cantharis
Sunburn	Belladonna, Calendula (as local application)
Community care–wide application for district nursing in the treatment of wounds and leg ulcers and care of the elderly	
Post-operative wounds	Arnica, Staphysagria
Leg ulcers	Calendula, Flouric acid
Care of the chronically and terminally ill, including pain management and emotional distress	
Terminal illness with restlessness	Arsen alba
Pain associated with tumours	Euphorbium
Distressed relatives, e.g. shock and grief reactions	
Shock	Gelsemium, Aconite
Grief	Ignatia
Endoscopic procedures	
Pre-general anaesthetic	Phosphorus
Apprehensive patients	Gelsemium, Argentum nitrate
Pre and post surgical management including dental surgery, before any surgical procedure	Arnica
Stress and phobias including anticipation and fear of unpleasant investigations and surgical procedures	
Phobic states	Phosphorus, Argentum nitrate
Anticipatory fear	Gelsemium
Accident and emergency and first aid, including road traffic accidents, air, sea and mountain rescue	
Sudden collapse	Carbo veg
Acute injuries	Arnica
Injured nerves	Hypericum

Contraindications for use

Homeopathic treatments are safe and can be used alongside conventional medicines. Yet some homeopaths feel that treatment may be less effective if combined with steroid preparations. Rankin-Box (1995) outlines contraindications to be aware of:

- Patients known to have milk product sensitivity should inform their homeopath as lactose is often used as a tablet base for the homeopathic medicine. Remedies may then be prescribed in a water and alcohol base in the form of drops.
- Diabetics should inform the homeopath that lactose based medicine is not suitable. A non-sugar based medication can be prescribed.
- Young babies may not be able to metabolize alcohol so medicines should be alcohol free. Alcohol free medicines may be dissolved in water and given in the feeding bottle.
- Homeopaths should work in partnership with doctors and should never attempt to treat a patient with a serious illness whose diagnosis is unclear without consultation with a patient's GP

Homeopathy cannot be used in isolation. The patient must not only comply with the prescription, but perhaps make changes in his or her lifestyle (e.g. stop drinking coffee while taking the medicines) and make time for relaxation and recuperation.

Aromatherapy

Aromatherapy is an individual treatment designed to help, heal or cure by the correct use and application of essential oils obtained from plants (Price, 1987). Cure in this context involves stimulating the body's natural healing mechanisms – no therapist can ever claim to 'cure' an illness or disease. The Aromatherapy Organizations Council (1996) definition states 'Aromatherapy is the systematic use of essential oils in holistic treatments to improve physical and emotional well being. Essential oils possess distinctive therapeutic properties which can be utilized to improve health and prevent disease. Their physiological and psychological effects combine well to promote positive health.'

Aromatology is both the precursor and an extension of aromatherapy. In the 1920's full body massage was not used to introduce essential oils into the body. Popular methods of this time were inhalation, mouth and throat washes, compresses and internal use (for example pessaries, suppositories (Price, 1998)). Aromatherapy was introduced into the UK via the beauty profession hence the common application of essential oils via massage (Price, 1998). It is probably the fastest growing complementary therapy discipline in the UK (Tisserand and Balacs, 1995). The national promotion of health and the gradual realization that the treatment of illness and the maintenance of well being are a personal responsibility has led to growth in over-the-counter sales of natural remedies such as essential oils (Tisserand and Balacs, 1995).

Essential oils

Essential oil essences are volatile, odorous molecules held within glandular pockets or canals within a plant and are known as a plant's 'life force' or energy. During extraction by distillation using heat, air or water their composition alters and they become known as essential oils (Price, 1987; McGilvery et al., 1997). Essential oils are 70 times more concentrated than the plants from which they are extracted, and as minute quantities of oil are held within plants this makes some pure essential oils expensive (Price, 1987). For example, approximately 20 rose heads produce only one drop of pure rose oil making it one of the most expensive essential oils.

The potency of essential oils will deteriorate if kept in poor storage conditions. Essential oils should be purchased in small quantities (i.e. 5–10 mL) in a dark bottle (i.e. normally brown, green or blue), kept cool around 5°C and in the dark. Life expectancy in these conditions is approximately one year (Price, 1987). The three main factors responsible for degradation of essential oils are:

- atmospheric oxygen
- heat
- light (Tisserand and Balacs, 1995).

Atmospheric oxygen may change the chemical composition of essential oils by interacting with some of their components – a process known as oxidation. This is more common in essential oils containing high amounts of terpenes such as lemon and pine (Tisserand and Balacs, 1995). This process happens more quickly in the presence of heat and light, hence the reason for storing in the dark, purchasing in a dark bottle, and keeping cool. Keeping the lid firmly closed will reduce the amount of air entering the bottle which again will reduce the speed of oxidation (Tisserand and Balacs, 1995).

A serious implication of essential oil degradation is that chemical change can make them hazardous. Terpene degradation in some oils can lead to compounds being formed which make the oils potential skin sensitizers. Degradation in types of citrus oils leads to chemical production which are weakly carcinogenic in mice (Tisserand and Balacs, 1995). Although this is unlikely to affect humans it does emphasize the importance of using good quality essential oils, which have been stored correctly, for aromatherapy treatments.

Historical use

The use of aromatic oils dates back as far as 2000 years BC, the Egyptians used them both as cosmetics and for embalming their dead to delay decomposition (Tisserand, 1992).

Benefits of aromatherapy

Aromatherapy may be used in a variety of ways prescribed to meet individual needs. The oils work on three distinct yet inter-related levels. Firstly, odour stimuli in the limbic system of the brain set off a cascade of neurotransmitters including enkephalins, endorphins (which reduce pain), serotonin (which stimulates relaxation) and noradrenaline (norepinephrine) (a stimulant) (Lawless, 1994; Worwood, 1992a). Secondly, aromas may play an important role in improving mental performance, enhancing memory, inducing relaxation and influencing mood (Worwood, 1992b). Thirdly, aromatherapy massage has physiological benefits by improving the circulation of blood and lymph, thereby helping to eliminate toxins from the body, slowing the pulse rate, lowering blood pressure, relaxing muscle tension, toning flaccid and weak muscles and relieving cramp (Price and Price, 1995).

Although not easy to evaluate, psychological effects play a significant role in the holistic healing effects of relaxing and calming an apprehensive mind, improving mild depression, relaxing panic or anger and most importantly giving the recipient the feeling of being cared for (Price, 1987).

Aromatherapy according to its clients, does make them 'feel better' and 'feeling better' may have a tremendous effect on physical symptoms, similar to those induced by exercise (Morrissey, 1997). There is no doubt that a type of 'placebo effect' is achieved which may be linked to the therapist giving the client their time, attention and interest whilst giving treatment. Also, as suggested by Vickers (1996) knowing someone 'cares' is a great comfort.

Essential oils may, when used with massage, 'balance' the subtle energy flows within the body in a similar way to acupuncture (Tisserand, 1992). Essential oils have a variety of properties the most popular being lavender, which aids sleep and relaxation (Cannard, 1996). Other properties are summarized in Table 18.3.

Table 18.3 Properties of essential oils (Davies, 1995)

Essential Oil	*Properties*
Lavender *(Lavender officinalis)*	Analgesic, antiseptic, anti-bacterial, sedative, hypotensive, anti-inflammatory, relaxant especially in severe anxiety states, antidepressant
Bergamot *(Citrus bergamia)*	Antidepressant, antiseptic, antiviral
Jasmine *(Jasmine officinale)*	Antidepressant, sedative, muscle relaxant
Geranium *(Pelargonium odarantissimum)*	Antiseptic, antidepressant, detoxifier, diuretic
Roman Chamomile *(Anthemis Noblis)*	Anti-inflammatory, muscle relaxant, analgesic, antidepressant, diuretic
Juniper *(Juniper communis)*	Antiseptic, diuretic, detoxifier
Black Pepper *(Piper nigrum)*	Rubefacient (heat producing), antispasmodic, diuretic, stimulant of the spleen and kidneys, analgesic
Ginger *(Zingiber officinalis)*	Antispasmodic, rubefacient (heat producing) antiseptic, analgesic
Eucalyptus *(Eucalyptus globulus)*	Decongestant, bactericidal, anti-viral, antiseptic, analgesic

Application and use of essential oils

Essential oils may be blended and applied in a number of ways to meet the individual needs of clients (Westwood, 1992). Massage is one of the most effective ways to reduce symptoms of stress and anxiety such as tension, tachycardia, hypertension and muscle stiffness in clientele who can tolerate touch (Walsh and Morrissey, 1998) A 2–3% blend of pure essential oils must be diluted within a carrier oil which may be of vegetable, nut or seed origin. Many carrier oils have therapeutic properties of their own. Sweet almond oil, for example helps reduce itching, dryness and inflammation in sensitive irritated skin (Westwood, 1992).

An aromatic bath is a simple way of helping induce relaxation. A 2–3% blend of pure essential oils in a small quantity of base oil (to aid adherence to the skin on leaving the water) may be added to the bath water. Relaxing for ten minutes in the water will aid absorption through the skin and promote relaxation as the fragrance is inhaled. Soap must not be used as it acts as an antidote and negates the effects of the essential oils.

Inhalation of essential oils affects the limbic system of the brain, as discussed earlier, and can help to relax and sedate the client (Price and Price, 1995). A 1–2% dilution of pure essential oils in a dish of water vaporized into the chosen atmosphere for 3–6 hours is desirable (Price and Price, 1995).

Following any of the above treatments clients should be advised to:

- Keep warm, allowing the essential oils to penetrate the skin and so be absorbed into the circulation.
- Drink 1–2 glasses of water or fruit juice (not tea or coffee due to their tannin and caffeine content) to extract toxins and essential oil residue via the kidneys.
- Leave the oils on the body for up to 12 hours to ensure that they penetrate and are absorbed by the skin, enter the circulation to detoxify (i.e. to promote excretion of uric and lactic acid) and to stimulate the immune system and the skin's natural healing mechanisms.
- Rest, to allow the oils to induce relaxation and calming effects, especially before bed.

It is quite natural within the first two or three days for symptoms to deteriorate as the oils stimulate deep-seated emotions and feelings. This is often referred to as a 'healing crisis' (Davis, 1995).

Essential oil dosage

Great care must be taken with the amounts of essential oils used in aromatherapy. A safe guide is:

- Body massage – 6–8 drops in total of up to three pure essential oils
- Facial massage – 1–2 drops in total of one pure essential oil (due to the delicate nature of the facial tissue)
- Bath oil – 6–8 drops in total of up to three pure essential oils
- Vaporizer/diffuser – 2–4 drops in total of 1–2 pure essential oils diluted in water

The quantity of essential oil absorbed into the body from an aromatherapy massage depends on:

- The percentage dilution of the essential oil
- The total quantity of oil applied
- The total area of skin to which the oil is applied (Tisserand and Balacs, 1995).

Frequency of use

Frequency of application is as important as the dosage used. A small dose of a toxic essential oil if applied daily for several months may cause slight tissue damage in the liver or kidneys (Tisserand and Balacs, 1995). The effects of toxicity over a long period of time may not be recognized by the individual, as the symptoms are relatively minor and commonplace.

Adverse effects and toxicity

Essential oils must be treated with great care and caution at all times. Toxicity includes skin reactions such as allergies and photosensitivity hazards in pregnancy and cancer. The individual's health status also needs to be explored such as age, blood pressure, liver dysfunction and conditions such as epilepsy, heart conditions and any medication being taken (Tisserand and Balacs, 1995). Toxicity is dose dependent, so that the more essential oil used the greater the risk of harm (Tisserand and Balacs, 1995). This may seem rather shocking as aromatherapy is often promoted as a 'natural' way of promoting health and well-being. However, 'natural' does not mean 'safe'.

Essential oils may be sold in a wide variety of outlets from chemists to health food shops and market stalls. The majority of oils do not have guidelines for use, contra-indicators or safe dilution advice. Typically, (but not in all cases) bottles state:

- Dilute to 5% or less in a carrier oil before skin application
- Keep out of eyes
- Do not swallow

This advice in itself may be hazardous:

- Does the average person know what a 5% dilution is and how to achieve it?
- If oils should come into contact with the eyes how should they be removed and with what?
- If oils are swallowed what should the person do?

Retailers on market stalls and health food shops may not have the knowledge to store the oils safely or advise people with health problems which oils not to buy to avoid adverse reactions.

Information on essential oil toxicity is available from Guy's Hospital specialist poisons unit in London. The unit advises doctors on substances which patients have swallowed or allowed to come into contact with the skin. Only a few enquiries received by the unit are essential oil related; yet as aromatherapy is becoming more and more popular this may change (Tisserand and Balacs, 1995).

The severity of toxicity depends on the route of application. Oral consumption of essential oils carries the highest risk especially if taken undiluted. Six cases of wintergreen oil poisoning in adults have been documented. Three people died from ingesting 15 mL, 30 mL and 80 mL and three survived after ingesting 6 mL, 16 mL and 24 mL. None received medical attention (Tisserand and Balacs, 1995).

Eucalyptus pure essential oil appears to be fatal in amounts between 30 mL and 60 mL which is rather daunting as it is one of the most common oils used for treating colds and flu and is perhaps one of the oils most aromatherapy lovers would buy.

Camphor essential oil has been reported to cause serious poisoning, usually in young children. Accidental ingestion of 60 mL of camphorated oil (not an essential oil) by a pregnant woman probably caused the death of her full term foetus (Riggs et al., 1965 cited in Tisserand and Balacs, 1995).

Cinnamon oil poisoning occurred in a 7-year-old boy who drank 60 mL of the oil as a dare by a friend. He experienced a burning sensation in the mouth, chest, and stomach, dizziness, double vision and nausea. He vomited and collapsed. Medical opinion felt that had he not vomited the dose may have been fatal (Philapil, 1989 cited in Tisserand and Balacs, 1995). Other pure essential oils, which may cause toxicity, include hyssop, pennyroyal, sassafras, wormseed and sage.

It must be remembered that documented cases of toxicity may be shocking but they are the only reliable way of recording adverse effects in humans as most of the toxicity testing of essential oils is performed in laboratory conditions using rats and mice. Although this research is useful it is problematic as the skin and metabolism of rats and mice are different to humans making direct application impossible.

Lack of published research

Research into the value and effects of aromatherapy in illness and disease has been rather superficial, with a tendency to be anecdotal. Where clinical trials have been reported they have been small scale, often poorly carried out and not reported in English (Stevenson, 1994b).

Vickers (1996) reviewed available research literature and was critical of numerous studies due to their poor standards, methods and small numbers involved. Essential oils are not classed as medicines and therefore do not come under the Medicines Control Agency or the Medicines Act 1968. Customer protection is extremely haphazard; this offers the opportunity for manufacturers to sell poorly produced aromatherapy products.

The lack of research evidence may make it difficult for nurses registered as aromatherapists to justify claims for the therapeutic properties of essential oils. This may result in nurses being unable to incorporate aromatherapy into their professional practice regardless of having obtained informed consent from the consultant/GP, patient and/or relatives (Stevenson, 1994b).

Who can practise?

Qualified and unqualified nurses who use essential oils within their nursing practice as either a bath oil or massage oil without aromatherapy registration are breaking their UKCC Professional Code of Conduct (1992) and may be reported for misconduct. Additionally, as aromatherapy oils penetrate the skin, their use may be classed as an assault.

The advent of nurse prescribing focuses responsibilities even more as it raises the issue about appropriate, recognized training as a nurse prescriber not about competence and confidence as a qualified nurse alone. Nurse prescribing training emphasizes the maintenance of high standards of accountability and professional responsibility (Sadler, 1995). Aromatherapy practice in the NHS should be restricted to qualified aromatherapists only, and only when informed consent has been obtained as discussed earlier.

Aromatherapy training recommended by the Aromatherapy Organisation Council (AOC) requests aromatherapists should have met at least the basic training standards of:

- 180 class hours, comprising of 80 hours aromatherapy, 60 hours of massage and 40 hours of anatomy and physiology, plus 10–15 case studies over 50 treatment hours over no less than 9 months.
- All therapists must be insured for both public and professional liability in the region of £1 000 000

The AOC, formed in 1991, is the governing body for the aromatherapy profession in the UK and currently holds membership of 11 professional aromatherapy associations. It aims to:

- Unify the professions by bringing together its various organizations.
- Establish common standards of training and ensure that all organizations registered with the Council provide appropriate standards of professional practice and conduct for their members.
- Act as a public watchdog.

- Provide for all organizations within aromatherapy a collective voice through which to initiate and sustain political dialogue with government, civil and medical bodies; in order to enhance the best interest of professional aromatherapy.
- Offer a mediating and arbitration service in any disputes involving aromatherapy organizations.
- Initiate support or sponsor research into aromatherapy (Diamond, 1998).

Complementary therapies will continue to grow in popularity and therefore standards of practice must be upheld and continually developed. Only with investment in well-conducted clinical trials similar to those used for conventional medications will the potential benefits and adverse effects of complementary therapies be identified. This will allow therapists and patients to make fully informed choices about which therapies they utilize.

References and further reading:

Aromatherapy Organizations Council (1996) Core curriculum. Market Harborough: Aromatherapy Organizations Council

British Medical Association (1993) Complementary medicine – new approaches to good practice. Oxford: Oxford University Press

Cannard G (1996) The effects of aromatherapy in promoting relaxation and stress reduction in a general hospital. Complementary Therapies in Nursing and Midwifery 2: 38-40.

Davis P (1995) Aromatherapy An A-Z. Cambridge: CW Daniel Company Ltd.

Diamond B (1998) The legal aspects of complementary therapy. A guide for healthcare professionals. Edinburgh: Churchill Livingstone

Ernst E (1999) Second thoughts about the safety of St John's wort. Lancet 354: 2014-5

Faculty of Homeopathy (1993) Non-medically qualified practitioners of homeopathy. British Homeopathic Journal 82: 200-3

Horrigan C (1991) Complementary cancer care. International Journal of Aromatherapy 3: 15-17

Hudson R (1996) The value of lavender to rest and activity in the elderly patient. Complementary Therapies in Medicine 4: 52-7

Lawless J (1994) Aromatherapy and the Mind. London: Thorsons

Livingston R (1991) Homeopathy evergreen medicine. Jewel in the Medical Crown. Poole: Asher.

Lundie S (1994) Introducing and applying aromatherapy within the NHS. The Aromatherapist 1:283

Machin A (1989) Advanced cancer. International Journal of Aromatherapy 2:19

McGilvery C, Reed J, Melita M (1997) The Encyclopaedia of Aromatherapy Massage and Yoga. Bristol: Paragon

Millar B (1996) Complementary therapies find a welcome home. Healthiness 28:20-2.
Morrissey M (1997) Exercise and mental health: A qualitative study. Mental Health Nursing 17: 6-8
Price S (1987) Practical aromatherpy. 2nd edn. London: Thorsons
Price S (1998) Using essential oils in professional practice. Complementary Therapies in Nursing and Midwifery 4:144-7
Price S and Price L (1995) Aromatherpy for Health Professionals. Edinburgh: Churchill Livingstone
Rankin-Box D (1995) The Nurses Handbook of Complementary Therapies. London: Churchill Livingstone.
Rowe L (1989) Anxiety in a coronary care unit. Nursing Times 85: 61
Sadler C (1995) Stretching the limits. Health Visitor 68: 403-4
Stevenson C J (1994a) The psychophysical effects of aromatherapy massage following cardiac surgery. Complementary Therapies in Medicine 2:27-35.
Stevenson L (1994b) Aromatherapy: The essentials. RCN nursing update 10. Nursing Standard 9: 3-8
Tisserand R and Balacs T (1995) Essential Oil Safety for Health Care Professionals. Edinburgh: Churchill Livingstone
Tisserand R (1992) The Art of Aromatherapy 13th impression. Essex: Daniel Company Ltd.
Trounce J (1997) Clinical Pharmacology for Nurses. 15th edn. Edinburgh: Churchill Livingstone
UKCC (1992) Code of Professional Conduct. London: UKCC
Vickers A (1996) Massage and Aromatherapy – a Guide for Health Professionals. London: Chapman and Hall.
Walsh D and Morrissey M (1998) Aromatherapy: An approach to managing symptoms of stress. Mental Health Nursing 8: 23-7
Westwood C (1992) Aromatherapy: A Guide for Home Use. Great Britain: Amberwood Publishing Ltd
Worwood VA (1992a) The Fragrant Mind – Aromatherapy for Personality Mood and Emotion. London: Doubleday Publishers
Worwood VA (1992b) The Fragrant Pharmacy. London: Bautian Books

Part 3
The Practice – 12
Case studies

Chapter 19
Assessment issues

Inaccurate diagnosis

Case study

Gertrude Stacey, a 78-year-old widow who lives alone, went to see her practice nurse because the scratch that she had received from her cat two months ago had got worse. The nurse took a full clinical history and then assessed Mrs Stacey's wound. She found that Mrs Stacey had a shallow 3 cm diameter sloughy ulcer on her left leg above the lateral malleolus, which was producing a moderate amount of exudate. The skin around the ulcer was hyperpigmented, and Mrs Stacey showed signs of varicose veins and pitting oedema. The nurse looked and found, after a little searching, a pedal pulse in both feet. The nurse also carried out a finger prick test and found Mrs Stacey's blood sugar was 8.7 mmol/L; she measured Mrs Stacey's blood pressure and found it to be 180/85 mmHg. The practice nurse diagnosed Mrs Stacey as having a venous leg ulcer and she applied a four-layer compression bandage. The practice nurse also identified that Mrs Stacey was hypertensive, and referred her to the GP. The GP examined Mrs Stacey and diagnosed mild left ventricular failure, for which he prescribed captopril 12.5 mg twice daily and furosemide (frusemide) 40 mg in the morning. Mrs Stacey was asked to return to the surgery in a week's time to have her bandages reapplied.

Mrs Stacey was a very compliant lady and wore the bandages as she has been told to, although she found them very uncomfortable. Mrs Stacey found that after she started on her new tablets that she had to get up at night to go to the toilet and she was quite worried by this. She suffered from osteoarthritis, found it difficult to move fast enough to get to the toilet and so was very worried that she would wet herself. She therefore decided to cut down the amount she drank, especially in the evening.

The next night when going to bed Mrs Stacey felt a bit faint and dizzy. She fell in the hall and broke her leg. She was unable to move and lay on the cold floor all night until the milkman saw her through the glass when delivering the milk the following morning and called an ambulance. Mrs Stacey was admitted to hospital with a fractured neck of femur and hypothermia, from which she did not recover.

Questions:

- Mrs Stacey was diagnosed as having venous ulceration and hypertension. How could the assessment of her condition have been improved upon?
- What was the underlying cause of Mrs Stacey's death?
- How could have Mrs Stacey's drug regimen have been improved upon?

Answers:

The practice nurse correctly took a full clinical history and then assessed the wound looking at the wound itself and the surrounding skin. All the symptoms that Mrs Stacey demonstrated supported a diagnosis of a venous ulcer. The nurse tried to rule out arterial disease by checking pedal pulses and looking for diabetes. However, two large studies have shown respectively that 67% and 37% of limbs with some degree of arterial disease have palpable foot pulses (Callam et al., 1987a; Moffat and O'Hare, 1995). Venous and arterial disease can, and often do, coexist in the same individual, and consequently signs of venous disease are insufficient to rule out some degree of arterial disease (Scriven et al., 1997). Thus the RCN (1998) recommend in their clinical practice guidelines that all patients presenting with a leg ulcer should be screened for arterial disease with Doppler measurements of the ankle/brachial pressure index. This is especially the case when compression therapy is to be used, because if applied to patients with arterial disease the resulting ischaemia can result in necrosis and worsening of the ulcer (Callam et al., 1987b).

Most elderly people with raised blood pressure have isolated systolic hypertension, defined as a systolic pressure greater than 140 mmHg and a diastolic pressure of less than 90 mmHg (Bennet, 1994). Looking at the readings for Mrs Stacey, she appears to fit in with this definition. As recent large clinical trials have shown that antihypertensive treatment in elderly patients is highly protective against stroke and myocardial infarction (Strandgaard and Paulson, 1994), it therefore appears to make sense to start Mrs Stacey on treatment immediately. However, when screening the elderly for hypertension extra care must be taken to ensure the correct diagnosis. Firstly, blood pressure readings are far more variable in the elderly, so more readings need to be taken before a diagnosis is made (Bennet, 1994). In any age group more than one blood pressure reading is required, and the British Hypertension Society recommends that in older patients with isolated systolic hypertension, but no target organ damage, measurements should be made over 3–6 months (Sever et al., 1993). Secondly, blood pressure should be measured in both the sitting and standing positions. This is because there is frequently (30% in the NHANES II Survey) a drop of 20 mmHg in standing blood pressure in patients with a sitting pressure of 160 mmHg (NHANES, 1986 cited Bennet, 1994). Standing blood pressure measurements should be used to guide treatment decisions. If standing blood pressure is not utilized to guide treatment decisions, there is a danger that the postural hypotension will be made worse, leading to falls and the serious consequences that they entail.

Mrs Stacey died from a fall caused by postural hypotension. As already identified, it is not clear that Mrs Stacey actually had hypertension, but even if she did, the drug therapy needs to be reconsidered. The elderly have increased sensitivity to antihypertensives and diuretics (Rajaei-Dehkordi and McPherson, 1997), probably because of their changing physiology, which makes maintaining homeostasis more difficult. Thus, in the elderly, cerebral circulation does not auto-regulate very efficiently and peripheral autonomic responses can be sluggish in response to hypotension. In addition, the elderly become easily hypovolaemic with diuretics or through not drinking and eating enough. Thus, when prescribing treatment for the elderly, the lowest possible doses should be used to commence treatment, and then the dose slowly titrated upwards against the symptoms. The doses of drugs prescribed for Mrs Stacey are not excessive, however, the British National Formulary (BMA and RPS, 1997) suggests that, when used in combination with a diuretic or in the elderly, the starting dose of captopril should be 6.25 mg twice daily. It also notes that profound first-dose hypotension is common when ACE inhibitors are introduced in patients with heart failure who are receiving loop diuretics, like furosemide (frusemide).

Mrs Stacey's problems were compounded by her not drinking. It is common for the elderly to worry about incontinence and they frequently respond by either not taking their drugs or not drinking. The ACE-inhibitors decrease the sensation of thirst (Jordan and Torrance, 1995) and so Mrs Stacey would not even feel the need to drink. Mrs Stacey should have been warned about this adverse effect and the implications discussed. Provision of a commode might have minimized the problem. It should certainly have been emphasized to her that she should not stop drinking. It must also be born in mind that one of the effects of compression therapy is to promote venous return, cardiac output and diuresis. Thus the combination of drugs and compression therapy would have increased her diuresis and hence the risk of dehydration.

Diagnosis failure

Case study

Margaret Fox is a 36-year-old married woman with carcinoma of the left breast. She had a mastectomy two years ago, followed by radiotherapy. A year later the cancer reoccurred, and despite chemotherapy the cancer broke through the skin as a fungating tumour. The wound produced large amounts of exudate and was extremely malodorous. Mrs Fox was very distressed by the malodour and sought advice from her GP who prescribed oral metronidazole. This effectively controlled the odour, which together with sheets of alginate dressing supplied by the district nurse made the wound manageable.

Mrs Fox had been losing weight for some time, and Mr Fox found this very distressing. He was an excellent cook and spent all his spare time making Mrs Fox little delicacies to tempt her appetite. He mentioned his concern to a friend who was a dietitian at the local hospital, and she recommended sherry before meals as an appetite stimulant. Mr Fox took his friend's advice and started encouraging his wife to have a glass of sherry before meals. Mr Fox also started adding whisky to his wife's bedtime drink in order to help her to sleep.

Mrs Fox's condition deteriorated and she developed severe pain as well as nausea and vomiting. She consequently became very distressed and depressed. She went to see her GP and she prescribed amitriptyline.

Questions:

- Why is Mrs Fox vomiting?
- How could the GP's management of Mrs Fox be improved?
- How else could the odour from the wound be controlled?
- Is amitriptyline a good choice of drug for Mrs Fox?

Answers:

It is common for cancer patients to develop nausea and vomiting, and there is a variety of possible reasons for this. These include psychological factors such as anxiety, gastrointestinal factors such as constipation and obstruction, side-effects of drugs including morphine and cytotoxics, environmental factors such as strong odours, raised intracranial pressure due to tumour within the brain, hypercalcaemia due to bony metastases, and radiotherapy (Williams, 1994). Not all of these factors apply to Mrs Fox, but several of them can be seriously considered. However, as well as the factors listed above, another possible cause could be a drug interaction. Metronidazole when taken with alcohol has what is called an 'Antabuse effect'. Disulfiram (Antabuse) is a drug given to alcoholics to encourage them to stop drinking. If they take both disulfiram and alcohol, or in Mrs Fox's case metronidazole and alcohol, the two chemicals interact causing severe nausea and vomiting.

To manage Mrs Fox more effectively, the GP should not assume that the nausea and vomiting is the result of cancer, but should take a history to try and find out when the nausea and vomiting started. Once he has identified that Mrs Fox is drinking alcohol to improve her appetite, and knowing of the interaction between metronidazole and alcohol, the GP has two lines of action open to him. One is to encourage Mrs Fox to stop drinking alcohol, while the second is for her to stop using the metronidazole. If she does the latter, then the GP will need to find some other way to control the odour from the wound. It thus may appear that the simple solution is for Mrs Fox to stop drinking the alcohol. However, this may not be the best solution as the use of alcohol is allowing the couple to take some control of Mrs Fox's disease, and having control can be very important for people suffering with a malignancy. Thus, other solutions should be carefully examined before banning alcohol is considered. Other methods of odour control may be utilized, and these include use of charcoal dressings such as Actisorb Plus™ and Carboflex™ (Thomas, 1989), or the use of room deodorizers, or the application of aromatherapy oils such as bergamot, clary sage, cypress, eucalyptus, lavender and neroli (Davis, 1995). Another possibility is to continue with metronidazole but to use it topically in the form of Anabact or Metrotop (Grocott, 1999). In both the topical and rectal formulation metronidazole does not interact with alcohol, but acts very effectively to control odour by killing the anaerobic bacteria growing within the wound which produce the malodour (Newman et al., 1989; Bower et al., 1992). It might be argued that after reading Chapter 14 the use of topical antibiotics should be avoided, especially such an important antibiotic as metronidazole, due to the dangers of resistance developing (Hampson, 1996). However, although the widespread use of topical metronidazole should be avoided, the small risk of resistance developing, especially in a patient's own home, is outweighed by the psychological trauma of a malodorous wound.

If Mrs Fox is suffering from depression, then prescribing an antidepressant may be a useful course of action. However, if the depression is the result of the underlying problems of nausea, vomiting and pain, then an antiemetic and analgesic are more appropriate. It is better to treat the cause of the problem rather than the symptom. However, if the doctor has diagnosed that depression is a problem in its own right, then an antidepressant might be useful. The major advantage that low doses of a non-sedative tricyclic antidepressants, like amitriptyline or imipramine, have is that as well as being antidepressants they are also useful in treating the superficial burning pain seen in neuropathic conditions. Neuropathic pain as well as occurring with peripheral nerve damage, such as diabetic neuropathy or herpes zoster (shingles), and central nervous disorders, such as stroke and multiple sclerosis, is a component of cancer pain. This form of pain is difficult to control with conventional analgesics, but can be helped by drugs like amitriptyline. However, it is important that when patients present with neuropathic pain and they are given an antidepressant as a treatment that they are informed of the value of this class of drug in pain relief. If not informed, there is a danger that the patient thinks that he or she is being 'fobbed off' and so does not bother to take the drug.

Self-assessment

Case study

Karin Lord is a 39-year-old mother of two children. She has experienced plaque psoriasis for 20 years. She feels it was triggered by the sudden death of her father to whom she was very close. At the time of consultation she was experiencing considerable stress as her 15-year-old son was playing truant from school and her husband had been made redundant and was feeling very low in mood.

Plaque psoriasis affected both her knees and elbows severely, and plaques had started to appear on her back. Karin found her tar and emollient treatments increasingly unacceptable, particularly as they were staining her skin.

She consulted an aromatherapist wishing to achieve a different treatment regime to help her psoriasis and hoped to achieve some relief from her stress. A full health assessment was taken of her previous health history, diet, sleep pattern, exercise and lifestyle.

A 3% blend of bergamot, geranium, sandalwood mysore, lemon and jasmine pure essential oils in a carrier blend of 25% evening primrose oil and 75% sweet almond oil was prescribed. This blend was to be applied to the affected areas twice a day and she was asked to add 6–8 drops of the blend to her bath water, use no soap and relax for ten minutes.

A week later Karin noticed a reduction in the inflammation and redness of her skin, minimal itching, and healing at a faster rate than usual for her. She reported having slept much better than in a long while and feeling much more relaxed. This improvement continued and four weeks later Karin's plaques were noticeably smaller and the redness as well as the dryness of her skin had improved.

Karin's friend was very impressed with her improvement, particularly as she had severe eczema and borrowed some of Karin's prescription. Within 48 hours of application Liz was aware of burning sensations and her skin had become 'tight', dark red and her eczema was weeping.

Questions:

- Why do you think Liz's eczema deteriorated having used Karin's prescription for psoriasis?
- What are the dangers of sharing aromatherapy prescriptions?

Answers:

A combination of factors led to Liz's eczema deteriorating after she applied Karin's psoriasis oil.

Firstly, some of the essential oils in the psoriasis oil are undesirable in eczema. Bergamot, despite being antiseptic and antiviral, was probably too concentrated for Liz's irritated and damaged skin, being part of the 3% dilution of the pure essential oils for psoriasis.

Bergamot oil is also phototoxic; after its application, exposure to sunlight within 12 hours increases the skin's reaction to sunlight, making sunburn more likely. As Liz's skin was already damaged and irritated by her eczema this only increased the likelihood of burning (Davis, 1995). Lemon essential oil, despite having the ability to stimulate the white corpuscles to aid defence against infection and being a powerful bactericide, is also a mild bleach useful for stimulating a healthy-looking complexion, but if applied to cracked and irritated skin will irritate the skin further causing it to weep, itch and become inflamed in appearance (Davis 1995).

Liz also had a very sensitive skin, being allergic to many cosmetic products. As Liz had not consulted an aromatherapist no full health assessment had been taken to identify these important factors which meant no patch testing had taken place, a useful way of predicting adverse skin reactions to essential oils (Tisserand and Balacs, 1995). The concentration of Karin's blend of essential oils for her psoriasis at 3% dilution was far too concentrated for Liz's sensitive skin. In eczema 1–2% dilution is often the most concentrated blend which may be tolerated.

Finally, a key principle to consider is synergy. Essential oils appear to enhance the action of other essential oils when used together, while this was the desired effect in the prescription for Karin for her psoriasis, it was disastrous for Liz having borrowed Karin's prescription, and led to the symptoms she experienced (Price, 1998). Sharing aromatherapy prescriptions may be as hazardous as sharing NHS prescriptions.

Aromatherapy prescriptions are a blend of pure essential oils that are individually made for one person following a full half hour consultation which assesses lifestyle, diet, exercise, previous and present health conditions, allergies to certain plants, pollens, foods, drugs, etc. as the essential oil is 70 times stronger than the original source. Therefore for example if germanium flowers cause a person to sneeze and develop a rash on contact, geranium essential oil will cause an extremely severe reaction! Sensitivity of the internal organs to an essential oil may lead to adverse effects. Ylang-ylang essential oil for example is prescribed for high blood pressure to soothe and lower both systolic and diastolic pressures, whereas Rosemary essential oil is a stimulant and will increase blood pressure which may sensitize a heart already under pressure (Davis, 1995). Another negative property of Rosemary is that it is contraindicated in epilepsy because it may stimulate seizures (Davis, 1995). Patch testing on the skin is required where sensitivity is known to determine possible adverse reactions to essential oils (Tisserand and Balacs, 1995).

Essential oils are very powerful and need a great deal of respect. Sharing and self-dabbling in oils guided by books, which may contradict each other, is a rather dangerous activity (Vickers, 1996). Consultation with a trained and registered aromatherapist is always desirable to avoid adverse reactions such as that Liz experienced.

References and further reading:

Bennet NE (1994) Hypertension in the elderly. Lancet 34: 447-9

Bower M, Stein R, Evans TRJ, Hedley A, Pert P, Coombes RC (1992) A double-blind study of the efficacy of metronidazole gel in the treatment of malodorous fungating tumours. European Journal of Cancer 28A: 888-9

British Medical Association and Royal Pharmaceutical Society of Great Britain (1997) British National Formulary. London: Pharmaceutical Press

Callam MJ, Harper DR, Dale JJ, Ruckley CV (1987a) Arterial disease in chronic leg ulceration: an underestimated hazard? Lothian and Forth Valley leg ulcer study. British Medical Journal 294: 929-31

Callam MJ, Ruckley CV, Dale JJ, Harper DR (1987b) Hazards of compression treatment of the leg: an estimate from Scottish surgeons. British Medical Journal 295: 1382

Davis P (1995) Aromatherapy. An A-Z. Cambridge: C W Daniel Company Ltd

Grocott P (1999) The management of fungating wounds. Journal of Wound Care 8: 232-4

Hampson JP (1996) The use of metronidazole in the treatment of malodorous wounds. Journal of Wound Care 5: 421-6

Jordan S, Torrance C (1995) Bionursing: explaining falls in elderly people. Nursing Standard 9: 30-2

Moffat CJ, O'Hare L (1995) Ankle pulses are not sufficient to detect impaired arterial circulation in patients with leg ulcers. Journal of Wound Care 4: 134-7

Newman V, Allwood M, Oakes RA (1989) The use of metronidazole gel to control the smell of malodorous lesions. Palliative Medicine 3: 303-5

Price S (1998) Using essential oils in professional practice. Complementary Therapies in Nursing and Midwifery 4: 144-7

Rajaei-Dehkordi Z, McPherson G (1997) The effects of multiple medication in the elderly. Nursing Times 93: 56-8

Royal College of Nursing (1998) Clinical Practice Guidelines. The Management of Patients with Venous Leg Ulcers. London: Royal College of Nursing

Scriven JM, Hartshorne T, Bell PRF, Naylor AR, London NJ (1997) Single-visit venous ulcer assessment clinic: the first year. British Journal of Surgery 84: 334-6

Sever P, Beevers G, Bulpitt C, Lever A, Ramsay L, Reid J, Swales J (1993) Management guidelines in essential hypertension: report of the second working party of the British Hypertension Society. British Medical Journal 306: 983-7

Strandgaard S, Paulson OB (1994) Cerebrovascular consequences of hypertension. Lancet 344: 519-21

Thomas S (1989) Treating malodorous wounds. Community Outlook October: 27-30

Tisserand R, Balacs T (1995) Essential Oil Safety for Health Care Professionals. Edinburgh: Churchill Livingstone

Vickers A (1996) Massage and Aromatherapy - A Guide for Health Professionals. London: Chapman and Hall

Williams C (1994) Causes and management of nausea and vomiting. Nursing Times 90: 38-41

Chapter 20 Drug interactions

Polypharmacy

Case study

Martha Philips is a 91-year-old widow who was found stumbling in the street in her dressing gown late in the evening. She was taken to the local hospital and admitted to an Elderly Care ward with a diagnosis of confusion. Mrs Philips' daughter Anne was telephoned to inform her that her mother had been admitted. Anne was very surprised to hear that her mother had been admitted with confusion as when she had seen her mother a few days previously she had been her usual alert, sprightly self. Anne was asked if she would bring in all of Mrs Philips' drugs when she came to visit her mother.

The drugs that Anne brought into the ward, together with Mrs Philips' hospital notes and a full assessment, allowed a holistic picture of Mrs Philips to be built up. It transpired that a cardiologist was treating Mrs Philips for congestive cardiac failure and atrial fibrillation. She had been prescribed digoxin 62.5 g daily together with bendroflumethiazide (bendrofluazide) 2.5 mg daily. Her cache of drugs also revealed that she was taking Aprinox 2.5 mg daily.

Four years ago Mrs Phillips had had a stroke and this had left her with a very slight right-sided weakness, together with epilepsy, which was being managed by a neurologist using phenytoin 150 mg daily. Mrs Philips also suffered with rheumatoid arthritis for which she was under the care of a rheumatologist. She had been prescribed indometacin (indomethacin) 50 mg three times a day as necessary. The indometacin (indomethacin) gave Mrs Philips indigestion, which she self-medicated with cimetidine, bought from the chemist.

Her drug collection also revealed an old bottle of dihydrocodeine, which Anne said her mother took when the pain was particularly bad. There was also a bottle of nitrazepam – 10 mg to be taken at bedtime – for Mrs Philips to take when she had difficulty sleeping, magnesium sulphate to take as necessary for constipation, and a bottle of calcium supplements which Mrs Philips used to keep osteoporosis at bay.

Two days prior to her admission, Mrs Philips had gone to see her GP complaining of severe dysuria. Urine analysis confirmed a urinary tract infection and the GP had prescribed co-trimoxazole 480 mg twice daily.

Questions:

- What are the problems with Mrs Philips' drug regimen?
- Why might she be suffering with confusion?

Answers:

Including her over-the-counter medications, Mrs Philips is taking a total of ten different drugs, and has a double prescription for one of them, i.e. bendroflumethiazide (bendrofluazide) is the generic name for Aprinox. She is a classic case of the phenomenon known as polypharmacy. This term does not simply mean that a patient is taking many drugs; instead, it implies that more drugs are being given than is clinically justified. The characteristics of polypharmacy are shown in Table 20.1, and Mrs Philips illustrates several of them.

Table 20.1 Indicators of polypharmacy (French, 1996)

- Use of duplicate medications in the same drug category
- Using a drug to treat an adverse effect
- Prescribing drugs contraindicated for use among the elderly
- Prescribing medications that have no apparent indication
- Ordering inappropriate dosages
- Concurrent use of interacting medications
- Clinical improvement following discontinuation of medications

Firstly, Mrs Philips is taking the same diuretic twice. This error occurs because drugs have both a generic and a proprietary name, and because patients, in particular the elderly, have multiple care providers. Mrs Philips is under the care of her own GP, as well as a cardiologist, rheumatologist and neurologist. This can be a major issue for patients with multiple problems as each specialist prescribes for the problems he deals with, and respects the clinical judgement of the other specialists. No specialist feels able to discontinue another doctor's prescription. Consequently, the patient receives prescriptions from each clinician without anyone rationalizing the prescriptions as a whole. In the case of Mrs Philips, poor communication resulted in her being prescribed Aprinox by her cardiologist and bendroflumethiazide (bendrofluazide) by her GP. As the drugs have different names Mrs Philips assumed that they were two different drugs. If Mrs Philips had taken both the drugs as prescribed, she would have suffered from dehydration. However, as the drugs made her visit the toilet so often, she had halved the dose of the tablets, demonstrating what Weintraub (1981) terms 'intelligent non-compliance'. This is where 'patients alter prescribed therapy usually by decreasing the prescribed dose or by not taking their medications at all, yet do not suffer any adverse effects'.

One major reason for inappropriate polypharmacy is the 'prescribing cascade', in which a drug is prescribed that causes a side-effect, another drug is prescribed to combat the side-effect, and the second drug causes further side-effects (Reid and Crome, 1997). Constipation, nausea, confusion, headaches, and dizziness are all symptoms that are frequently the result of medication rather than new disease. In Mrs Philips' case, she was treating the indigestion that was caused by her indometacin (indomethacin), with cimetidine. She had seen this 'antacid' as she described it advertised on the television and so had bought it. It would have been more useful for the rheumatologist to prescribe ibuprofen, which has fewer adverse upper gastro-intestinal effects than indometacin (indomethacin), and does not have the added risk of aggravating Mrs Philips' seizures (see Halligan et al., 1993). The current drive to encourage patients to self-treat minor ailments with over-the-counter medications compounds the problem of polypharmacy (Coppel and Law, 1997).

Mrs Philips occasionally takes dihydrocodeine for her pain, and that causes her to become constipated. For this she has been prescribed magnesium sulphate, another example of the 'prescribing cascade'. It would be more appropriate to treat the constipation using non-pharmacological methods such as increased fluids and fibre. Alternatively, the original prescription could be reviewed, especially as an overdose of magnesium can be lethal, particularly if the patient has some degree of kidney failure (Qureshi and Melonakos, 1996; Trehan et al., 1996).

In one study of 416 successive admissions of elderly patients to a teaching hospital 11.5% were on drugs that were absolutely contraindicated and 27% could have had one or more drugs discontinued without harm (Lindley et al., 1992). Although Mrs Philips is not on any absolutely contraindicated drugs she is on nitrazepam, which could certainly be discontinued without harm. The use of hypnotics should be avoided in the elderly as their brains are particularly sensitive to their effects, and because the half-lives of the benzodiazepines can be prolonged up to threefold in the elderly (Grahame-Smith and Aronson, 1992). The side-effects of benzodiazepines are serious and include confusion and ataxia, which can lead to falls. The normal half-life of nitrazepam is 16–40 hours, and if Mrs Philips really does require a hypnotic, one with a shorter half-life would be more appropriate, such as lorazepam or temazepam. Furthermore, the recommended dose of nitrazepam for the elderly is 2.5–5 mg at bedtime, rather than the 10 mg prescribed for Mrs Philips.

Mrs Philips is taking three drugs that interact and probably account for her symptoms of drowsiness and poor coordination. Cimetidine inhibits the hepatic metabolism of phenytoin, as does co-trimoxazole. The latter may also displace it from its plasma protein-binding site (Planchock and Slay, 1996). Therefore, the concentration of the total, and the free active, phenytoin increases. Toxicity manifested by hypotension, ataxia and nystagmus may result. With a decreased serum albumin concentration, common in the chronically ill, there may be a further increase in the free fraction of the drug, while dehydration will decrease the volume of distribution and add to the problem.

Finally, Table 11.2 lists several drugs that may lead to confusion, and as can be seen six of Mrs Philips medications have the potential to cause confusion, i.e. cimetidine, digoxin, dihydrocodeine, indometacin (indomethacin), nitrazepam, and phenytoin. So the question is not why is Mrs Philips suffering from confusion, but why have the symptoms just appeared! It would appear that the addition of the co-trimoxazole was the 'final straw' that precipitated her into her confusional state.

Over-the-counter medications

Case study

Ernest Saunders is an independent 74-year-old widower who lives alone. While out walking his neighbour's dog, he twisted his ankle. The ankle was quite painful, so utilizing the information in his First Aid manual, Mr Saunders strapped his left ankle from toe to knee and spent the following week with his leg raised on a wooden footstool. At the end of the week he removed the strapping and found that he was able to walk comfortably, although his calf ached and was a bit tender. However, as Mr Saunders was due to go on holiday to the south coast he did not dwell on the discomfort.

On the first day of his holiday, while he was walking along the promenade, Mr Saunders became a little breathless and felt unwell. He returned to the guesthouse where he was staying, and his landlady insisted on calling out the doctor. The doctor suspected a pulmonary embolism and Mr Saunders was admitted to the local hospital where the diagnosis was confirmed and he was treated initially with heparin, and then stabilized on warfarin. On discharge, Mr Saunders was given a warfarin information card and a supply of warfarin tablets, and he returned to the guesthouse where he was staying to complete his holiday. Before the end of his holiday, Mr Saunders returned to the local hospital to check his clotting times. The doctor informed Mr Saunders that he was pleased with his progress and arranged an outpatient appointment for him at the hospital in his home town.

Shortly after getting home, Mr Saunders got soaked while out walking his neighbour's dog. He developed a feverish cold and took to his bed. His neighbour was concerned and called out the GP, who was not Mr Saunders normal GP but a locum. The doctor was in a hurry and after a quick examination, he assured Mr Saunders that it was only a cold, but that he would give him a prescription for antibiotics. The neighbour kindly got the prescription of erythromycin for Mr Saunders, and while she was in the chemist, she picked up some Beecham's™ powders for his cold. Mr Saunders accepted his neighbour's kindly administrations. The next day when she called she found him lying in a pool of blood, and promptly called an ambulance.

Questions:

- Why did Mr Saunders develop a pulmonary embolism?
- Why was Mr Saunders treated with both heparin and warfarin?
- What is meant by the term 'narrow therapeutic index'?
- What is the International Normalized Ratio (INR)?
- Why was it inappropriate for the GP to prescribe antibiotics?
- Why did Mr Saunders awake in a pool of blood?

Answers:

After Mr Saunders twisted his ankle, he applied strapping from toe to knee. Unfortunately, as self-application of strapping is quite difficult, especially with arthritic joints, instead of applying the bandage with graduated compression from ankle to knee, Mr Saunders had a low bandage pressure at his ankle and a high pressure at his knee. Therefore, venous return was impeded. Furthermore, the footstool on which Mr Saunders rested his leg on was not well padded and applied further pressure to his calves. Consequently, Mr Saunders developed a deep vein thrombosis, the signs of which are minimal and consist of slight pain and swelling in the calf, and a low-grade fever.

When Mr Saunders went on holiday, the increased exercise of his energetic stroll along the promenade dislodged the thrombus, which then travelled in the veins back to the heart, through the right atrium and ventricle to lodge in one of the branches of the pulmonary artery, causing a pulmonary embolism. The common symptoms of a pulmonary embolism are dyspnoea, cyanosis, and chest pain, with a cough and haemoptysis being a later symptom. However, in some cases, as with Mr Saunders, small emboli give rise to breathlessness on exertion without obvious pain or haemoptysis.

Mr Saunders was admitted and treated initially with heparin. This works by enhancing the interaction between antithrombin III and both thrombin and the factors that are involved in the intrinsic clotting cascade. Heparin also inhibits fibrin induced platelet aggregation. Thus heparin does not break down clots, but prevents them from getting bigger while allowing the body's fibrinolytic system to break them down. Warfarin takes longer to begin to exert its effects than heparin because it inhibits the production of the clotting factors prothrombin, VII, IX, and X. Consequently, the effect of warfarin is not seen until the clotting factors already present in the blood are removed. Thus it is conventional to start patients on intravenous heparin, which begins to act immediately, and oral warfarin. After the warfarin has begun to exert its effect, the heparin can be discontinued and the patient can continue on the more convenient warfarin tablets.

An individual's response to warfarin is very variable. As warfarin has a narrow therapeutic index, i.e. the difference between the dose that gives a therapeutic effect and that which gives a toxic effect is very small, it is important to monitor the patient's response to treatment closely. This is achieved by measuring the time the patient's blood takes to clot, or the prothrombin time as it is termed. Blood is taken from the patient, thromboplastin is added to it, and the time taken to clot measured. Because the thromboplastin used in the test varies with the laboratory, an attempt has been made to standardize prothrombin time measurement internationally by the issue of a standard thromboplastin to all laboratories. Each laboratory then calibrates its own thromboplastin against the standard and translates the test results obtained with its own thromboplastin into the equivalent International Normalized Ratio (INR). In the treatment of deep vein thrombosis and pulmonary embolism an INR of 2.0–3.0 is the aim.

When Mr Saunders got home he developed a cold. When the locum came to see him Mr Saunders did not tell him about his admission to hospital, as it was not his own doctor. Furthermore, the discharge letter from the hospital where Mr Saunders has been treated had not reached his notes; thus the locum was unaware that Mr Saunders was being treated with warfarin. The failure of medical information to follow a patient is a major problem, and as this case study illustrates it can result in severe adverse effects. Possible solutions to this problem are being developed. One solution is the utilization of Smart cards. These are cards the size of credit cards that contain microchips holding the patient's medical history. The patient carries the card with him and it is updated each time he makes contact with the health care service. An alternative solution, which does not leave the patient with the responsibility of looking after his own medical records, is for both hospital and community services to become computerised and for patient summaries to be e-mailed between the different services. This would overcome many of the problems and delays of the manual system.

The locum in his hurry failed to observe one of the first rules of drug administration, which is identify what other medications a patient is taking. Although Mr Saunders' notes might be expected to contain information on prescribed medications, it will not include information on hoarded medications, borrowed ones, or those purchased by the patient. Thus it is imperative before prescribing any medication to assess exactly what drugs the patient is presently taking. The doctor could also have prevented the adverse effects that occurred to Mr Saunders by not prescribing any medication at all, and instead simply advising him to keep warm, rest and drink plenty of fluids. Mr Saunders had a cold, which is a viral infection, for which antibiotics are ineffective, as they only work against bacteria. If antibiotics are prescribed not only may the patient suffer needless adverse effects, but also inappropriate prescribing can encourage the development of bacterial resistance.

Warfarin is a highly protein-bound (99%) drug and can be displaced from its albumin binding sites by some drugs, e.g. sulphonylureas, phenytoin, leading to increased free drug and possibly haemorrhage. Some warfarinized patients given erythromycin have also haemorrhaged. However, the mechanism involved is believed to be a metabolic one rather than drug displacement. Erythromycin can stimulate the liver enzymes to produce metabolites that bind to cytochrome P450 to form inactive complexes and reduce the metabolism of warfarin. Its effects are thereby increased (Bachmann et al., 1984). Why it only happens to a few individuals is not clear. A similar effect has been noted with miconazole gel (Table 20.2) and metronidazole.

Table 20.2 Potentiation of warfarin by miconazole oral gel

Miconazole is a synthetic imidazole with broad-spectrum activity against pathogenic fungi and Gram positive bacteria. When given systemically it inhibits several microsomal P450 enzymes, including the enzyme responsible for inactivating warfarin. As it is poorly absorbed from the gut it was assumed that it was poorly absorbed from the oral mucosa, and hence this formulation is available over-the-counter. However, there have been several cases where use of miconazole gel has potentiated oral anticoagulants, which suggests that it is absorbed sufficiently to interact with other drugs (Ariyaratnam et al., 1997).

Acute illness tends to reduce serum albumin levels in the elderly (Moore and Beers, 1992), and this combined with the fact that Mr

Saunders has not been eating for the past two days because of his sore throat, may increase his free warfarin levels significantly. On their own the interaction between the two drugs and Mr Saunders' lowered albumin levels, in combination with the trauma to his nasal mucosa from sneezing and blowing his nose, could explain Mr Saunders' haemorrhage. However, the picture is more complicated. Mr Saunders was also taking a cold remedy, i.e. Beecham's Powders™ that contains 600 mg of aspirin per sachet. Aspirin interacts with warfarin synergistically as it inhibits platelet stickiness and so inhibits haemostasis. Mr Saunders had been given the normal advice about the do's and don'ts of warfarin therapy, and was fully aware that he was not to take aspirin while he was taking the warfarin (Table 20.3). However, he did not realize that the cold remedy he was taking contained aspirin. This demonstrates the importance of highlighting the problems of cold cures to patients.

Paracetamol is frequently recommended to patients on warfarin as an analgesic agent and antipyretic because it does not inhibit platelet function. However, a study by Hylek et al. (1998) demonstrated that an intake of paracetamol equivalent to seven or more tablets a week can raise the INR above 6.0, although the actual

Table 20.3 Advice that should be given to patients taking anticoagulants

- Take your dose at the same time every day; in order to keep your blood concentration of the drug stable
- If you miss a dose take it as soon as you remember it. Do not double the next dose
- Do not miss the blood tests that your doctor will arrange for you
- Do not drink alcohol without checking with your doctor. Alcohol may affect the blood test used to determine if your anticoagulant is effective
- Report any abnormal bleeding to your doctor, e.g. nosebleeds, bleeding from your gums, unusual bruising or tiny bruises that resemble a rash, discoloration of your urine, dark tarry stools, so that he can adjust your drug dose accordingly
- Avoid changing your eating habits substantially. In particular avoid increasing your intake of foods that are high in vitamin K, e.g. green leafy vegetables, cauliflower, chickpeas, beef and pork liver, green tea
- Do not take any other drugs in combination with your anticoagulants, including those that you buy without a prescription, without checking with your doctor or pharmacist, as other drugs may interfere with the action of your anticoagulant
- Inform your dentist that you are receiving anticoagulants
- Always carry identification that indicates the anticoagulant you are taking, the dose and the name of your doctor

mechanism by which paracetamol potentiates warfarin is not clear. The research also found that the effect of warfarin was potentiated by advanced malignancy, recent diarrhoeal illness and decreased oral intake. Higher vitamin K intake and habitual alcohol intake of from one drink every other day to two drinks a day was associated with decreased effect.

Social and complementary drugs

Case study

Geraldine Flood is an 18-year-old girl who lives at home with her parents. She has grand mal (tonic-clonic) epilepsy, which was originally diagnosed 10 years ago and which is well controlled with phenytoin. Geraldine and her parents have not allowed the epilepsy to handicap her in any way and she leads a full and active life. She is an athletic young lady and particularly enjoys team sports including netball and hockey, as well as skiing. She works hard at her studies and is preparing to go to university to read art and design. She has numerous friends, many who know about her epilepsy, and she likes to party and disco with them until the early morning at the local pub. She loves animals and has her own chinchilla and parrot. Geraldine is also a vegetarian, but her mother worries that she does not get a balanced diet and so encourages her daughter to take multivitamin tablets and garlic.

After Geraldine finished her A-levels, she went to Saudi Arabia to stay with a friend for a holiday. While she was out there she ran out of phenytoin tablets and went to see her friend's doctor who prescribed some more tablets for her, but of a different brand. Geraldine read the data sheet that went with the tablets and found that phenytoin can induce folate deficiency, which may result in megaloblastic anaemia. She therefore decided to add folic acid to the rest of her dietary supplements, in order to protect against this adverse effect. A few days later Geraldine had a grand mal fit and was admitted to hospital.

Questions:

- Are there any aspects of Geraldine's lifestyle that might increase her risk of having a fit?

- What might have caused Geraldine's epilepsy to become uncontrolled, leading her to have a grand mal fit?

Answers:

Geraldine has a very active life, which is to be recommended, and her epilepsy should not handicap her. However, she must be careful not to put herself in danger, as she does not know when she will next have a fit. However, the facts that she is not a loner and that her friends know that she suffers with epilepsy means that the danger to her is reduced. However, she would be advised to choose carefully the discos that she attends as the use of strobe lighting can induce a fit.

One possible explanation for why Geraldine has had a fit on holiday is that in the excitement of being away from home she has forgotten to take her medication. However, the fact that she ran out of medication and had to see the local doctor to get further supplies suggests that she is probably taking her drugs, especially as she has shown herself to be reliable with her medication in the past. A more likely explanation is that Geraldine is taking a different brand of phenytoin to that she was taking at home. Research has identified that there can be significant variations in the bioavailability of different oral formulations, e.g. capsules, tablets, syrups, and between different brands of phenytoin (Melikian, 1977). The reason for the difference in bioavailability is illustrated by a problem that developed in 1968 when one of the companies manufacturing phenytoin changed one of the bulking agents in their tablets from calcium sulphate to lactulose, for reasons of convenience. The result was that quite a few patients taking the medication suddenly started to show signs of toxicity, e.g. poor coordination and fits. The reason for these effects was that the calcium sulphate in the original tablets inhibited absorption of the drug. When this was changed to lactulose more active drug was absorbed, giving the patients the equivalent of an overdose. This occurs because the therapeutic index of the phenytoin is small and the margin for error is small (Torrance and Jordan, 1995a).

Another possible reason for Geraldine's fit is a drug interaction. It has been indicated in the case study that Geraldine is a partygoer and that she loves her nightlife. This might mean that Geraldine consumes a significant amount of alcohol. Alcohol interacts with phenytoin in the liver where it competes for the same microsomal enzymes. In chronic ingestion of alcohol, the microsomal enzymes are induced, and the increase in hepatic enzymes increases the rate of metabolism of phenytoin. A study which compared the phenytoin levels 24 hours after the last dose in a group of drinkers and controls, found that phenytoin levels in the drinkers were about half those found in the controls, and that the half-life of phenytoin was reduced by 30% (Torrance and Jordan, 1995b). This effect may be more marked if alcohol intake is decreased and the enzymes which would have metabolized the alcohol are now free to metabolize the phenytoin instead. Geraldine's alcohol intake might have decreased when she went to stay with her friend in Saudi Arabia.

A fourth possibility is that the drug interaction is not between alcohol and phenytoin, but between folic acid, the nutritional supplement which Geraldine takes, and phenytoin. Concurrent use of folic acid and phenytoin has resulted in increased seizure frequency and decreased phenytoin levels in some patients (Berg et al., 1983). For example, Glazko (1975) took four healthy volunteers, administered 300 mg of phenytoin daily, and measured their blood phenytoin levels for 10 days. The study group was then started on folic acid 10 mg daily for 15 days, and further blood tests demonstrated that their blood levels of phenytoin had decreased by 15–45% within 10 days of starting the folic acid. Why folic acid should have this effect on phenytoin is not clear. Several studies indicate that folic acid supplementation increases the metabolism of phenytoin in the liver (Glazko, 1975; Makki et al., 1980), while Andreasen et al. (1971) suggests that folic acid changes the rates of the different elimination pathways of phenytoin, resulting in decreased phenytoin levels. Alternatively, animal data suggest that folic acid can provoke seizures directly. MacCosbe and Toomey (1983) suggest that the controlled studies which demonstrated no significant effect of folate on seizure frequency in patients controlled with phenytoin, may not have been conducted over a sufficient time period since cerebrospinal folate concentrations may take several months to rise.

References and further reading:

Andreasen PB, Hansen JM, Skovsted L, Siersbaek-Nielsen K (1971) Folic acid and the half-life of diphenylhydantoin in man. Acta Neurologica Scandinavia 47: 117-119

Ariyaratnam S, Thakker NS, Sloan P, Thornhill MH (1997) Potentiation of warfarin anticoagulant activity by miconazole oral gel. British Medical Journal 314: 349

Bachmann K, Schwartz J, Forney R, Frogameni A, Jauregui (1984) The effect of erythromycin on the disposition kinetics of warfarin. Pharmacology 28: 171-6

Berg JM, Fischer LJ, Rivey MP, Vern BA, Lantz RK, Schottelius (1983) Phenytoin and folic acid interaction: a preliminary report. Therapeutic Drug Monitoring 5: 389-94

Coppel A, Law J (1997) Avoiding the increasing problem of polypharmacy. Prescriber 8: 88-90

French DG (1996) Avoiding adverse drug reactions in the elderly patient: issues and strategies. Nurse Practitioner 21: 90-105

Glazko AJ (1975) Antiepileptic drugs: biotransformation, metabolism, and serum half-life. Epilepsia 16: 367-91

Grahame-Smith DG, Aronson JK (1992). Oxford Textbook of Clinical Pharmacology and Drug Therapy 2nd edn. Oxford: Oxford University Press.

Halligan A, Nan A, DeChazal R, Taylor D (1993) Indomethacin-induced maternal convulsion in the treatment of preterm labour. European Journal of Obstetrics, Gynecology and Reproductive Biology 52: 71-2

Hylek EM, Heiman H, Skates SJ, Sheehan MA, Singer DE (1998) Acetaminophen and other risk factors for excessive warfarin anticoagulation. Journal of the American Medical Association 279: 657-62

Lindley CM, Tully MP, Paramsothy V, Tallis RC (1992) Inappropriate medication is a major cause of adverse drug reactions in elderly patients. Age and Ageing 21: 294-300

MacCosbe PE, Toomey K (1983) Interaction of phenytoin and folic acid. Clinical Pharmacology 2: 362-9

Makki KA, Perucca E, Richens A (1980) Metabolic effects of folic acid replacement therapy in folate-deficient epileptic patients. In: Johannessen SI, Morselli PI, Pippenger CE, Richens A, Schmidt D, Meinardi H (Eds). Antiepileptic Therapy: Advances in Drug Monitoring. New York: Raven Press 391-6

Melikian AP, Straughn AB, Slywka GWA, Whyatt PL, Meyer MC (1977) Bioavailability of 11 phenytoin products. Journal of Pharmokinetic Biopharmaceutics 5: 133-46

Moore AA, Beers MH (1992) Drug interactions in the elderly. Hospital Medicine. May: 88-102

Planchock NY, Slay LE (1996) Pharmacokinetic and pharmacodynamic monitoring of the elderly in critical care. Critical Care Nursing Clinics of North America 8: 79-89

Qureshi T, Melonakos TK (1996) Acute hypermagnesemia after laxative use. Annals of Emergency Medicine 28: 552-4

Reid J, Crome P (1997) Polypharmacy: causes and effects in elderly patients. Prescriber 8: 83-6

Torrance C, Jordan S (1995a) Pharmacology in the bionursing model. Nursing Standard 9: 27-9

Torrance C, Jordan S (1995b) Bionursing: the role of hepatic enzymes. Nursing Standard 10: 31-3

Trehan S, Rutecki GW, Whittier FC (1996) Magnesium disorders: what to do when homeostasis goes awry. Consultant 36: 2485-97

Weintraub M (1981) Intelligent noncompliance with special emphasis on the elderly. Contemporary Pharmacy Practice 4: 8-11

Chapter 21
Drug misuse

Misuse for self-harm

Case study

Tanya Sparrow, a 19-year-old undergraduate, went to the local Friday night disco with her fiancé Tom. They had a row and Tanya stormed out. She went back to her flat where she took a large number of paracetamol tablets. The following morning Tom rang Tanya, apologized for the night before, and offered to take her out on Saturday and Sunday to make up for the previous evening. Tanya felt very foolish. As she did not appear to have any after effects other than a bit of gastro-intestinal cramping, nausea and diarrhoea, which she put down to the previous night's vegetarian curry, she did not tell anyone about her paracetamol overdose.

On Monday morning, Tanya did not feel very well in lectures. She felt tired and anorexic, she was itching, and she started vomiting. She went to see the Occupational Health Nurse, who noticed that Tanya looked jaundiced, and, on gentle probing, Tanya admitted to her overdose. The nurse immediately took Tanya to the local hospital where she was admitted to a medical ward. Over the next few days Tanya's condition deteriorated as she developed hepatic and renal failure, and encephalopathy. As a suitable liver donor could not be found, Tanya went into a coma, and died a week after the overdose.

Questions:

- Why did the paracetamol tablets kill Tanya?
- Could anything else have contributed to Tanya's death, other than the paracetamol?

- How could her death have been prevented, despite her taking the overdose?
- How could death from paracetamol overdose be prevented altogether?

Answers:

The paracetamol tablets killed Tanya because of enzyme saturation. When paracetamol is taken in therapeutic doses, the hepatic enzymes inactivate it safely, mainly by conjugation, to give the glucuronide or sulphate metabolites. However, at higher doses these enzymes become saturated. The paracetamol consequently has to be metabolized by a second pathway in which the drug is oxidized by the mixed function oxidases to form toxic intermediates. These intermediate metabolites can be rapidly inactivated by conjugation with glutathione, to give an inactive soluble metabolite, which can be excreted. However, in the case of paracetamol overdose the glutathione becomes depleted. Consequently, the toxic intermediates cannot be inactivated and so they accumulate, in particular n-acetyl p-benzoquinone. The toxic intermediates interact with the cells of the liver through a variety of mechanisms (Budden and Vink, 1996) and in massive acute overdose (10–15 g per day) can lead to hepatocellular necrosis or fulminate hepatic failure (Artnak and Wilkinson, 1998). Fulminate hepatic failure can lead to encephalopathy, renal failure, cerebral oedema and death, as occurred with Tanya.

Whether anything else contributed to Tanya's death, other than the paracetamol, is difficult to know, as her case history is not very detailed. However, long-term antiepileptic therapy and chronic alcohol ingestion both potentiate paracetamol poisoning by activating the P450 oxidases and increasing the production of toxic paracetamol intermediates. Chronic alcohol ingestion also depletes glutathione stores, making it difficult for the body to inactivate the toxic intermediates formed from paracetamol metabolism. Malnutrition has a similar effect, especially a diet containing insufficient sulphur-containing amino acids. Although it is unlikely that that Tanya is an alcoholic or suffering from malnutrition, her alcohol intake may still be sufficient to activate the P450 oxidases, and she may well not be taking a well-balanced diet.

In the case of paracetamol overdose, damage to the liver can be prevented by intravenous administration of acetylcysteine, preferably within 15 hours of the overdose, although protective effects have been reported when administered as long as 24 hours after ingestion (Parker et al., 1990). The acetylcysteine substitutes for the body's depleted glutathione, and it also enhances peripheral glutathione synthesis. Acetylcysteine is also reported to improve oxygen delivery and consumption by increasing cardiac output and blood pressure (Harrison et al., 1991), as well as reducing free radical damage (Aruoma et al., 1989). Oral methionine can also be administered as an antidote, but again it needs to be administered as soon as possible after the overdose, and its use is normally limited to the first 24 hours after ingestion (Vale and Proudfoot, 1995).

As with any poisoning, it is helpful not just to use an antidote to the toxin, but also to try to prevent absorption of the poison from the gut, if it was taken orally. Administration of activated charcoal can be used to reduce paracetamol absorption (Davis, 1991), and this treatment (Carbomix™ to drug ratio 10:1) has been shown in a comparative trial to be significantly more effective than ipecacuanha-induced vomiting and gastric lavage (Underhill et al., 1990). Although it is best administered within 60 minutes of ingestion of the paracetamol, it has been observed to reduce urinary recovery of the drug's metabolites even when administered 2 hours after ingestion. Krenzelok and Dunmire (1992) suggest combining the activated charcoal with a purgative such as sorbitol in order to reduce absorption further. Although not as effective as activated charcoal, ipecacuanha-induced vomiting is effective at reducing paracetamol absorption, provided the patient is not too drowsy to maintain a gag reflex. In patients without a gag reflex gastric lavage within 6 hours of the overdose may be useful, although Kulig (1985) suggests that it is only effective in the first hour after ingestion of the poison.

Recent research efforts have been directed towards other strategies to reduce the toxic effects of paracetamol. One possibility is to inhibit the cytochrome P450 system responsible for the generation of the toxic metabolites. The H_2-histamine antagonist cimetidine does this and when used clinically its effects appear to be additive to those of acetylcysteine (Rolband and Marcuard, 1991). Another possibility is to use calcium-channel blocking agents, e.g. verapamil, and antagonists of calcium calmodulin, e.g. chlorpromazine, to decrease intracellular calcium. One of the main effects of paracetamol's toxic intermediates is to increase membrane permeability to calcium, resulting in calcium accumulating in the nucleus and causing DNA fragmentation. Animal studies would seem to indicate that this strategy is of value and that cellular damage is decreased (Ray et al., 1993).

Paracetamol is a cheap and easily available product, which is kept in the majority of homes in order to treat minor aches and pains. Not only is it available in pharmacies, where at least its use can be supervised to some extent, but also in a multitude of other retail outlets. Not surprisingly paracetamol is readily to hand when overdose is contemplated, and the general public still seem unaware of its significant toxic effects on the liver (MacConnachie, 1998). In September 1998, regulations were passed which limit the sale of paracetamol tablets to 32 tablets or capsules from pharmacies and 16 tablets from other retail outlets. It is hoped that these regulations will go some way to decreasing paracetamol overdose. However, the toxic effects of paracetamol could be nullified by inclusion of methionine within the formulation, and this is available as Paradote™. However, the use of this preparation is not promoted, and its cost compared with conventional paracetamol dissuades the public from purchasing it.

Accidental misuse

Case study

Marjorie Price is an 84-year-old widow who lives by herself in a small bungalow. Ten years ago, she was diagnosed as having diabetes. She became quite upset when she was told this, especially as her nephew had recently died from renal failure due to diabetes. Her GP reassured Marjorie that she only had a mild form of diabetes and that she would not have to inject herself with insulin. Marjorie was much less agitated when told this and agreed to see the dietitian and the diabetic specialist to discuss her diet and control of her blood sugar level. Marjorie was very 'laissez-faire' about managing her diabetes, and her blood sugar level remained elevated despite further educational input from the diabetic nurse specialist. Consequently, the GP prescribed Marjorie oral chlorpropamide 250 mg at breakfast, and this seemed to maintain Marjorie's blood sugar at around 8–10 mmol/L.

Recently Marjorie's eyes became inflamed and her vision blurred, making it difficult for her to get around the cottage. A neighbour called out the GP who diagnosed an eye infection and prescribed 0.5% chloramphenicol eye drops, which the neighbour very kindly got from the chemist for Marjorie. Due to her rheumatoid arthritis Marjorie had difficulty putting the drops in her eyes and ended up putting in more than prescribed at each application. As the drops relieved the discomfort of her eyes, Marjorie also used them more frequently than prescribed.

The next day when the neighbour called round to see Marjorie she found that she was still in bed, her supper untouched. When she tried to rouse Marjorie the neighbour was unable to do so. She called an ambulance and Marjorie was admitted to the local hospital, where her blood sugar was found to be 3 mmol/L.

Questions:

- What possible reasons are there for Marjorie's blood sugar level being so low on admission to hospital?
- What error did the GP make when dealing with Marjorie?
- How should diabetes be managed when a patient is unwell?

Answers:

A person's blood sugar level is the result of the interaction between her hormonal levels, her diet, the amount of exercise that she undertakes and any drugs that she takes. In the case of Marjorie, the fact that she has type II diabetes means that she is not producing sufficient 'effective' insulin. This does not necessarily mean that her blood insulin levels are low, although this certainly may be the case. Her insulin levels may be normal or elevated, but her cells are resistant to the circulating insulin (Brown, 1998a). The effect of this would be to raise her blood sugar levels, giving her hyperglycaemia.

Insulin is not the only hormone having an effect on Marjorie's blood sugar levels. She has an infection, and the response of the body in this stressful condition is to produce glucocorticoids. These hormones live up to their name and serve to increase the blood sugar level. Their effect under physiological conditions is not as great as that observed when steroids such as prednisolone are given therapeutically, but they have a small effect nonetheless.

Marjorie has an eye infection and so is not eating a great deal, as she does not feel very well. In fact, as pointed out in the case study, she did not eat her supper, and had had only numerous cups of unsweetened tea all that day. Lack of nutritional intake will serve to lower Marjorie's blood sugar levels and may account partially for her lowered blood sugar on admission. However, when blood sugar levels fall, the pancreas responds by producing glucagon and this should have raised Marjorie's blood sugar level.

Exercise utilizes energy and so serves to lower the blood sugar level. However, exercise also leads to a decrease in insulin production and an increase in glucagon production, so it is likely that the overall effect on blood sugar levels will be minimal. This is certainly true in Marjorie's case as her normal exercise consists of simply pottering around the cottage and the walk to the corner shop. This pattern will not have changed significantly with her eye infection, other than to decrease slightly.

Marjorie is taking two drugs. The first is chlorpropamide, a sulphonylurea that serves to lower blood glucose (Table 21.1). Because the sulphonylureas stimulate insulin secretion they can cause hypoglycaemia. The risk is greatest when the drug has a long half-life, if the drug has a prolonged action on the ß-cells (e.g. glibenclamide), or if the patient has renal impairment and the drug is cleared mainly by the kidneys (e.g. glibenclamide) (Amiel, 1993). Chlorpropamide has a long half-life, and consequently its duration of action is 24–72 hours (Brown, 1998b). Because of this, chlorpropamide is not a good choice of drug for the elderly, and should be replaced with drugs of a shorter half-life such as gliclazide or tolbutamide. The dose prescribed by the GP is 250 mg daily, which might seem quite acceptable, as the maximum dose is 500 mg. However, the recommended daily dose for the elderly is 100–125 mg (BMA & RPS, 1997).

Table 21.1 Actions of the sulphonylureas

- increasing ß-cell sensitivity to glucose and so increasing insulin release by the pancreas
- increasing the number of insulin receptors on the surface of body cells and so increasing glucose uptake
- stimulating lipogenesis with decreased plasma free fatty acids

The second drug Marjorie is taking is chloramphenicol eye drops. Studies in diabetics have shown that 2 g oral daily doses of chloramphenicol can approximately double the half-lives of tolbutamide (Christensen and Skovsted, 1969) and chlorpropamide (Petitpierre et al., 1972). Other studies using 1 g oral daily doses of chloramphenicol similarly showed that serum levels of tolbutamide could be doubled and blood sugar levels reduced by an average of 24% (Brunova et al., 1977). This effect occurs because chloramphenicol inhibits the enzymes that metabolize tolbutamide, and probably chlorpropamide as well, leading to their accumulation in the body. This is reflected in prolonged half lives, reduced blood sugar levels, and occasionally acute hypoglycaemia.

Marjorie is taking her chloramphenicol topically as her eye drops, and so it might be anticipated that their systemic effects are negligible. This may be the case if they are used correctly, but Marjorie is using them in excessive quantities, partly due to problems of administration, and partly for reasons of non-compliance. The problem is that the eye drops run through the naso-lacrimal duct into the nasal cavity where they are absorbed into the general circulation, and so may have a systemic effect. However, despite the fact that Marjorie is using her eye drops incorrectly, short of using a bottle a day, she is not going to approach the doses describe in the literature as causing hypoglycaemia. Nevertheless, the amount of chloramphenicol she is absorbing, together with her poor nutritional intake, and high dose of chlorpropamide, in combination may account for her hypoglycaemia.

As indicated above the GP did not choose the best drug or dose of drug to deal with Marjorie's diabetes. However, he made a mistake before this in informing Marjorie that she had 'mild' diabetes. This served to reduce her agitation in the short term, but did not promote good management in the long term. Marjorie convinced herself that if her diabetes was only mild she did not have to stick to the prescribed diet, and could adopt a relaxed attitude to her disease. If the doctor had conveyed to Marjorie the true seriousness of her disease she might have had more reason to comply with her diet, and this alone might have controlled her blood sugar level so that she did not require the oral hypoglycaemic agent.

Marjorie's hypoglycaemic attack might have been prevented if the need to take food even when she did not feel hungry or when she was unwell had been impressed upon her. This is needed in order to counterbalance the effect of the oral hypoglycaemic agent. Thus, Marjorie should have been advised to add sugar to her tea, or take sweet drinks such as Ribena™ and Lucozade™ to replace the sugars she would normally take in her diet.

Intentional misuse

Case study

Dawn Pearl is a 28-year-old single mother of three. She lives with her children in a small council flat in Peterborough, and works as a research assistant whilst the three children are at school during the day. She is a hard working and proud woman, who does not like to ask for help, or to admit that she is finding it difficult to make ends meet financially.

Dawn has been suffering from a gnawing, burning pain in her upper abdomen, which comes on within 20 minutes of eating and which is putting her off eating. On occasion Dawn has been woken up at night by the pain, and it has been so severe as to cause her to vomit. She has had these symptoms for several months, and they are beginning to make her snappy with the children. Her mother, who lives nearby and who helps Dawn look after the children, suggests that she goes to see her GP in order to get the problem investigated and treated. Dawn is seen by the GP who is clearly in a hurry as he has a large surgery, which is already running late because he was called out on an emergency. Based on Dawn's classic symptoms, the GP diagnoses gastric ulcer and prescribes treatment regimen A (Table 21.2). He tells her to take the full course of tablets and then dismisses her.

Dawn goes to the chemist to collect her prescription and is horrified to have to pay over £17.00 for it, as this would feed the family for at least three days. She starts to take the medication, and after 3 days, her ulcer symptoms resolve. However, Dawn is finding that the drugs are making her feel nauseated. She therefore decides to stop taking them and carefully puts them at the back of the pantry for future use.

Questions:

- Why was Dawn given antibiotics and omeprazole to treat her gastric ulcer?

Table 21.2 Recommended treatment regimens for the eradication of *Helicobacter pylori* (MacConnachie, 1997)

Treatment A	A proton pump inhibitor (e.g. omeprazole 20 mg or lansoprazole 15 mg) twice daily + amoxicillin (amoxycillin) 500 mg three times daily + metronidazole 400 mg three times daily
Treatment B	A proton pump inhibitor (e.g. omeprazole 20 mg or lansoprazole 15 mg) twice daily + amoxicillin (amoxycillin) 500 mg three times daily + clarithromycin 250 mg three times daily
Treatment C–if patient allergic to penicillin	A proton pump inhibitor (e.g. omeprazole 20 mg or lansoprazole 15 mg) twice daily + metronidazole 400 mg three times daily + clarithromycin 250 mg three times daily

Take for 7 days, and then continue proton pump inhibitor for one week in patients with active duodenal ulcer or three weeks in active benign duodenal ulcer

- Why do you think that Dawn was not compliant with her treatment?
- How could the doctor have promoted her compliance?
- What are the possible repercussions of Dawn's non-compliance?
- As well as giving Dawn advice about compliance with her medication, the doctor should have advised her about something else. What did he omit to discuss with her?

Answers:

Over 90% of duodenal ulcers and 70% of gastric ulcers are associated with infection with the Gram-negative bacterium *Helicobacter pylori* (Marshall, 1994). However because the incidence of *Helicobacter pylori* infection is much greater than the incidence of gastrointestinal-related disease, other factors may be necessary for the disease to develop, e.g. environmental and genetic factors (Garnett, 1998).

Helicobacter pylori is an S-shaped bacterium has four to six flagella at one end of the cell, which allow it the motility to burrow below the mucosal layer of the antrum of the stomach. The bacterium produces urease, an enzyme that converts urea in gastric juice to ammonia and carbon dioxide. The urea acts as an energy source for the bacteria whilst the ammonia produces an alkaline environment which protects the bacteria from the stomach's powerful acid. Pathogenic strains of the bacterium produce toxins which result in an inflammatory response and inhibit the release of the gastroduodenal hormone somatostatin (MacConnachie, 1997). This hormone is an important inhibitor of gastric acid secretion, with over-secretion leading to gastritis and ulceration. The presence of the bacteria can be confirmed by a simple serological test which can be performed in the GP's surgery and which gives results within 10 minutes (Johnson, 1996). Dawn should perhaps have had this test. The rationale behind her drug therapy is that the antibiotics will kill the bacteria whilst the proton pump inhibitor will prevent acid secretion and so allow ulcer healing (Kelly, 1994).

There are many reasons why Dawn might not have been compliant with her drug regime. Once the symptoms of her ulcer had resolved she may not have seen the need, nor understood why she needed to carry on taking the drugs. It is a commonly held belief that you take drugs to relieve symptoms, and once the symptoms have resolved there is no need to carry on taking the medication. Poulton (1991) identified that immediately after a consultation roughly 40% of what is said is forgotten by patients, so although she was told to take the full course of drugs, Dawn might not remember being advised to do so. Alternatively, Dawn might have remembered what the doctor said about taking the full course of treatment, but decided to ignore his advice. This might be because she did not have a very positive image of him after her brief consultation, or because she believes that doctors tend to be over careful in their advice.

Probably the main reason Dawn stopped taking her medication was that she found the side-effects unacceptable. Patients often carry out a cost benefit analysis to identify the advantages of pursuing a line of treatment compared with the disadvantages. In Dawn's case the treatment had cured her symptoms so as far as she could see there were no benefits to continuing treatment. If she stopped taking her medication she would not have to endure the drugs' side-effects, and she would prudently have a supply of drugs in case the symptoms reoccurred in the future.

The doctor could have promoted Dawn's compliance by giving her more information about the course of treatment that he was prescribing for her. Table 17.4 identifies the information patients should ideally be given about any drug that they are prescribed. In particular the GP should have explained to Dawn why it was so important that she take the full course of drugs. The doctor should also consider his treatment of Dawn's peptic ulcer. His use of three drugs to combat *Helicobacter pylori* provides 90% eradication after a seven-day course (Axon et al., 1997). From a medical perspective this is to be recommended. However, the cost for the patient in prescription charges can be unacceptable. It is known for patients to arrive at the pharmacy and to ask which of their prescribed drugs is most important as they can only afford one of the items prescribed. The GP must therefore be aware of such issues and consider alternative regimes, which although perhaps not as effective, are more likely to be adhered to. The combination of omeprazole (20 mg twice daily) and clarithromycin (500 mg three times daily) for 14 days has an 80% cure rate (Logan et al., 1992; Anon, 1996). It is a simpler regimen which is more acceptable to patients in terms of both fewer side-effects and improved compliance (Cottrill, 1996; Podolski, 1996). It is however, an expensive drug combination for the health service, and a cheaper combination would be omeprazole with amoxicillin (amoxycillin), which based on intention-to-treat analysis has eradication rates of between 68% and 82%, depending on the dose of omeprazole (Penston, 1994). If a single drug regimen is used clarithromycin is the most effective single therapy with cure rates of up to 40%.

One possible repercussion of Dawn's non-compliance is that the ulcer reoccurs. As with any infection the full course of antibiotics should be taken in order to ensure that all the microorganisms are destroyed. If a few organisms survive the antibiotics, as can occur when the patient does not take the full course of treatment, then once the antibiotics are discontinued the few remaining bacteria can start to multiply and re-infect the patient. A second repercussion of failure to complete a course of antibiotics is the development of antibiotic resistant microorganisms. When a patient starts taking a course of antibiotics the most susceptible microbes will be killed first, followed by the more resistant. If the patient does not take the full course of antibiotics these more resistant organisms are the ones that survive, and consequently the patient is actually helping to select for the most resistant microbes. *Helicobacter pylori* readily become resistant to metronidazole, tinidazole, and clarithromycin when given as the sole antibiotic, or with a proton pump inhibitor (Goodwin et al., 1997), which is why a triple therapy is the preferred drug regimen.

Other repercussions are that one of the children may find the tablets hidden in the pantry, and assume that as they are in there that they are sweets. If one of the children takes all the tablets, he may suffer toxic effects. Unused drugs should be stored in a locked cabinet out of the reach of children. Even if one of the children does not take them, there is a danger to Dawn that she stores the drugs for several years before remembering she has them, and when she takes them they have begun to decay and produce adverse effects. For example, the degradation products of tetracycline can cause proximal tubular defects resembling a reversible Fanconi's syndrome.

As discussed in Chapter 2, one of the adverse effects of some antibiotics is that they can interact with the bacteria in the gut that are important in keeping the oral contraceptive active. Consequently the contraceptive is less effective and pregnancy can result. The GP should therefore have checked whether Dawn was taking the pill and if she was he should have advised her to take extra precautions if she had sexual intercourse whilst she is taking the antibiotics.

References and further reading

Amiel SA (1993) Hypoglycaemia in diabetes mellitus. Medicine International 21: 279-81

Anon (1996) Want to improve H. pylori therapy? Follow this HMO's initiative. Disease State Management 2: 121-4

Artnak KE, Wilkinson SS (1998) Fulminant hepatic failure in acute acetaminophen overdose. Advanced Practice Nursing 17: 135-44

Aruoma OI, Halliwell B, Hoey BM, Butler J (1989) The antioxidant action of N-acetylcysteine: its reaction with hydrogen peroxide, hydroxyl radical, superoxide, and hypochlorous acid. Free Radicals & Medicine 6: 593-7

Axon ATR, O'Morain CA, Bardhan JD, Crowe JP, Beattie AD, Thompson RPH, Smith PM, Hollanders FD, Baron JH, Lynch DAF, Dixon MF, Tompkins DS, Birrell H, Gillon KRW (1997) Randomised double blind controlled study of recurrence of gastric ulcer after treatment for eradication of Helicobacter pylori infection. British Medical Journal 314: 565-8

British Medical Association and Royal Pharmaceutical Society of Great Britain (1997) British National Formulary. London: Pharmaceutical Press

Brown AM (1998a) Diabetes mellitus (1) The disease. The Pharmaceutical Journal 60: 704-6

Brown AM (1998b) Diabetes mellitus (3) Management of non-insulin-dependent diabetes mellitus. The Pharmaceutical Journal 60: 905-8

Brunova E, Slabochova Z, Platilova H, Pavlik F, Grafnetterova J, Dvoracek K (1977) Interaction of tolbutamide and chloramphenicol in diabetic patients. International Journal of Clinical Pharmacology 15:7-12

Budden L, Vink R (1996) Paracetamol overdose: pathophysiology and nursing management. British Journal of Nursing 5: 145-52

Christensen LK, Skovsted L (1969) Inhibition of drug metabolism by chloramphenicol. Lancet 2: 1397-9

Cottrill MRB (1996) Helicobacter pylori. Professional Nurse 12: 46-8

Davis JE (1991) A consideration not to be overlooked. Activated charcoal in acute drug overdose. Professional Nurse 6: 710-14

Garnett WR (1998) Is curing peptic ulcer disease an oxymoron? A focus on Helicobacter pylori. The American Journal of Managed Care 4(4 Suppl.): S281-99

Goodwin CS, Mendall MM, Northfield TC (1997) Helicobacter pylori infection. Lancet 349: 265-9

Harrison PM, Wendon JA, Gimson AES, Alexander GJM, Williams R (1991) Improvement by acetylcysteine of hemodynamics and oxygen transport in fulminant hepatic failure. New England Journal of Medicine 324: 1852-7

Johnson DA (1996) Helicobacter pylori and GI disease. Consultant 36: 1911-23

Kelly J (1994) Drug therapy and peptic ulceration. British Journal of Nursing 3: 1129-34

Krenzelok EP, Dunmire SM (1992) Acute poisoning emergencies. Postgraduate Medicine 91: 179-86

Kulig K, Bar-Or D, Cantrill SV et al. (1985) Management of acutely poisoned patients without gastric emptying. Annals Emergency Medicine 14: 562-7

Logan RP, Gummet PA, Hegarty BT, Walker MM, Baron JH, Misiewicz JJ (1992) Clarithromycin and omeprazole for H. pylori. Lancet 340: 239

MacConnachie AM (1998) Paracetamol poisoning. Accident and Emergency Nursing 6: 43-4

MacConnachie AM (1997) Eradication therapy in peptic ulcer disease. Intensive and Critical Care Nursing 13: 121-2

Marshall BJ (1994) Helicobacter pylori. American Journal of Gastroenterology 89: 5116-28

Parker D, White JP, Paton D, Routledge PA (1990) Safety of late acetylcysteine treatment in paracetamol poisoning. Human & Experimental Toxicology 9: 25-7

Penston JG (1994) Helicobacter pylori eradication - understandable caution but no excuse for inertia. Alimentary Pharmacology and Therapeutics 8: 369-89

Petitpierre B, Perrin L, Rudhart M, Herrera A, Fabre J (1972) Behaviour of chlorpropamide in renal insufficiency and under associated drug therapy. International Journal of Clinical Pharmacology, Therapy & Toxicology 6:120

Podolski JL (1996) Recent advances in peptic ulcer disease: Helicobacter pylori infection and its treatment. Gastroenterology Nursing 19: 128-36

Poulton B (1991) Factors influencing patient compliance. Nursing Standard 5: 3-5

Ray SD, Kamendulis LM, Gurule MW, Yorkin RD, Corcoran GB (1993) Ca2+ antagonists inhibit DNA fragmentation and toxic cell death induced by acetaminophen. The FASEB Journal 7:453-63

Rolband GC, Marcuard SP (1991) Cimetidine in the treatment of acetaminophen overdose. Journal of Clinical Gastroenterology 13: 79-82

Underhill TJ, Greene MK, Dove AF (1990) a comparison of the efficacy of gastric lavage, ipecacuanha and activated charcoal in the emergency management of paracetamol overdose. Archives of Emergency Medicine 7: 148-54

Vale JA, Proudfoot AT (1995) Paracetamol (acetaminophen) poisoning. Lancet 346: 547-52

Chapter 22
Empowerment

Allowing choices

Case study

Rose Darling is a 52-year-old married women who works as a biology teacher. She started her menopause two years ago and has been suffering with hot flushes ever since. She finds these flushes acutely embarrassing when they occur in the middle of a lecture and at night she has such severe sweats that her husband has started sleeping in the spare room. Rose is also worried about the long-term effects of the menopause. Her mother suffered from severe osteoporosis which gave her a very unsightly dowager hump, and Rose is desperate not to end up like her mother.

Rose reads a lot of women's magazines which all seem to be extolling the virtues of hormone replacement therapy (HRT). Rose decided that this was the solution to her predicament, and consequently made an appointment to see her GP.

When Rose arrived at the surgery it was clearly very busy, and she had to wait a long time to see her doctor. She explained her problems to the GP, and he took her history. When the GP discovered that Rose's mother had died from breast cancer, he stopped the interview and told her that she could not have HRT. Instead, he advised her that the hot sweats would wear off soon and he told her to increase her calcium intake and to take plenty of exercise in order to ward off osteoporosis. Rose left the GP feeling very angry and disappointed.

Questions:

- What is hormone replacement therapy?
- Was the GP right to deny Rose HRT? On what grounds have you made your decision?

Answers:

Hormone replacement therapy usually consists of natural oestrogens, and progestogen. The oestrogen is given for the relief of menopausal symptoms and for the long-term protection of the skeletal and cardiovascular systems. If given alone to a women who has an intact uterus, i.e. has not had a hysterectomy, long-term oestrogen therapy will cause endometrial proliferation which increases the risk of endometrial cancer, not only during therapy but also for many years subsequently (Whitehead et al., 1990). Giving progestogen significantly reduces the risk of this occurring, but it does mean that the women now has withdrawal bleeding, which can be unacceptable to some women, especially the more elderly ones. Furthermore, progestogens can have an adverse effect on lipid and lipoprotein metabolism.

The oestrogen component of HRT is given continuously, and is available for administration by the oral, transdermal, subcutaneous and vaginal route. Non-oral therapies avoid first pass metabolism which may be important in women with such medical conditions as diabetes, thrombosis, hypertension and previous liver disease (Abernethy, 1997a). Progestogen can be administered orally, transdermally or via an intrauterine device, and may be given continuously, cyclically, or tricyclically (Gangar and Penny, 1995).

Whether the GP should have withheld HRT from Rose is open to debate. As Table 22.1 indicates HRT has a number of advantages and disadvantages.

Starting with the advantages, HRT is effective in reducing the perimenopausal symptoms which occur in 75% of women (Khaw, 1992). These symptoms, which include hot flushes and sweats, may appear to be insignificant, and some people argue that they should just be lived through. However, for the women suffering the symptoms they can be very incapacitating both physically and psychologically. As can be seen with Rose, the night sweats are causing a rift in her relationship with her husband not to mention a lot of extra washing.

As well as the short-term effects of HRT there are some very significant long-term effects, especially in relation to osteoporosis and heart disease. Five years' use of oestrogen therapy is associated with a halving in the risk of hip fractures (Paganini-Hill et al., 1981) and a reduction in vertebral fractures (Ettinger et al., 1985) in white

Table 22.1 The advantages and disadvantages of hormone replacement therapy

Advantages	*Disadvantages*
Reduces perimenopausal symptoms of the menopause, e.g. hot flushes/ sweats, insomnia, formication, lack of concentration, irritability	Short term side-effects of HRT include breast tenderness, leg cramps, oedema, and nausea due to the oestrogen component
Reduces vaginal atrophy and dyspareunia	Increased risk of endometrial cancer
Effective in prevention and treatment of osteoporosis	Increased risk of breast cancer
Lowers incidence of heart disease	Menstruation and pre-menstrual symptoms due to the progestogen component
May delay onset or reduce risk of Alzheimer's	Pill popping – medicalizing a natural process (Greer, 1991)
Improved wound healing (McCarthy, 1997b)	Small increased risk of thrombosis (Daly et al., 1996; Jick et al., 1996)

women. To put this benefit in context, it must be appreciated that one in every two women over 70 years of age can expect to get an osteoporosis fracture, and one in every ten beds in NHS hospital is taken up by osteoporosis-related fractures. In 1987, Howie estimated the cost of these fractures to the health service as £165–£180 million.

Although it is never too late to start HRT, for maximum protection against osteoporosis, women should start taking HRT at or soon after the menopause and continue therapy for years, rather than months. Women with a family history of osteoporosis may be advised to consider HRT even if they are not experiencing menopausal symptoms (Abernethy, 1997b). In the case of black women, the risks of osteoporosis are considerably reduced, and the value of HRT has not been ascertained as all studies have been conducted on white women (Litchtman, 1991).

In the UK, heart disease is the most common cause of mortality in women over the age of 50 (DoH, 1994). Studies have demonstrated that oestrogen is protective of the cardiovascular system and that among groups of women of the same age post-menopausal women are at a higher risk of heart disease than women with functioning ovaries (Gordon et al., 1978; Rosenberg et al., 1981). The use of HRT after the menopause appears to reduce the risk of heart attacks (Stampfer and Colditz, 1991; Mijatovic and Pines, 1995) and strokes (Finucane et al., 1993). It is unclear why oestrogen has such beneficial effects, but possible explanations include:

- beneficial changes in the blood lipid, i.e. an increase in high density lipoproteins (HDLs) and a decrease in low density lipoproteins (LDLs)
- a direct effect on the blood vessel wall
- positive influence on insulin metabolism
- positive effects on clotting factors.

As well as having positive effects on the skeletal and cardiovascular systems there is mounting evidence that HRT has positive effects on other body systems. Studies by Paganini-Hill and Henderson (1994) and Tang et al. (1996) suggest that the increased incidence of Alzheimer's in older women may be due to oestrogen deficiency and that oestrogen therapy may be useful for preventing or delaying the onset of this dementia. It is suggested that oestrogens may have this effect through their synergistic action with nerve growth factor in maintaining the cholinergic neurones in the basal forebrain (Holloway, 1992).

The main concern about using HRT is the increased risk of developing breast cancer. However, the results of research studies are controversial. Litchman (1991) reviewed 20 studies on HRT and breast cancer and found:

- 6 studies showing no adverse effect
- 3 studies showing a possible protective effect
- 2 studies showing a possible beneficial effect on prognosis
- 9 studies showing adverse effects.

The consensus suggests that taking HRT for up to five years does not increase the risk of breast cancer. Using HRT for more than eight years does increase the risk when compared with women who have never used HRT (Colditz et al., 1995), but the extent to which the risk is increased needs further assessment. Studies are ongoing to ascertain the level of risk for women with a family history of breast cancer.

It is generally agreed HRT is totally contradicted for only a very small number of women. The main contraindications are pregnancy, breast or endometrial cancer, undiagnosed abnormal vaginal bleeding, severe active liver disease and porphyria (Hillard, 1996). There are also some oestrogen-dependent conditions such as endometriosis and fibroids, where oestrogen might worsen the condition.

So, where does this leave Rose? The evidence for and against HRT is voluminous and often contradictory and unclear (Litchman, 1991). As the evidence for and against the use of HRT is so ambiguous it is not right for the GP to make a decision on Rose's behalf. In doing so he is being paternalistic. Instead, he should provide Rose with the current knowledge about the advantages, disadvantages, and unknowns of HRT. He should be able to respond to her questions, and allow her to make the decision as to what is best for her. Each individual has his or her own fears about particular diseases, e.g. for some the fear of a stroke far outweighs the fear of breast cancer. Only the individual patient knows what risks they are prepared to take for what benefits.

Fighting for change

Case study

Jeremy Blake is a 54-year-old businessman who lives alone in a flat in London. Six years ago, he was diagnosed as suffering from multiple sclerosis, but otherwise he is fit and healthy. He follows the opera and ballet, and spends a lot of his spare time reading or fly-fishing. The main problems that he has with his multiple sclerosis are painful muscle spasms and blurred vision, neither of which have responded effectively to conventional medicine. A couple of years ago he read a report about a trial in which 112 patients with multiple sclerosis self-administered cannabis and found that they had 90% fewer muscle spasms (Shamash, 1998). On reading the report, Jeremy sought out some of his friends from university days until he found one who was able to supply him with some cannabis. Jeremy smoked the plant and found that not only did it reduce his spasms, but it improved his vision. Since that time Jeremy has continued to use cannabis to relieve his symptoms.

Two years ago the police caught Jeremy with a small amount of cannabis on his person and cautioned him about the illegality of being in possession of the drug, even if it was for personal use. He has now been caught again in possession of a small amount of cannabis and this time has been charged, found guilty and given a 6-month prison sentence.

Questions:

- Cannabis is at present an illegal substance, which is why Mr Blake was sent to prison. Is the judgement fair, and what are your reasons?
- Should cannabis be legalized for recreational purposes, and what are your reasons?

Answers:

Cannabis is the most widely used illicit drug in many countries, with more than 30% of teenagers using it in some urban areas (Luke, 1997). Currently in Britain, it is a class B agent under the 1971 Misuse of Drugs Act and a schedule 1 drug according to the 1985 Use of Drug Regulations. It is categorized as having no therapeutic value, and only under special circumstances can cannabis derivatives such as nabilone be prescribed.

Preparations of the drug are mainly derived from the female plant of *Cannabis sativa.* When leaves and flower heads are dried this is referred to as marijuana, while hashish refers to the extracted resin. The primary psychoactive constituent is δ-9-tetrahydrocannabinol (THC), which binds to specific receptors in the brain involved with cognition, memory, reward, and pain perception and motor coordination. These receptors respond to an endogenous ligand, anandamide, which is much less potent and has a shorter duration than THC.

Cannabis is used as a recreational drug because it promotes a feeling of relaxation and well being bordering on euphoria, and there is a perception of increased sensory awareness affecting sight and hearing (Campbell, 1999). Cannabis is also used for medicinal purposes. Table 22.2 indicates some of the conditions that it is claimed to be effective in treating. However, there is only anecdotal evidence and case studies of cannabis' effectiveness in treating these

Table 22.2 Possible therapeutic applications of cannabis

- Anorexia and wasting syndrome of AIDS and cancer
- Antiepileptic for epilepsy
- Depression and other mood disorders
- Intraocular pressure of glaucoma that can cause blindness
- Muscle relaxant for multiple sclerosis and other neurological impairments
- Nausea and vomiting induced by chemotherapy and radiotherapy for cancer
- Pain–including menstrual cramps, labour, migraines, phantom limb pain after amputation, cancer
- Pruritus

conditions. Nevertheless, it must be noted that for many of the conditions identified alternative treatments are often inadequate.

Like all drugs, cannabis has adverse effects and these are indicated in Table 22.3. Just as the evidence for the effectiveness of cannabis is poor, so is some of the evidence of its adverse effects, and there is considerable debate as to whether the evidence has been

Table 22.3 Suggested adverse effects of cannabis

Acute adverse effects of cannabis
- Short-term memory and attention, motor skills, reaction time, and skilled activities are impaired whilst the person is intoxicated, making driving and operating machinery dangerous
- Acute epiglottitis due to thermal injury from high burning temperature of marijuana
- Anxiety and panic reactions

Adverse effects due to chronic usage
- Chronic bronchitis, increased respiratory infections and decreased lung function
- Cannabis smoke may be carcinogenic and increase risks of cancers of the oral cavity, pharynx, larynx, oesophagus, and lung
- Prostatic and cervical cancer
- Impairment of memory, attention, and cognitive function similar to that found with heavy alcohol use
- Increased risk of psychosis in those with a personal or family history
- Dependency syndrome in which individuals have difficulty controlling their use and continue to use the drug despite experiencing adverse personal consequences, i.e. a psychological dependence
- Withdrawal syndrome including symptoms of anxiety, depression, irritability, insomnia, tremor and chills (Smith and Seymour, 1997)

distorted for political reasons (McCarthy, 1997a; Anon, 1998a). Hall and Solowij (1998) present a summary on the most probable adverse effects of cannabis use, acknowledging where appropriate the uncertainty that remains. Their rationale for presenting this information is so that doctors can advise their patients of the most likely ill-effects of cannabis use.

So, was the judgement to send Jeremy to prison fair? It was certainly correct from a legal perspective, but the law should be about justice, and not about following the law to the letter. Jeremy had a medical problem for which there is no current accepted treatment, and having tried all the treatments offered to him was still suffering from muscle spasm and blurred vision. He had found an effective treatment in cannabis and was fully aware of the adverse effects of the drug. He had thus made an informed choice. His use of the drug was not doing anyone else any harm, in fact his use of cannabis had cut down on the number of days he was having off sick, and so had made him a more productive member of society. Many people would support Jeremy's use of cannabis. On the 11th November 1998 a committee of the House of Lords recommended that clinical trials be carried out on the effects of cannabis in multiple sclerosis and in chronic pain. They also recommended that the UK government should reclassify cannabis so that doctors can prescribe it in certain circumstances

The second question is should cannabis be legalized for recreational purposes? This question engenders considerably more debate than the issue over whether or not to legalize cannabis for medicinal purposes. The full debate cannot be addressed here and the reader is directed to the items already referenced in this section. However, one of the main arguments for legalizing cannabis for recreational purposes is that cannabis would appear to be less of a threat to health than alcohol and tobacco, products which in many countries are not only tolerated and advertised but provide a valuable source of tax revenue. It is the contrast between the benefits and detriments of cannabis versus tobacco, and the starkly different levels of government control, which irks so many advocates who want to legalize therapeutic cannabis and eliminate any use of the latter.

In conclusion, on the medical evidence available, moderate indulgence in cannabis has little ill-effect on health, and decisions to ban or legalize cannabis should be based on other considerations (Anon, 1998b).

General education

Case study

Peter Hancock is a muscular 45-year-old executive who works on the stock exchange in London. He is married and lives in Essex with his wife and two children. He works long hours, smokes 20 cigarettes a day and drinks 30 units of alcohol a week. Peter suffers with a stress-related ulcer, and despite considerable advice from his GP and from the staff at the hospital, he refuses to change his life style to minimize his risk factors.

One evening whilst at home Peter has gastro-intestinal haemorrhage and has to be rushed to hospital by his wife. He is admitted to the medical unit and is commenced on six hourly intravenous cimetidine 300 mg.

Peter complains to the admitting doctor that he finds it difficult to sleep in hospital and asks for a sleeping tablet to be prescribed. The doctor prescribes the benzodiazepine alprazolam 250 g at bedtime as necessary. However, what Peter failed to tell the doctor was that due to work related worries he had not been sleeping well at home for the last couple of nights and so had been taking his wife's sleeping tablets, which also happened to be alprazolam.

Two days after admission Peter started to become confused and aggressive, and the following day whilst walking to the day room to ring his wife he fell and fractured his wrist. The fracture was quite severe and required Peter to have surgery, after which he was transferred to the orthopaedic ward. Here he continued to receive intravenous cimetidine and alprazolam, together with 10 mg of intramuscular morphine four hourly for pain.

On the second day on the orthopaedic ward, Peter suddenly deteriorated. His pulse was 110 beats a minute, his blood pressure was 80/40 mmHg, respiratory rate was 10 and he was unresponsive to his name. The doctor was called, but before he arrived, Peter had a respiratory arrest. Though he recovered fully after prompt emergency intervention, his family took legal advice and attempted to sue the hospital for negligence.

Questions:

- What is one of the main problems with the benzodiazepines, including alprazolam?
- How does cimetidine interact with alprazolam?
- If a benzodiazepine were to be prescribed as a hypnotic for a patient, which ones would have been a better choice?
- Other than receiving general emergency treatment for respiratory arrest, what special treatment would Peter have received?
- Does Peter have a case for suing for negligence? On what do you base your decision?
- Bearing in mind the title of this chapter and section, what is the important message for health professionals and the general public?

Answers:

Like most benzodiazepines, alprazolam has a long half-life of 12–15 hours. Consequently, by the time Peter took his first dose in hospital some of the drug, which he had taken from his wife, had already begun to accumulate in his system. Compounding this problem is the fact that cimetidine inhibits the enzymes in the liver which break down alprazolam. Therefore the alprazolam is not metabolized and eliminated and so blood levels of the drug rise, explaining Peter's confusion and aggressive behaviour.

Benzodiazepines can act as both hypnotics and anxiolytics, and the British National Formulary (BMA and RPS, 1997) classifies alprazolam as the latter. The benzodiazepines used as hypnotics include nitrazepam, flunitrazepam and flurazepam. These however have a prolonged action and so can lead to residual drowsiness the following day. Loprazolam, lormetazepam and temazepam act for a shorter time and so have little or no hangover effect. Withdrawal symptoms can however be more of a problem with the short-acting benzodiazepines. The Committee on Safety of Medicines suggests that 'benzodiazepines should be used to treat insomnia only when it is severe, disabling and subjecting the individual to extreme distress' (BMA and RPS, 1997).

As the respiratory arrest is likely to be drug-induced, Peter is likely to receive an antidote to the causative agent. Peter is taking two drugs that could be the cause of his respiratory depression namely morphine and alprazolam. If the former is the cause Peter will be given intravenously the opioid antagonist naloxone, 1 mg every two to three minutes up to a maximum of 10 mg. As the dose of morphine, which Peter is receiving, is not excessive and as the half-life of morphine is only four hours, the morphine is unlikely to be the cause of his respiratory depression. The more likely cause is the build up of alprazolam, and for this, he will be given the benzodiazepine antagonist flumazenil, 0.2 mg intravenously over three seconds. The response to flumazenil is rapid, but it has a half-life of around an hour, compared with the half-life of 12–15 hours of alprazolam. Thus, it is likely to need to be re-administered, possibly within the hour, in order to prevent re-sedation.

Peter's family tried to sue the hospital for negligence. If you look at Table 15.5 you will see the criteria for negligence. The answer to question one is yes, the hospital did owe Peter a duty of care. The answer to question two was debated at length in court with some doctors claiming that the choice of alprazolam was quite reasonable, and others saying that it was not a reasonable choice of sleeping tablet. The answer to question three is dependent on the answer to question two, as the alprazolam was the cause of Peter falling and sustaining a fracture. As to whether the injuries were foreseeable, it was argued that they were not as Peter had withheld information, although the prosecutor argued that the effect of combining alprazolam and cimetidine was foreseeable. However, although Peter's injuries could be compensated for by financial payment from the hospital (question 5), Peter's case was unsuccessful because he had not disclosed the fact that he was self-medicating with his wife's sleeping tablets and so was seen to have contributed to his injuries.

The essential message of this case study, and the entire book, is that drugs are a two-edged sword. They can cure many diseases, control unpleasant symptoms, and improve the quality of our life. However, it must be appreciated that their ability to do harm is equal to their ability to do good, especially if used incorrectly or inappropriately. Thus, the main message of this book is to learn as much as possible about the drugs that you are giving to your patients, or which you are using yourself, so that you can use them safely and keep adverse effects to a minimum.

References and further reading

Abernethy K (1997a) The menopause and hormone replacement therapy. Nursing Standard 11: 49-53

Abernethy K (1997b) Hormone replacement therapy. Professional Nurse 12: 717-9

Anon (1998a) Marijuana. A safe high? New Scientist 157: 24-9

Anon (1998b) Dangerous habits. The Lancet 353: 1565

British Medical Association and Royal Pharmaceutical Society of Great Britain (1997) British National Formulary. London: Pharmaceutical Press

Campbell J (1999) Cannabis: the evidence. Nursing Standard 13: 45-7

Department of Health (1994) On the State of Public Health. London: HMSO

Colditz GA, Hankinson SE, Hunter DJ, Willett WC, Manson JE, Stampfer MJ, Hennekens C, Rosner B, Speizer F (1995) The use of estogens and progestins and the risk of breast cancer in postmenopausal women. The New England Journal of Medicine 332: 1589-93

Daly E, Vessey MP, Hawkins MH, Carson JL, Gough P, Marsh S (1996) Risk of venous thromboembolism in users of hormone replacement therapy. Lancet 347: 977-80

Ettinger B, Genant HK, Cann CE (1985) Long-term oestrogen replacement therapy prevents bone loss and fractures. Annals of Internal Medicine 102: 319-24

Finucane FF, Madans JH, Bush TL, Wolf PM, Kleinman JC (1993) Decreased risk of stroke among postmenopausal hormone users. Archives of Internal Medicine 153: 73-9

Gangar E, Penny J (1995) Advances in hormone replacement therapy. Nursing Standard 9: 23-5

Gordon T, Kannel WB, Hjortland MC, McNamara PM (1978) Menopause and coronary artery disease. Annals of Internal Medicine 89: 157-61

Greer G (1991) The Change: Women, Ageing and the Menopause. London: Hamish Hamilton

Hall W, Solowij N (1998) Adverse effects of cannabis. Lancet 352: 1611-6

Holloway M (1992) The estrogen factor. Scientific American 266: 11

Hillard A (1996) Hormone replacement therapy. Nursing Standard 10: 51-4

Howie C (1987) Sparing the flushes. Nursing Times 9: 51-3

Jick H, Derby L, Myers MW, Vasilakis C, Newton K (1996) Risk of hospital admission for idiopathic venous thromboembolism among users of postmenopausal oestrogens. Lancet 348: 981-3

Khaw K (1992) Epidemiology of the menopause. British Medical Bulletin 48: 249-61

Litchman R (1991) Perimenopausal hormone replacement therapy. A review of the literature. Journal of Nurse-Midwifery 36: 30-48

Luke C (1997) Weed control. Nursing Times 93: 40-1

McCarthy M (1997a) Oestrogen accelerates wound healing in postmenopausal women. Lancet 350: 1301

McCarthy H (1997b) Gray matter (not even the page is black and white!). Rehabilitation Education 11: 127-35

Mijatovic V, Pines A (1995) Menopause-induced changes in cardiovascular functions and HRT. European Menopause Journal 2:4-9

Paganini-Hill A, Henderson VW (1994) Estrogen deficiency and risk of Alzheimer's disease in women. American Journal of Epidemiology 140: 256-60

Paganini-Hill A, Ross RK, Gerkins VR, Henderson BE, Arthur M, Mack TM (1981) Menopausal estrogen therapy and hip fractures. Annals of Internal Medicine 95: 28-31

Rosenberg L, Hennekens CH, Rosner B, Belanger C, Rothmans KJ, Speizer FE (1981) Early menopause and risk of myocardial infarction. American Journal of Obstetrics and Gynaecology 139: 47-51

Shamash J (1998) Purely medicinal. Nursing Standard 12:12

Smith DE, Seymour RB (1997) Cannabis and cannabis withdrawal. Journal of Substance Misuse 2: 49-53

Stampfer MJ, Colditz GA (1991) Estrogen replacement therapy and coronary heart disease: a quantitative assessment of the epidemiologic evidence. Preventive Medicine 20: 47-63

Tang M, Jacobs D, Stern D, Marder K, Schofield P, Gurland B, Andrews H, Mayeux R (1996) Effect of oestrogen during menopause on risk and age of onset of Alzheimer's disease. Lancet 348: 429-32

Abbreviations and Glossary

Abbreviations

BMA – British Medical Association
BNF – British National Formulary
DoH – Department of Health
DHSS – Department of Health and Social Services
GP – General Practitioner
MRC – Medical Research Council
RCN – Royal College of Nursing
RGN – Registered General Nurse
UKCC – United Kingdom Central Council for Nursing, Midwifery and Health Visiting

Glossary

Absorption is the passage of a drug from the site of administration to the blood or plasma.

ACE inhibitors are drugs which inhibit the action of angiotensin-converting enzyme (ACE), preventing the conversion of angiotensin I to angiotensin II.

Active transport is an energy or ATP requiring process that moves particles across a cell membrane, usually against the particles' concentration gradient.

Adrenoceptors are receptors for adrenaline (epinephrine).

Adverse effects are any unwanted drug effects. They range from minor side-effects through to harmful or seriously unpleasant effects.

Affinity refers to a drug's tendency to bind to receptors or other binding sites.

Agonist is a drug that binds to a receptor and activates the receptor on binding, bringing about a response.

Agranulocytosis refers to the complete absence of circulating neutrophils.

Allergic reaction is any immunological response to a drug or its metabolites that results in adverse effects.

Anabolic refers to synthetic reactions, which usually involve the utilization of energy in the form of ATP.

Angio-oedema is swelling due to fluid leaking out of blood vessels.

Antagonist is a drug that binds to a receptor without activating it.

Arachidonic acid is derived from phospholipids, for example those in cell membrane, and converted into a variety of chemicals involved with inflammation.

ATP (adenosine triphosphate) is the energy source of the cell.

Bacteriophages are viruses that infect bacteria.

Bioavailability is the amount of drug that reaches the systemic circulation. It is related to the route of administration, absorption, and any presystemic metabolism.

Blood-brain barrier refers to the relatively impermeable capillaries that supply the brain and inhibit the passage of chemicals from the blood into the brain tissues.

Bound drug refers to the proportion of drug that is carried in the blood attached to carrier proteins such as albumin.

Catecholamines are a group of amine derivatives of catechol which act as hormones or neurotransmitters. They include noradrenaline (norepinephrine), adrenaline (epinephrine) and dopamine.

Catabolic refers to the processes involved in the breakdown of molecules in order to provide energy in the form of ATP.

Cations are positively charged particles, such as a sodium or calcium ion.

Chelation is the process by which a substance binds the molecules of a metal. Chelating agents can be used to aid the excretion of metals in cases of poisoning.

Clearance is the elimination of a drug from the body. It is the sum of clearance by the kidney and all other routes of elimination.

Complement is a group of serum proteins involved in the control of inflammation, the activation of phagocytes and the lysis of cell membranes. They are so called because they 'complement' the rest of the immune system.

Cytoplasm is the cellular material surrounding the nucleus and enclosed by the cell or plasma membrane.

Cytosol is the viscous, semitransparent fluid in which the other elements of the cell are suspended.

Diffusion is movement of particles from a high concentration to a low concentration.

Distribution is the movement of the drug from the blood to its site of action.

Divalent refers to a charged particle.

Down-regulation occurs when the number of receptors in a cell membrane decreases because have they have been moved into the cytoplasm. This results in a loss of sensitivity.

Dyscrasia is an abnormality in the development of blood cells.

Electrochemical gradient refers to both the concentration and electrical gradients that exist for charged particles across a membrane.

Endocytosis is a form of bulk transport utilized by cells, which requires the utilization of energy in the form of ATP. It involves the cell engulfing external particles such as bacteria (phagocytosis), fluid droplets (pinocytosis) or bound membrane receptors (receptor mediated endocytosis).

Endoplasmic reticulum is an extensive system of interconnected parallel membranes that coil through the cytoplasm, enclosing fluid-filled cavities.

Enterohepatic recirculation is the process in which a drug or its metabolite is excreted into the bile and hence into the intestine, before being reabsorbed and returned to the liver for secretion into the bile again.

Enzyme induction occurs when there is an increase in the amount and activity of an enzyme following exposure to various chemicals.

Eosinophilia refers to an increase in circulating eosinophil, a type of white blood cell.

Excretion is the movement of a drug or its metabolites from the tissues and out of the body, the main routes being through the kidney and liver.

Facilitated diffusion is the movement of particles from a high concentration to a low concentration across a cell membrane with the aid of a transmembrane carrier protein. It is also called carrier-mediated diffusion.

Filtration is the movement of water and solutes through a semipermeable membrane from a region of high hydrostatic pressure to a region of low hydrostatic pressure, i.e. along a pressure gradient.

First-pass metabolism occurs when a drug is metabolized before it enters the systemic circulation.

Free drug refers to the proportion of a drug that dissolves in the plasma and is available to interact with tissues, be metabolized and excreted.

Granulocytopenia refers to a reduction in white blood cell numbers, in particular neutrophils, eosinophils and basophils

Gynaecomastia is the abnormal accumulation of tissue in the male breast.

Half-life is the time necessary to decrease the serum concentration of a drug by half.

Hapten is a small molecule that will not stimulate an immune response by itself. However, if it becomes attached to a larger molecule it can stimulate antibody production.

Hypersensitivity reaction is any immunological response to a drug or its metabolites that results in adverse effects.

Idiosyncrasy implies a qualitative abnormal reaction to a drug, usually due to a genetic abnormality.

Intolerance is an undesirable pharmacological effect that occurs at sub-therapeutic drug dosages.

Intrathecal drug administration involves injection of the drug between the meninges of the spinal cord, and usually into the cerebrospinal fluid in the subarachnoid space.

Ions are charged particles. Because they conduct electricity when in solution, they are also referred to as electrolytes, e.g. sodium ($Na+$), calcium ($Ca\ 2+$), chloride ($Cl-$).

Isoenzymes are variant forms of an enzyme found within an organism. They have the same function, but differ in their structure.

Leucocytosis is an increase in number of circulating white blood cells.

Leukotrienes are derivatives of arachidonic acid which are involved with inflammatory processes, including asthma.

Ligands are small molecules such as drugs that bind to receptors, e.g. agonists or antagonists.

Lysosomes are structures found in the cell that contain powerful digestive enzymes.

MAOIs or monoamine oxidase inhibitors are drugs that inhibit the enzyme monoamine oxidase, which is responsible for the breakdown of noradrenaline (norepinephrine) in the presynaptic nerve terminal.

Metabolite is a substance that takes part in any of the processes of metabolism.

Nosocomial infections are hospital acquired, i.e. the patient is not admitted with the infection but develops it as a result of being in hospital.

NSAIDs is an abbreviation for non-steroidal anti-inflammatory drugs, e.g. aspirin, ibuprofen.

Nystagmus is a spasmodic involuntary movement of the eyeball.

Over-the-counter medications are drugs that are bought without the need for a prescription.

Oxidation is a metabolic reaction that involves the addition of oxygen or the removal of hydrogen from a drug or chemical.

Overdose effects are exaggerated but characteristic pharmacological effects produced by administering supratherapeutic doses of a drug.

Paracrine secretions are chemicals released by cells that act near to their site of release, i.e. local hormones.

Partition coefficient is a term that reflects the solubility of a drug molecule in a lipid relative to its solubility in water. The higher the partition coefficient the faster the drug molecule can diffuse across the lipid bilayer.

Pharmacodynamics describes the processes by which cell physiology is altered by a drug. It normally involves interaction with receptors, enzymes, ion channels or carriers.

Pharmacokinetics describes a drug's absorption, distribution, metabolism and excretion, with time

Pharmacological efficacy refers to the ability of a drug, once bound to a receptor, to initiate changes, which lead to effects.

Plasma membrane is the term used to describe the phospholipid bilayer and its embedded proteins, which makes up the cell membrane.

Polar molecules have a small positive charge at one end of the molecule and a small negative charge at the other end, e.g. water molecules.

Priapism is a persistent, usually painful, erection of the penis.

Pro-drugs are inactive drugs that rely on metabolism by the body to convert them into active substances.

Polypharmacy is administration of multiple medications to an individual client with the implication that more drugs are being given than is clinically justified.

Porins are protein channels in the outer cell membrane.

Prostaglandins are a group of hormone like chemicals that have a wide spectrum of activity. They are involved in the inflammatory response of damaged tissue, and are used therapeutically to induce abortion and labour.

Reduction is a metabolic reaction that involves the addition of hydrogen or the removal of oxygen from a drug.

Ribosomes are organelles found in cells that are the sites of protein synthesis.

Secondary effects are the indirect consequences of a primary drug action, e.g. opportunistic infections that may develop after antibiotic treatment. They are type A effects.

Side-effects are unwanted effects that occur as a result of the pharmacology of the drug. They are type A effects.

SSRIs or selective serotonin re-uptake inhibitors are drugs that prevent the neurotransmitter serotonin from being taken up into the pre-synaptic nerve terminal. The serotonin thus continues to be active on the post-synaptic membrane and this serves to improve mood.

Substrate is the chemical on which an enzyme acts.

Sympathomimetics are drugs that mimic the effect of the sympathetic nervous system, e.g. noradrenaline (norepinephrine).

Teratogens are drugs capable of producing developmental defects in the foetus.

Therapeutic efficacy refers to the effectiveness of a drug.

Therapeutic index is a ratio comparing the dose of a drug that is therapeutically beneficial with the dose that produces side-effects. Drugs with a narrow index are potentially dangerous as the difference between the therapeutic and toxic dose is small.

Thrombocytopenia refers to a reduction in platelet numbers.

Tolerance is the decreased physiological response to a drug as a result of prior exposure.

Toxic effects are exaggerated but characteristic pharmacological effects produced by administering supratherapeutic doses of a drug.

Type A or augmented effects are adverse effects that occur as a result of the pharmacology of a drug. They are also referred to as side-effects.

Type B or bizarre effects are unpredictable adverse effects that are not dose-related.

Type C or chronic effects are adverse effects that occur as the result of prolonged drug usage.

Type D or delayed effects are adverse effects that do not occur for years after treatment or that affect the next generation.

Type E or end-of-use effects are adverse effects that occur when the drug is stopped suddenly, i.e. withdrawal effects.

Up-regulation occurs when the number of receptors in a cell membrane increases because they have been moved from the cytoplasm to the cell membrane. This increases the cell sensitivity to the receptor's ligand.

Urticaria is a skin condition characterized by red raised patches that itch intensely, and is usually caused by allergic reactions. It is also called 'hives' and 'nettle rash'.

Volume of distribution is the volume of plasma that would contain the total body content of the drug at a concentration equal to that in the plasma.

Index